Plastic Surgery of the Lower Eyelids

Jeremiah P. Tao
Editor

Plastic Surgery of the Lower Eyelids

Springer

Editor
Jeremiah P. Tao
Gavin Herbert Eye Institute
University of California, Irvine
Irvine, CA, USA

Video Editors
Jenny N. Wang
Maria A. Belen Camacho
Sophia I. Strugnell

Illustrator
Michael M. Han

International Associate Editor
Roberto C. Limongi

ISBN 978-3-031-36174-6 ISBN 978-3-031-36175-3 (eBook)
https://doi.org/10.1007/978-3-031-36175-3

This Springer imprint is published by the registered company Springer Nature Switzerland AG
The registered company address is: Gewerbestrasse 11, 6330 Cham, Switzerland

Foreword

Dr. Jeremiah P. Tao is a formidable expert, with many contributions, in the field of ophthalmic plastic and orbital surgery. He has now turned his attention to a long-overlooked arena in mid-facial surgery: the lower eyelid. A surgical book dealing only with this topic is both unique in the surgical literature and quite possibly destined to become a classic.

The lower eyelid has been a source of trepidation for many surgeons who operate in the midface. The pursuit of best practice management of the lower eyelid has seen disagreements regarding anatomic understanding, best surgical approaches, and choices to avoid surgical complications. In this timely and important book, Dr. Tao and co-authors have addressed numerous relevant topics to guide surgeons through the surgical management of both cosmetic and reconstructive challenges in the lower eyelid and its approach to the inferior orbit.

Dr. Tao has assembled an impressive array of co-authors who comprise leading and experienced oculofacial plastic and orbital surgeons. They share their expertise on a wide variety of lower eyelid topics important to successful outcome and safety when approaching this challenging surgical anatomy. Their insights will help guide surgeons when surgical outcomes can either protect or endanger both cosmetic results as well as vision. Readers will find the chapters lucid, often enlightening, understandable, and a benefit to their patients.

All surgeons who delve into lower eyelid and inferior orbital surgery will appreciate and value this fine contribution to the medical and surgical literature. I highly recommend it to mid-facial surgeons of all disciplines and all experience levels.

William R. Nunery, M.D., FACS
Past President, American Society of Ophthalmic
Plastic and Reconstructive Surgery
Emeritus Professor, Department of Ophthalmology
and Visual Sciences
University of Louisville
Louisville, KY, USA

Preface

The lower eyelids are central on the face, both literally and figuratively, yet their important roles in oculofacial physiology are often under-appreciated. Often, the key roles of the lower eyelids in ophthalmologic and facial structure and function manifest after the lower eyelids are damaged. Impairments to the lower eyelids can lead to dry eye, tearing, ocular discomfort, as well as vision loss.

Most cosmetic patients aiming to improve their facial appearance have complaints related to their lower eyelids. Under-eye bags, wrinkles, and dark circles are common concerns. Unlike their upper eyelid counterparts that can be forgiving to poor technique or over-resection, the lower eyelids have some of the highest rates of complications in all facial surgeries.

The lower eyelids are highly visible and offer the opportunity to give patients great aesthetic improvements, yet there are many surgical challenges. Malposition, scars, and even the slightest irregularities can cause discomfort and distress. Ectropion, lagophthalmos, chemosis, and retraction are common negative results of attempts to rejuvenate the periocular area. Importantly, these complications can pose serious risks to the health of the eye.

The surgical skills in avoiding these poor outcomes, as well as the knowledge of how to repair them when they do occur, are paramount for any facial specialist. Many variables influence good lower eyelid position and function. These include surrounding orbital anatomy as well as the intricate, layered anatomy of the eyelid.

This textbook is uniquely dedicated to lower eyelid conditions and treatments. It offers a systematic approach to wide-ranging congenital, acquired, reconstructive, and aesthetic disorders of the lower eyelids, the surrounding canthi, and the midface. The authors provide a comprehensive discussion and step-by-step description of techniques. Expert eyelid surgeons contributed to this book that includes photographs, diagrams, and videos for efficient skills and knowledge transfer. The hope is that the reader is inspired to advance quality and safety of plastic surgery of the lower eyelids.

Jeremiah P. Tao, M.D., FACS
Professor, Department of Ophthalmology
University of California
Irvine, CA, USA

Contents

Clinical Anatomy of the Lower Eyelids

Stephanie H. Noh, Divya Devineni and Lilangi S. Ediriwickrema

Abstract

An understanding of anatomy is key to successful surgery of the lower eyelids. Relevant structures include not only the intricate layers of the eyelid itself but also the surrounding midface, extraocular muscles, and anterior orbit. This chapter details lower eyelid anatomy relevant to oculofacial surgery. (Lacrimal drainage anatomy is described in Chaps. "Canalicular and Tearing Considerations" and "Medial Canthal Surgery").

Keywords

Eyelid anatomy · Midface anatomy · Eyelid structure

1 Lower Eyelid Dimensions and Configuration

The lower eyelid measures 25–30 mm is curvilinear between the medial and lateral canthus. The lateral canthus is usually 2–3 mm higher than the lower eyelid. The central lower eyelid margin should meet the eyeball at or slightly above the inferior limbus. The eyelid should hug the eyeball throughout its course (Fig. 1).

Illustrations by Michael Han

S. H. Noh · D. Devineni · L. S. Ediriwickrema (✉)
Division of Oculofacial Plastic and Orbital Surgery, University of California, Irvine, Irvine, CA, USA
e-mail: lilangise@gmail.com

2 Lower Eyelid and Midface Surface Anatomy

The lower eyelid transitions to the cheek at the palpebromalar groove that blends medially with the nasojugal groove (a.k.a tear trough). The palpebromalar groove is formed by the orbitomalar (a.k.a orbicularis or orbital containing) ligament. Inferiorly a second groove known as the midface groove may be evident and formed by zygomaticocutaneous ligaments (Fig. 2).

3 Layers (Lamellae) of the Lower Eyelid

The lower eyelid structures can be divided into anterior, middle, and posterior lamella. The anterior lamella consists of the skin and orbicularis oculi muscle. The middle lamella consists of the orbital septum, orbital fat, and suborbicularis fibroadipose tissue. The posterior lamella consists of the tarsal plate and conjunctiva. The concept of lamella is useful in reconstructive contexts. The anterior lamella is reconstructed with skin or skin and muscle. The posterior lamella requires mucous membrane or other conjunctiva growth-promoting substrate.

J. P. Tao (ed.), *Plastic Surgery of the Lower Eyelids*,
https://doi.org/10.1007/978-3-031-36175-3_1

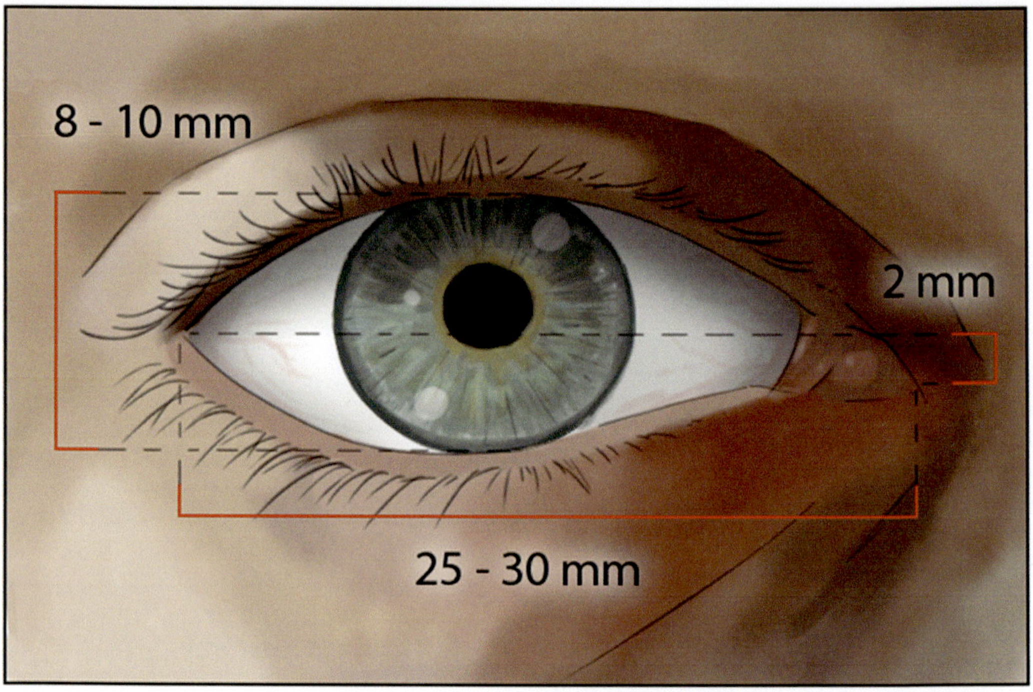

Fig. 1 Dimensions of a normal palpebral fissure. The lateral canthus sits slightly higher than the medial canthus

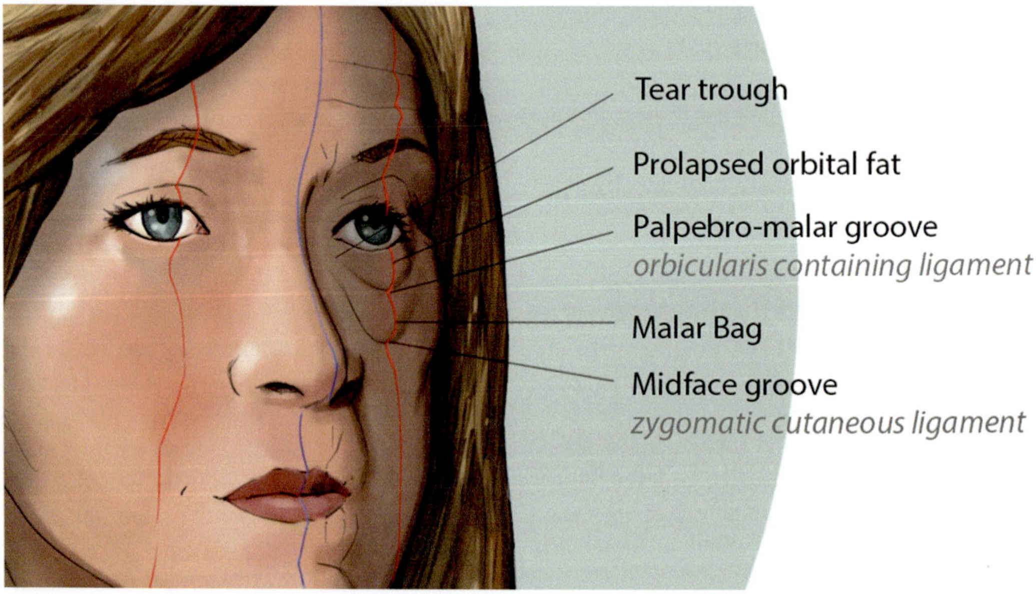

Fig. 2 Split face diagram demonstrating a smooth transition from the cheek to the eyelid in youth (image left, patient's right) and several grooves and surface contour alterations commonly seen with normal facial aging

4 Lower Eyelid Retractors

Compared to the upper eyelid, the lower eyelids have less excursion on eyelid opening and closing or eye movement. However, the lower eyelid contains retractors that pull the lower eyelid inferiorly in downgaze. This mechanism moves the lower eyelid inferiorly on downgaze and prevents visual axis occlusion. The lower eyelid retractors include the capsulopalpebral fascia (CPF) and inferior tarsal muscle. The CPF, as the name suggests, is fascial tissue that extends from the inferior rectus muscle to the inferior margin of the tarsus. It is analogous to the levator palpebrae superioris in the upper eyelid. The CPF begins as the capsulopalpebral head from the distal border of the inferior rectus muscle, then divides, encircles the inferior oblique muscle, and condenses anteriorly to form Lockwood suspensory ligament. From this point it extends further anteriorly to send strands to the inferior conjunctival fornix and inserts onto the inferior border of the tarsus after fusing with the orbital septum (Figs. 3 and 4).

The inferior tarsal muscle is smooth muscle that lies posterior to the CPF. These fibers are sympathetically innervated and are analogous to Muller's muscle in the upper eyelid. Because this muscle is often poorly defined, the inferior tarsal muscle and CPF are collectively referred to as the lower eyelid retractors.

5 Orbital Septum

The orbital septum is a sheet of fibrous tissue that demarcates the anterior boundary of the orbit, lying posterior to the orbicularis oculi and anterior to the orbital fat pads (Fig. 4). It originates from the arcus marginalis on the orbital rim.

6 Fat Pad Compartments

In the lower eyelid, there exist three orbital fat pad compartments named by their anatomic location: medial, central, and lateral. The inferior oblique muscle divides the medial and central fat pads. This is crucial to understand during lower eyelid blepharoplasty to prevent inferior oblique damage (Fig. 5). The central and lateral fat pads are separated by the arcuate expansion, which is continuous with the inferior oblique fascia and Lockwood ligament. As with the upper eyelid, orbital fat is an important anatomic landmark when identifying the lower eyelid retractors, as the fat pads will be anterior to them.

7 Lockwood Ligament

Lockwood ligament, also known as the suspensory ligament, functions as a hammock in supporting the position of the globe and preventing displacement (Fig. 3). There are three components as described by Kakizaki et al.: the inferior ligament, the main Lockwood ligament (analogous to Whitnall ligament in the upper eyelid), and the arcuate expansion. The inferior ligament supports the medial margin of the lower eyelid retractors. As discussed earlier, the arcuate expansion separates the central and lateral lower eyelid fat pads.

8 Vascular Supply

The blood supply to the lower eyelid is a plexus formed by the inferior medial palpebral and lateral palpebral arteries. They are branches of the facial, angular, infraorbital, zygomatico-orbital, transverse facial, and anterior branch of the superficial temporal arteries (Fig. 4). These arteries are branches of the external carotid artery. The internal carotid artery also supplies the palpebral arteries, which forms anastomoses via the lacrimal, dorsal nasal, anterior, and posterior ethmoid arteries. These arteries communicate through the ophthalmic artery.

Lower eyelid venous blood is drained through the superior and inferior ophthalmic veins to the cavernous sinus or pterygoid venous plexus. The junction near the cheek is drained through the angular and lateral nasal vein to the facial vein. Additional drainage pathways include the superficial temporal vein, supratrochlear vein, and supraorbital vein.

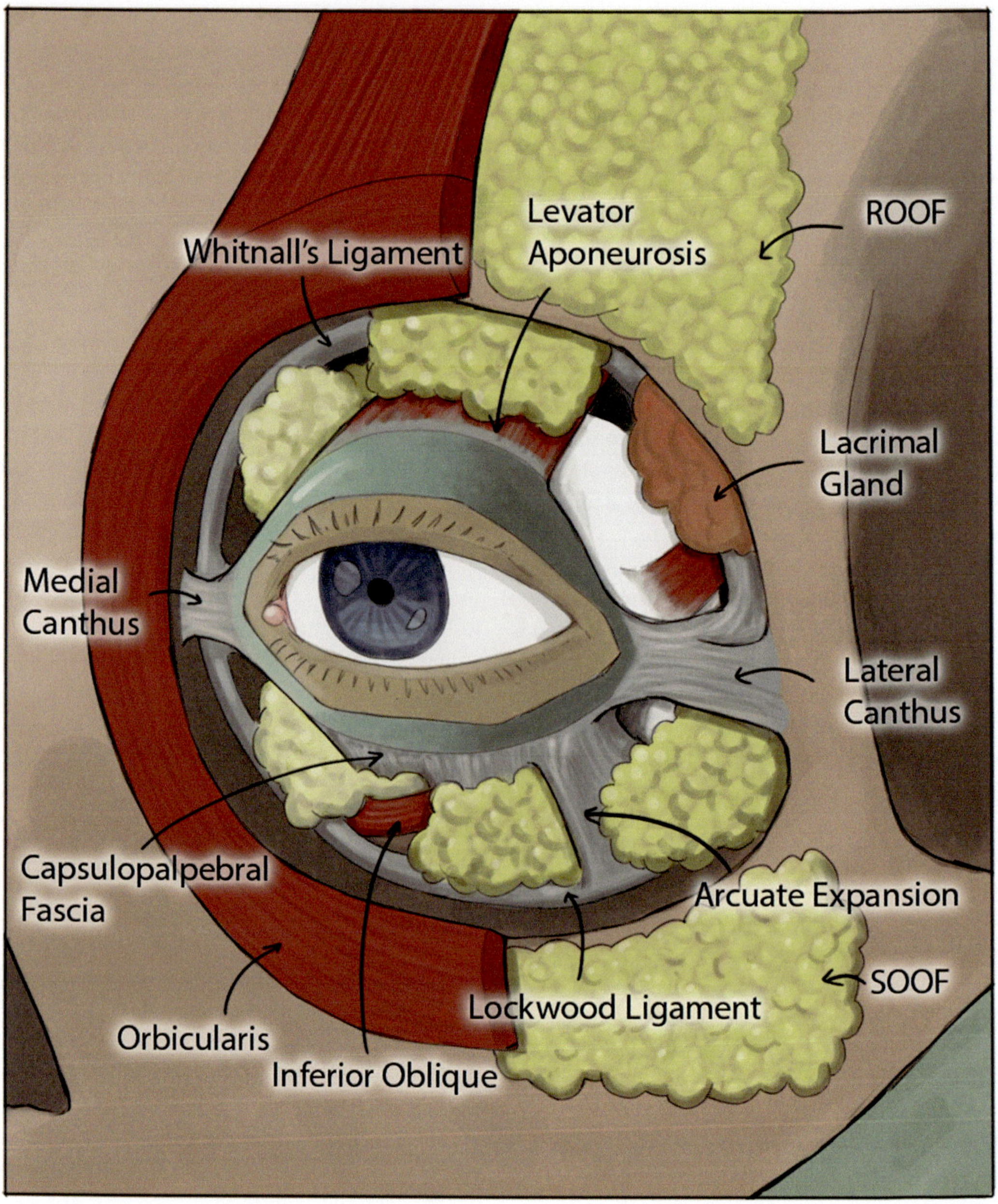

Fig. 3 Diagram of key inferior periorbital structures

9 Lymphatic Drainage

The lymphatic system drains from the medial portion of the lower eyelids to the submandibular lymph nodes, whereas the lateral portion drains to the preauricular and deep parotid lymph nodes. The deeper sections of the lymphatics drain the tarsal apparatus and the conjunctiva, whereas the superficial section drains the skin and orbicularis oculi muscle. These inferolateral drainage pathways are important to consider when designing incisions or

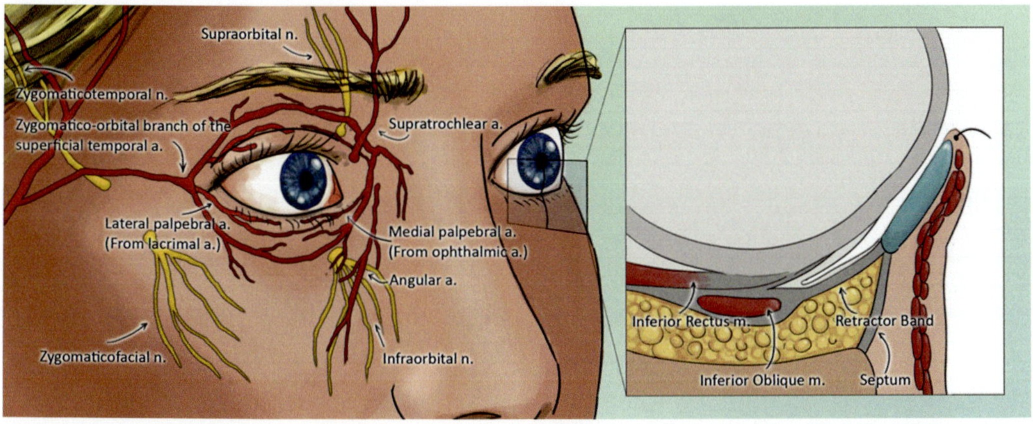

Fig. 4 Major acrteties and sensory nerves in the periocular region (left). Sagittal section of the lower eyelid (right)

flaps on the midface. Long, deep incisions or other trauma between the eyelids and these nodal basins may trap fluid in the eyelid as lymphedema.

10 Innervation

Most of lower eyelid sensation is by the infraorbital nerve, a branch of the maxillary nerve. It courses through the infraorbital foramen between the levator labii superioris and the levator anguli oris muscle. The infraorbital foramen is located above the zygomatic process of the maxilla, approximately 2–3 cm lateral to the vertical midline of the face. It is typically 0.7–1 cm inferior to the infraorbital margin. In most patients, the infraorbital foramen may be located on a line connecting the lateral canthus to the inferior nasal ala at the midline of the face (Fig. 6).

The medial portion of the lower eyelid is innervated by the infratrochlear nerve, a branch of the ophthalmic nerve. The lateral portion is supplied by the zygomaticofacial nerve, a branch of the maxillary nerve. All three of the major cutaneous nerves contain somatosensory fibers.

The orbicularis oculi's motor innervation is supplied by the buccal, zygomatic, and frontal branches of the facial nerve. For the lower eyelid retractors, motor supply is from the oculomotor nerve that simultaneously innervates the inferior rectus muscle.

11 Midface Anatomy

The midface is key in the aging face. Descent and deflation due to sagging tissue and loss of facial fat and bony remodeling are common age-related changes targeted in many rejuvenation procedures. Functionally, the midface supports the lower eyelid. Functional or aesthetic lower eyelid surgery, often requires attention to the greater anatomic structure of the midface.

The midface consists of five basic layers: (1) skin, (2) subcutaneous fat tissue, (3) superficial musculoaponeurotic system (SMAS), (4) deep fat tissue, and (5) deep fascia. The SMAS is a sheet of connective fibrous tissue that encases the muscles of facial expression and allows the facial muscles to function together as one cohesive unit. On the eyelids, there exists no subcutaneous fat and no SMAS (Fig. 7). Instead, the orbicularis oculi muscle is contiguous with SMAS of the midface and occupies the subcutaneous plane. Retaining ligaments extend through the SMAS (from periosteum to skin) and serve as supportive anchors. In the midface, these retaining ligaments are the orbitomalar, zygomatico-cutaneous, and upper masseteric ligaments.

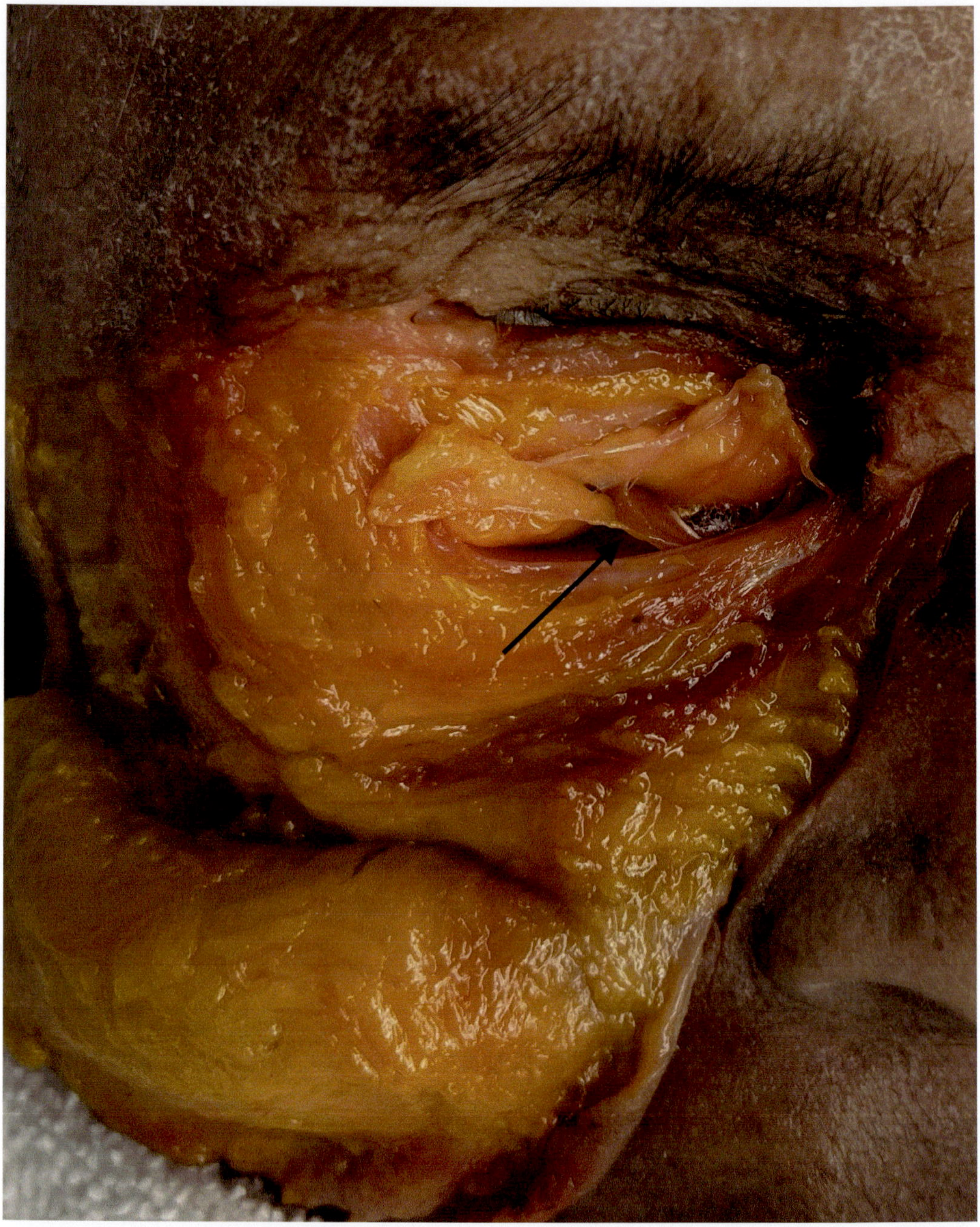

Fig. 5 Inferior oblique medial to to the central fat pad on cadaver dissection

The orbitomalar ligament originates from the periosteum of the inferior orbital rim and extends through the SMAS to insert onto the skin in a fan-like fashion. Because this ligament suspends the inferior periocular skin and subcutaneous tissue, as it loses its elasticity and starts to sag, it delineates the characteristic under eye bag that patients commonly notice with aging.

The most important retaining ligaments of the cheek are the zygomatico-cutaneous ligament and masseteric ligaments. The zygotomatico-cutaenous ligament is a curvilinear true

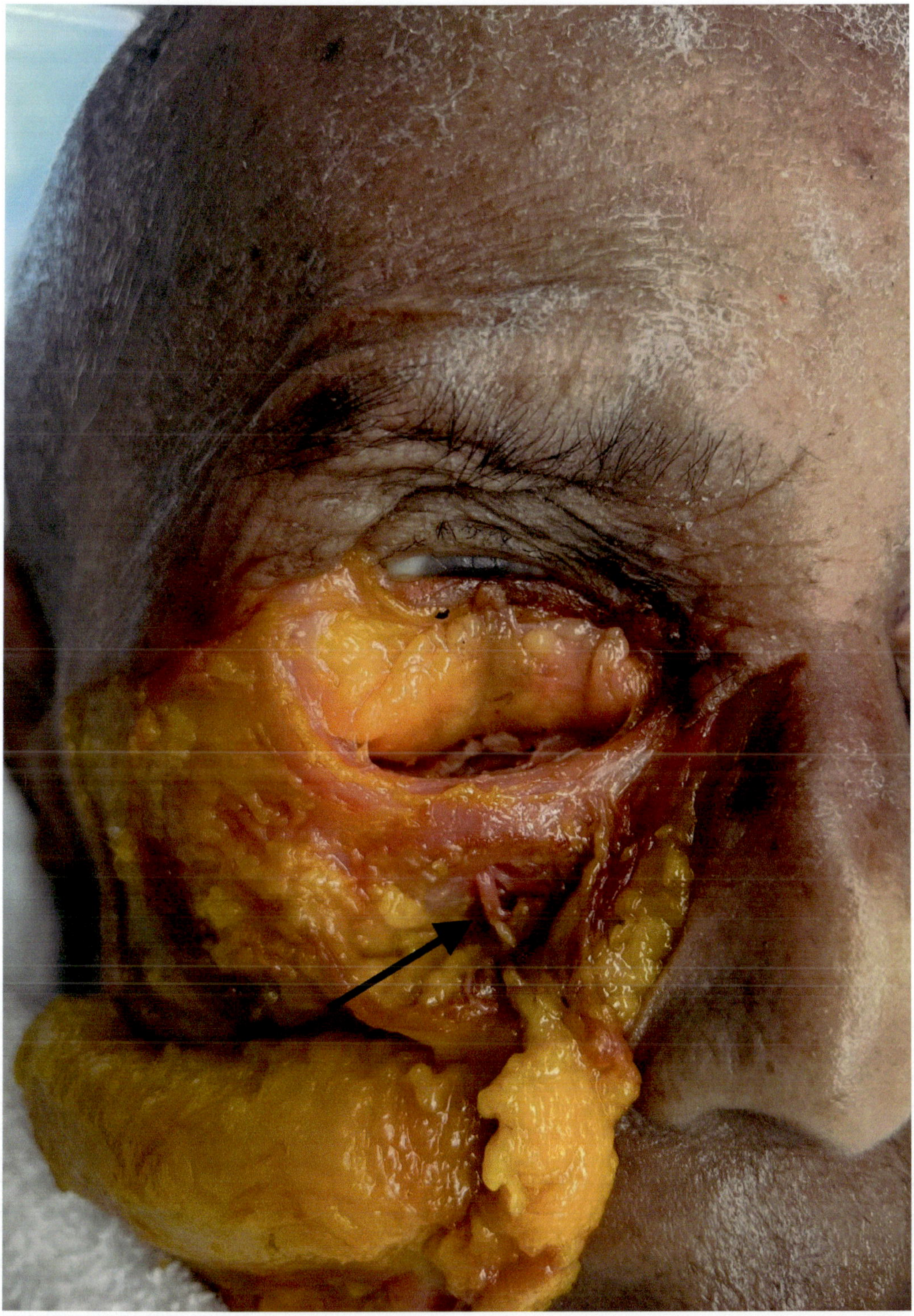

Fig. 6 Infraorbital nerve (arrow) demonstrated on a cadaver dissection

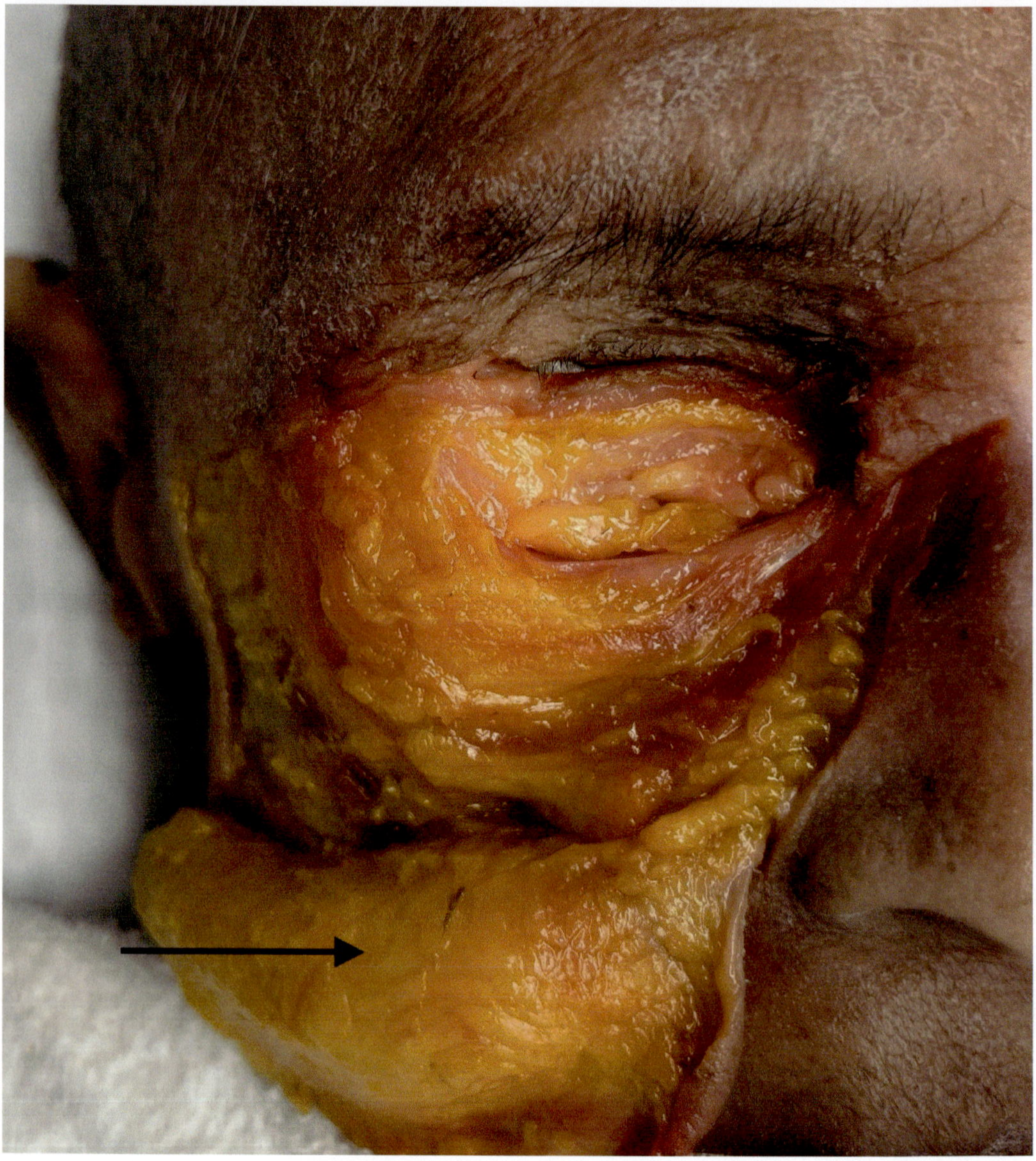

Fig. 7 Subcutaneous fat (arrow) deep to facial skin. On the eyelid, orbicularis oculi muscle occupies the layer directly beneath skin and orbital fat is deep to the muscle

ligament that originates at the inferior border of the zygomatic arch and extends anteriorly to the junction of the arch and body of the zygoma. The masseteric ligaments are condensations of masseter muscle that also suspend midface tissue.

12 Fat Pads

The facial fat pads should be distinguished from the orbital fat that herniates through the lower eyelid in the aging face. Facial fat can be divided into two categories: superficial and deep (in relation to the SMAS). The malar fat pad is a superficial fat pad located in the subcutaneous tissue anterior to the SMAS in the malar region. The deep facial fat pads in the midfacial region include the suborbicularis oculi fat (SOOF), buccal fat pad, and deep medial cheek fat. The SOOF is located deep to the orbicularis oculi and above the periosteum of the inferior orbital rim and can be further divided into medial and lateral components. The buccal fat pad is a large, deep fat pad that has three divisions: the anterior, intermediate, and posterior lobes.

13 Vascular Supply

The midface is a highly vascularized region and is mostly supplied by branches of the external carotid artery—more specifically, the angular artery (terminal part of the facial artery), transverse facial artery, and infraorbital artery (branch of the maxillary artery). These arteries and their branches form extensive anastomoses in the midface (Fig. 4).

Venous drainage occurs via the infraorbital vein which drains into the pterygoid plexus, as well as the facial vein.

14 Innervation

Motor function to the muscles of facial expression is supplied by the facial nerve (cranial nerve VII). The buccal branch provides most of the motor innervation to the midface, though the zygomatic branch also helps supply the lower orbicularis oculi. Sensory innervation is provided by the branches of the maxillary division of the trigeminal nerve (cranial nerve V2).

15 Lymphatic Supply

As with the lower eyelid, the medial compartments of the midface drain into the submandibular lymph nodes, whereas the lateral midface drains into the preauricular and deep parotid nodes.

16 Conclusion

The anatomy of the lower eyelid has important relationships to the underlying orbit and surrounding midface. Understanding these structures is key to successful eyelid and facial surgery.

References

1. Mojallal A, Cotofana S. Anatomy of lower eyelid and eyelid-cheek junction. Ann Chir Plast Esthet. 2017;62(5):365–74.
2. Kakizaki H, Malhotra R, Madge SN, Selva D. Lower eyelid anatomy: an update. Ann Plast Surg. 2009;63(3):344–51.
3. Whipple K, Oh S, Kikkawa D, Korn B, Chapter 1: Anatomy of the midface. In: Morris H, Wulc A, Holck D, editors. Midfacial rejuvenation. Springer; 2012. p. 1–14.
4. Nerad JA. Techniques in ophthalmic plastic surgery. London: Elsevier; 2010.
5. Wan D, Amirlak B, Rohrich R, Davis K. The clinical importance of the fat compartments in midfacial aging. Plast Reconstr Surg Glob Open. 2014;1(9): e92.
6. von Arx T, Tamura K, Yukiya O, Lozanoff S. The face—A vascular perspective. A literature review. Swiss Dent J. 2018;128(5):382–92.

Clinical Assessment of the Lower Eyelids

Abigail Jebaraj and Kian Eftekhari

Abstract

The lower eyelid examination is essential for surgical planning. It includes assessment of eyelid position, skin quality, midface anatomy, and the underlying orbit. Eyelid laxity and malposition is characterized by manual testing such as snap back test, distraction test, and forced traction testing. Photographic documentation is essential to document baseline findings as well as to chart progress. This chapter details keys of lower eyelid clinical assessment.

Keywords

Lower eyelid examination · Entropion · Ectropion · Eyelid retraction · Eyelid laxity · Eyelid malposition · Lower eyelid pre-operative assessment · Lower eyelid clinical examination

A. Jebaraj
Moran Eye Center, Salt Lake City, USA

K. Eftekhari (✉)
Eyelid Center of Utah, Salt Lake City, USA
e-mail: kianef@gmail.com

1 Introduction

Clinical assessment of the lower eyelids is multifaceted and requires a clear understanding of the patient's goals and expectations. The history and exam will guide appropriate management. An understanding of the anatomy and physiology of the lower eyelid is important to have in context with clinical findings.

2 History

The pre-operative assessment of a patient with lower eyelid complaints starts with the history. Important components of the history include:

- Chief complaint—what is their primary concern?
- Onset—an old, new, or smoldering problem?
- Prior treatment surgical or non-surgical—critical for surgical planning
- History of traumatic injury or facial cancer
- Impact on quality of life
- Mitigating or exacerbating factors—especially if the complaint is tearing or discomfort
- Relevant past medical or ocular history—dry eye or tearing
- Current medications—particularly anticoagul ants

J. P. Tao (ed.), *Plastic Surgery of the Lower Eyelids*,
https://doi.org/10.1007/978-3-031-36175-3_2

3 Physical Examination

The physical examination begins with observing the patient's entire face in room light. A handheld mirror is most useful so the patient can point out their issues.

The upper and lower eyelid height and position, anatomy of the midface, and symmetry are assessed. Measurements such as margin-reflex distance, or MRD, can be obtained by measuring the distance from the margin of the upper eyelid (MRD1) or lower eyelid (MRD2) to the pupillary light reflex. The normal MRD1 measurement is 4–4.5 mm and the normal MRD2 is 5 mm [1] (Fig. 1).

4 Eyelid Malposition

Eyelid malposition, once identified, should be further assessed for the underlying etiology. Entropion, or inward rolling of the eyelid margin, can be congenital, involutional, spastic due to contraction of the orbicularis oculi, or cicatricial due to scarring-induced shortening of the posterior lamella due to injury or inflammation. Ectropion, or outward rolling of the eyelid margin, can be congenital, involutional, paralytic due to facial paralysis, mechanical due to a mass or eyelid edema weighing down the eyelid, or cicatricial due to scarring-induced shortening of the anterior lamella secondary to trauma, prior surgery, chronic inflammation, or contracture from sun damage. Cicatricial changes to the posterior lamella may be present as well. The conjunctiva and fornix should be assessed by everting the eyelid (Fig. 2).

Lower eyelid retraction, or inferior displacement of eyelid margin without ectropion or entropion causing scleral show, should also be measured and an underlying cause sought out if one is not known. Measurement of lagophthalmos is essential in evaluation of the lower eyelid, as it may indicate prior palsy, trauma, surgery, or thyroid eye disease. It is also important to have a high index of suspicion for globe position and consider if proptosis may be causing lower eyelid malposition, which can occur in thyroid eye disease or if the clinician suspects

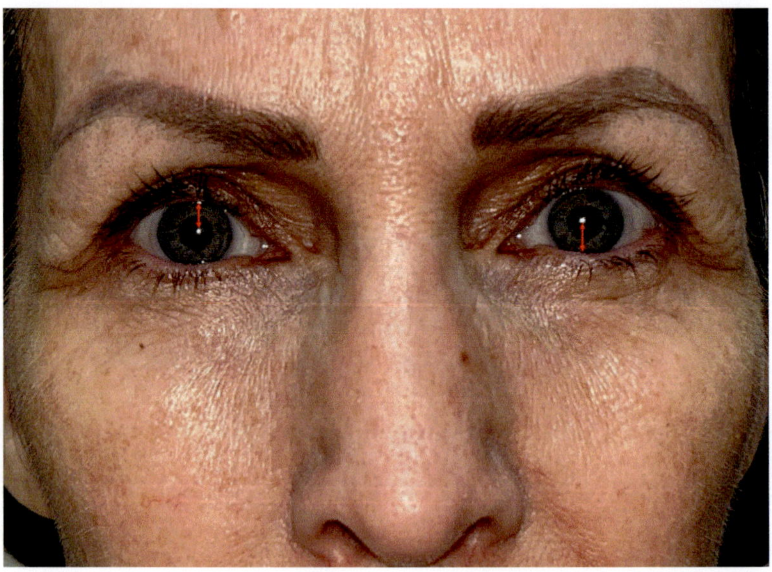

Fig. 1 Clinical image demonstrating margin-reflex distance (MRD) measurements. MRD1 is demonstrated by an arrow on the right eye as the distance from the margin of the upper eyelid to the corneal light reflection. MRD2 is demonstrated by an arrow on the left eye as the distance from the corneal light reflection to the margin of the lower eyelid

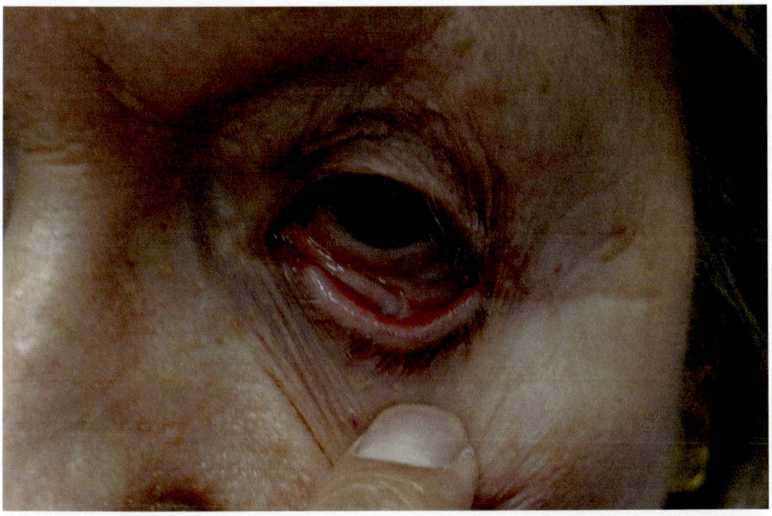

Fig. 2 Eyelid eversion demonstrating posterior lamella scarring after transconjunctival blepharoplasty

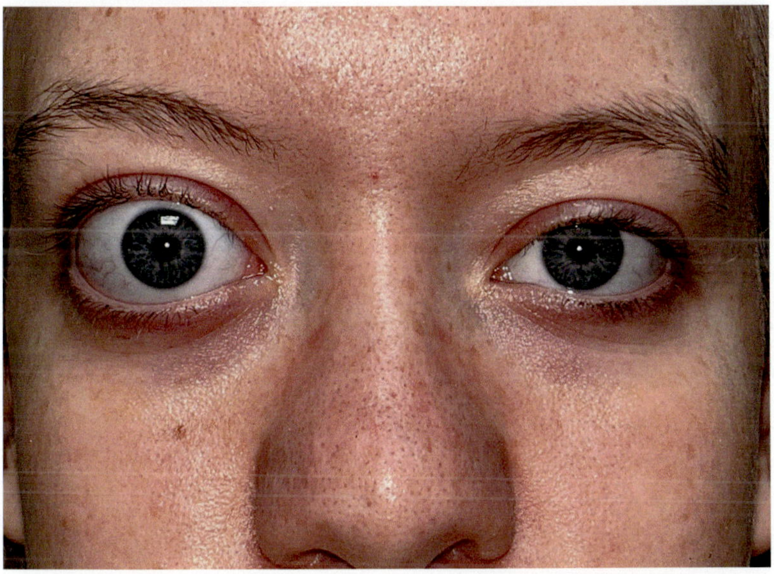

Fig. 3 Clinical image demonstrating right eye proptosis with significant eyelid retraction

an orbital mass (Fig. 3). With or without formal exophthalmometry, prominent eyes should be noted since lower eyelid repair generally require a more sophisticated approach and surgery is more prone to fail.

5 Aesthetic Elements of the Exam

Patients may also report lower eyelid aesthetic concerns such as baggy eyelids or a tired appearance. This may be caused by lower eyelid skin rhytids, dark circles, or fat prolapse. Other aesthetic issues in the lower eyelid may include malar mounds (chronic lower eyelid soft tissue swelling), lower eyelid festoons (folds of skin and orbicularis muscle associated with the lower eyelid), and malar edema [2]. These features are associated with the aging face (Fig. 4).

6 Skin

The surgeon should examine the health of the skin to determine the need for dermatologic procedures or postoperative healing considerations such as risk of cicatricial changes. Sun damage, cicatricial

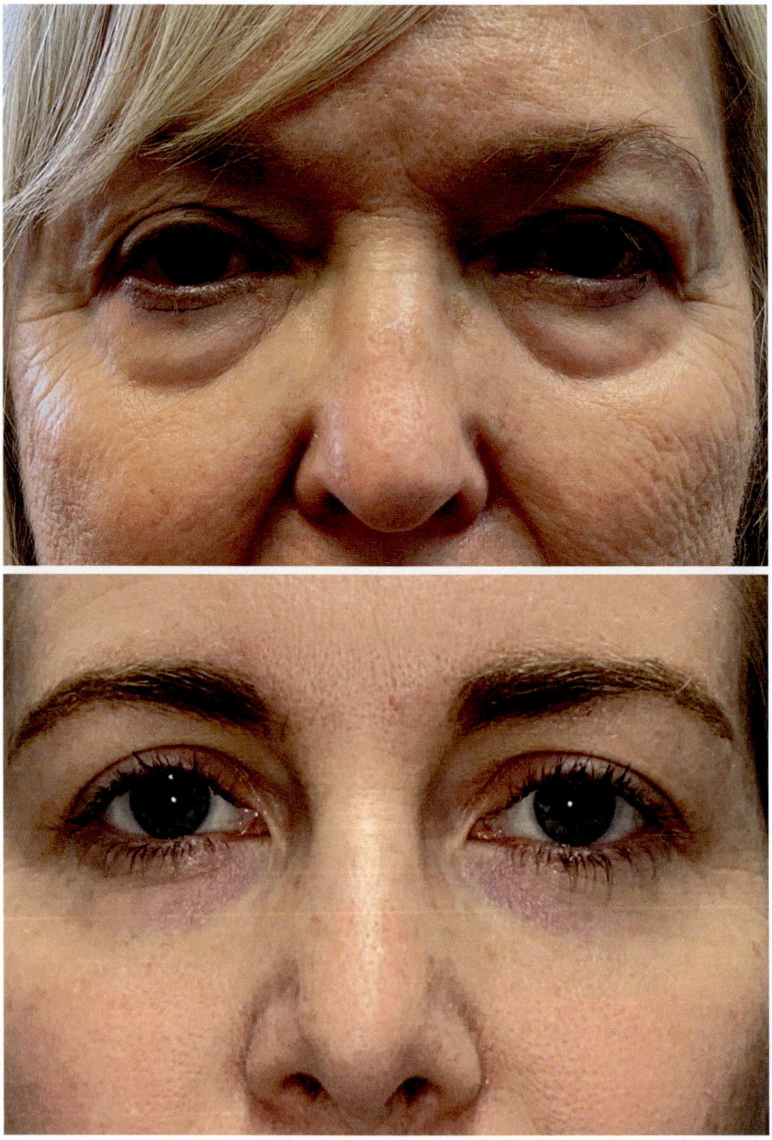

Fig. 4 Clinical images demonstrating the aging face (upper) compared to the young face (lower). The upper image demonstrates brow ptosis, dermatochalasis, prominent lower tear trough with malar mounds, midface descent, and lateral canthal lines

changes, pigmentation, rhytids, laxity, and edema may influence post-surgical healing and final appearance.

7 Muscle

Surgical planning should also involve observation of dynamic movement of the face and eyelids. Orbicularis oculi strength is tested by attempting to open the patient's closed eyelids, and it can reveal subtle facial nerve paralysis if abnormal or asymmetric. It is important to observe any involuntary or voluntary twitches or spasms of the eyelids or face including laterality, which may warrant further workup. Facial nerve paralysis may be obvious, but mild paresis can be overlooked. The patient's face should be assessed in various states of animation and while they are speaking to detect subtle paresis or relative tone imbalances between the two sides of the face.

8 Fat

Lower eyelid fat pads can contribute to tear trough deformities and a step off between the lower eyelid and upper cheek. Deflation or devolumization of the malar fat pads, particularly the medial malar fat pad, can occur. Orbital fat can protrude through weakened septum and orbicularis. Fat prolapse and fat atrophy can contribute to continued midface descent and less than desirable postoperative outcomes unless the midface is supported or fat is repositioned.

9 Midface

The lower eyelid clinical evaluation must include an analysis of the midface. Aging with gravitational changes and tissue weakening can lead to changes in eyelid position. Midface descent can be associated with loosening ligaments, resorption of bony structure, gravitational descent, and soft tissue deflation and laxity [3].

Midface anatomy is closely related to lower eyelid position. Vector analysis is essential for surgical planning, as this suggests stability of the midface. This is done by comparing the anterior projection of the globe in comparison to the malar eminence to assess midfacial support of tissues. If the cheek is more prominent than the globe, this is a positive vector, which lends to better tissue support. If the globe is more prominent than the cheek, this is a negative vector which leads to a higher risk of continued descent with time and postoperative eyelid malposition if surgical considerations are not taken into account, such as a need for fat repositioning or an implant. Evidence of midface descent includes a prominent tear trough, flat malar eminence, and volume loss in the medial malar fat pad [4].

10 Manual Examination Techniques

Manual palpation of the lower eyelid and surrounding tissues is essential. The tissues can be palpated and manipulated into the correct position to determine the amount of tissue available for reconstruction and effect on the midface. The snap back test and distraction test can characterize tissue tone. The snap back test evaluates orbicularis oculi tone and horizontal eyelid laxity by pulling the lower eyelid inferiorly and letting go to determine if the globe apposition is swift and appropriate in position (Fig. 5). The test is abnormal if the eyelid does not return to position against the globe or returns slowly [1].

The distraction test evaluates canthal tendon laxity by gently grasping and pulling the lower eyelid anteriorly away from the globe (Fig. 6). If the eyelid can be distracted over 8 mm, the test is abnormal [1]. Medial and lateral traction testing allows for the assessment of canthal laxity. Medial canthal laxity is tested by applying medial traction to the lower eyelid to determine the amount of displacement. Lateral canthal laxity is tested by applying lateral traction to the lower eyelid to also determine the amount of displacement.

Anterior lamellar shortage can be assessed by the patient looking up with their mouth open.

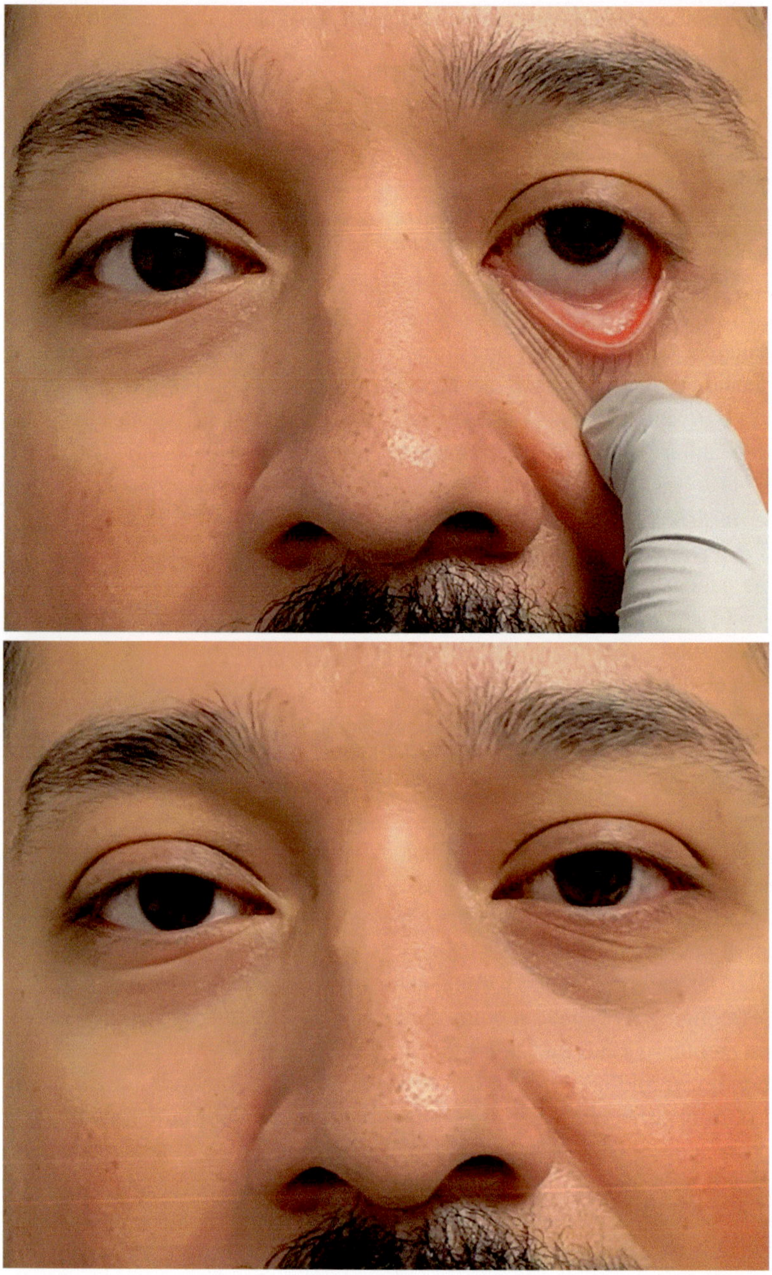

Fig. 5 Clinical images demonstrating a normal snap back test. The examiner gently pulls the lower eyelid inferiorly (a) and then lets go with resulting eyelid apposition to the globe that is swift and appropriate in position

A patient with anterior lamellar deficiency will demonstrate lower eyelid retraction or ectropion [5]. Forced traction testing can be utilized to assess for middle lamellar scarring in an eyelid that does not appear to have decreased skin. This is performed by the patient looking up with the examiner superiorly displacing the lower eyelid (Fig. 7). A normal test will result in the ability of the lower eyelid to stretch upwards, closing the eye. An abnormal test results in an inability to superiorly displace the lower eyelid and indicates scarring [5].

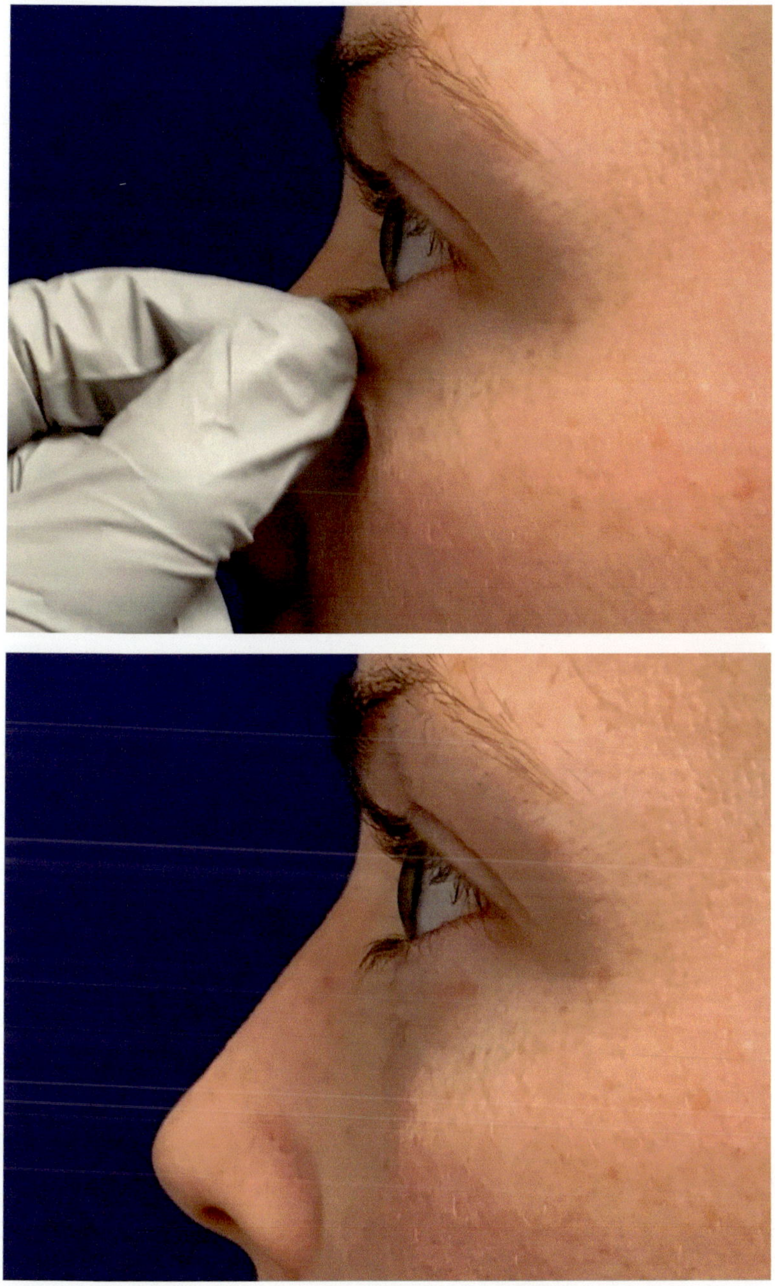

Fig. 6 Clinical images demonstrating a normal distraction test. The examiner gently grasps and pulls the lower eyelid anteriorly away from the globe. The distance of eyelid distraction is less than 8 mm, which is normal

In addition to assessing for eyelid laxity, digital manipulation can mimic the effects of aesthetic surgery (Fig. 8). These maneuvers can corroborate particular plans for midface lifting.

11 Masses

The surgeon should examine carefully for lesions, and note the extent of disruption to the normal architecture, such as irregular pigmentation, lash

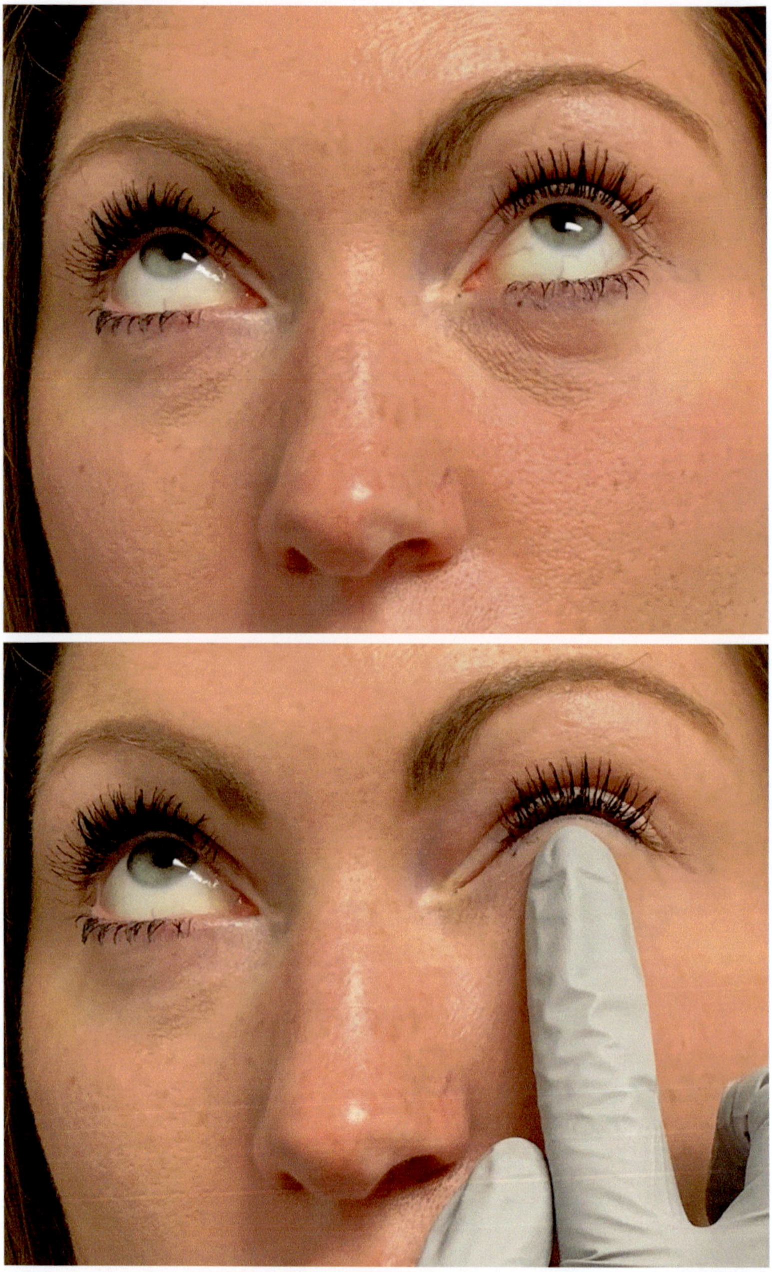

Fig. 7 Clinical images demonstrating a normal forced traction test. With the patient looking up, the examiner superiorly displaces the lower eyelid. The examiner is able to close the eye, which is normal

loss, ulceration, bleeding, or telangiectasias, as this can indicate a malignant lesion. Transillumination can help characterize cystic lesions. Tissue defects should be characterized as to the suspected etiology, if it is full or partial thickness, size of wound, and if the canthal or canalicular integrity is compromised. Careful measurement of dimensions of a lesion or defect is important for surgical planning. Additionally, assessing masses by palpation is important to determine if the mass is mobile or tethered to underlying tissue. Diffuse eyelid edema and erythema acutely may suggest

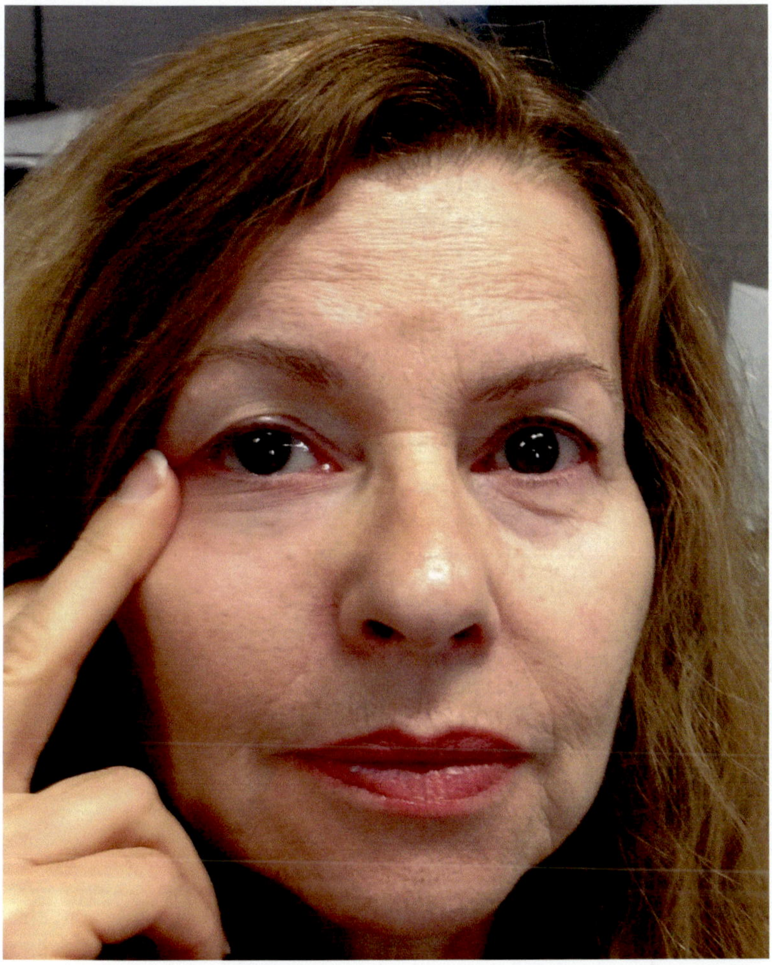

Fig. 8 Digital manipulation of the lower eyelid and cheek to eliminate under eye rhytids and to demonstrate potential of midface lifting

an infectious process, such as preseptal or orbital cellulitis, or an allergic type of reaction. Orbital cellulitis may exhibit signs such as pain with eye movement, restriction of eye movement, chemosis, decreased visual acuity, and afferent pupillary defect. If any of these signs are present, urgent further imaging and workup may be necessary.

12 Ophthalmologic Exam

Conjunctival injection on inspection and with eyelid eversion, tear height, and uniform and reflective corneal surface are methods of evaluating ocular surface health. If the patient has a history of or symptoms of dry eye syndrome, fluorescein staining and a Schirmer test can quantify the extent of disease. A baseline measurement of vision, assessment of pupils, measurement of intraocular pressure, visualization of motility, and assessment of visual fields to confrontation should be considered to assess baseline ocular health. Eyelid position and movement should be assessed in different positions of gaze. Infraduction should be associated with inferior movement of the lower eyelid through connections between the inferior rectus and capsulopalpebral fascia. Eye rotation up on eyelid closure (Bell reflex) should be assessed as it is an important protective mechanism for the cornea.

Meibomian gland health, blepharitis, and telangiectasias are evaluated by close inspection of the eyelid margin, which can also influence ocular surface health. Lash loss may suggest a destructive lesion such as malignancy. The eyelids should be examined for trichiasis, distichiasis, and punctal abnormalities such as erythema and edema, stenosis, or malposition. Epiphora or a high tear lake warrants further workup for nasolacrimal duct abnormalities.

13 Photography

Photographic documentation of the patient's baseline and clinical course is essential. The image background should be uniform in color and texture and not detract from the clinical image [6]. Different angles should be taken including full face, hemifacial, and focused on one eye at a time. The patient should have a neutral facial expression with a relaxed brow and mouth but additional photos with expressions may display pathology more clearly. Additional photos in various positions of gaze such as up and downgaze is also useful. Consistent lighting is key to avoid shadows that may enhance contours or overexposure which can minimize details. The camera lens and zoom should also be consistent as to not distort the ratios of facial features [6]. Additionally, consistent angles are important, particularly in comparing preoperative and postoperative photographs. To achieve an identical oblique angle, the photograph can be captured at the angle where the leading edge of the patients's nose meets the leading edge of the cheek. Videography can also be used to capture and document dynamic findings. Images should be of high quality to allow for detailed analysis of the eyelids and face. The various factors should all be reproducible to allow for clear comparison. Additionally, clinical images can be helpful if needed for medical-legal purposes or for education.

Photographic Considerations

- Uniform background and lighting
- Angles: full face, hemiface, centered around each eye, different positions of gaze, profile, oblique angle
- Expression: neutral, smiling
- Reproducible image factors for comparison throughout surgical course

14 Setting Expectations

Finally, in the pre-operative setting, the patient's expectations should be assessed and if a "perfect" result is desired or one that would not be achievable, a conversation about realistic goals in addition to a thorough informed consent regarding surgical risk is essential. Surgical candidacy should take into account body dysmorphic disorder and psychosocial issues [7]. Clear pre- and post-operative expectations and instructions should be conveyed.

15 Summary

The focus of the clinical exam should center around the patient's chief concern, but the surgeon should also observe the full face for any pathology or special considerations. Eyelid malposition such as entropion, ectropion, or eyelid retraction should be examined in detail to identify the pathology that drives a sound treatment plan.

References

1. Massry GG, Murphy MR, Azizzadeh B. Master techniques in blepharoplasty and periorbital rejuvenation. Springer Science + Business Media; 2011. p. 31–43.
2. Kpodzo DS, Nahai F, McCord CD. Malar mounds and festoons: review of current management. Aesthet Surg J. 2014;34(2):235–48. https://doi.org/10.1177/1090820X13517897.
3. Liao HT. Lower eyelid and midface rejuvenation: suborbicularis oculi fat lift. Facial Plast Surg Clin North

Am. 2021;29(4):497–509. https://doi.org/10.1016/j.fsc.2021.06.003.
4. Rohrich RJ, Pessa JE. The fat compartments of the face: anatomy and clinical implications for cosmetic surgery. Plast Reconstr Surg. 2007;119(7):2219–27. https://doi.org/10.1097/01.prs.0000265403.66886.54.
5. Griffin G, Azizzadeh B, Massry GG. New insights into physical findings associated with postblepharoplasty lower eyelid retraction. Aesthet Surg J. 2014;34(7):995–1004. https://doi.org/10.1177/1090820X14544306.
6. Cheney ML, Hadlock TA. Facial surgery: plastic and reconstructive. Taylor & Francis Group; 2015. p. 49–63.
7. Mauriello J. Techniques of cosmetic eyelid surgery: a case study approach. Lippincott Williams & Wilkins; 2004. p. 1–22.

Excision of Lower Eyelid Lesions

Davi Araf

Abstract

Eyelid lesions require excision for disfigurement, discomfort, or because they may be malignant. In this chapter, the author describes excision and repair techniques that minimize eyelid malposition and scars. Features of benign versus malignant lesions are also described.

Keywords

Lower eyelid · Lower eyelid lesion · Lower eyelid excision · Lower eyelid repair

1 Introduction

When excising lower eyelid lesions, many variables should be considered. These include suspicion for malignancy and attributes of the resultant defect.

In addition to defect size and depth, the amount of eyelid laxity can influence decisions on repair. Eyelid defects may be small (up to 25%), medium-sized (25 to 50%) and large (greater than 50%) [1]. The defect depth should also be considered. Anterior, posterior lamella, or a full thickness defects require different strategies. In addition, excision in the periorbital region may involve other important structures such as the canthal tendons, tear ducts and eyelashes.

In the excision of lower eyelid tumors, it is essential to differentiate between benign and malignant lesions, since this may guide the type and extent of excision that, in turn, determines the reconstruction needs. To this end, eyelid biopsy is important. Incisional and excisional biopsy techniques are described.

2 Incisional Eyelid Biopsy Techniques

In incisional biopsy, a portion of the tumor is sampled to confirm the clinical diagnosis. In excisional biopsy, the entire gross lesion is removed, with attempt to have margins of the sample free of tumor. Samples that are too small or damaged through electrocoagulation or crush artifact should be avoided since they may confound histopathologic analysis. The chief categories of lower eyelid incisional biopsy include

Supplementary Information The online version contains supplementary material available at https://doi.org/10.1007/978-3-031-36175-3_3.

D. Araf (✉)
Division of Oculoplastic Surgery, University of São Paulo Medical School, Cema Hospital, São Paulo, Brazil
e-mail: cppo@ig.com.br

J. P. Tao (ed.), *Plastic Surgery of the Lower Eyelids*,
https://doi.org/10.1007/978-3-031-36175-3_3

shave, punch, elliptical excision, and full thickness wedge resection.

Shave biopsy is the use of a blade to remove the elevated portion of a benign lesion. A seborrheic keratosis in the periocular area or nevus affecting the eyelid margin are common tumors amenable to a shave technique.

Punch biopsy is the use of a circular punch blade to cut perpendicularly and deepened into the skin with rotation movements, yielding a cylindrical core of tissue sample. It may be used to obtain full-thickness samples of the skin for incisional or excisional biopsy (small lesions). Punch biopsy may be used in the periocular region but owing to the highly visible nature of this zone, elliptical scalpel excisions with resultant scar within relaxed facial skin tension lines may be preferable to better camouflage the wound.

Elliptical excision describes using a scalpel or other cutting device to surround a lesion in an ellipse. This is also used for excisional biopsy. These are described in detail below.

Wedge resection is the removal of a full thickness segment of the eyelid. This is performed in cases where tumors affecting the eyelid margin cannot be sufficiently removed or sampled in one of the techniques above. This is also used for excisional biopsy and is described below.

3 Incision Placement

Incision design and placement are important in obtaining good functional outcomes and favorable cosmetic results. Whenever possible, incisions should be oriented parallel to skin tension lines, which correspond to lines and creases of the skin that can conceal a planned incision (Fig. 1). These lines are perpendicular to muscle fibers and corresponding to wrinkles or other skin creases. Incisions that traverse these creases tend to be more conspicuous (Fig. 2).

In addition to skin tension lines, incisions that fall in other facial contour lines are ideal. These are division lines in the junction from one region to the other, such as nasojugal and malar groove and dependence (i.e., due to the effect of gravity and fat tissue) such as base contour of fat bags in lower eyelids [2]. Previous scars may also be ideal locations to perform incisions.

Skin incisions in the eyelid region should be made with a scalpel blade (or energy based cutting device such as CO_2 laser or radiofrequency), positioned perpendicular to the plane in the vertical position to prevent margin beveling [3]. Natural skin folds or the malar groove on lower eyelids are ideal [4]. The following are other preferred lines or folds on the eyelid that may best conceal a scar:

Subciliary or infraciliary line/fold: 1–2 mm inferior to the eyelash line. Care should be taken to preserve the pretarsal orbicularis oculi muscle.

Subtarsal incision or mid-lower eyelid line/fold: approximately 4 to 7 mm below the eyelid margin and usually results in a more noticeable scar.

Infraorbital line/fold: the transition between the thickest portion of the cheek skin and the thin eyelid skin [4].

3.1 Incision and Drainage of Chalazion

A chalazion is one of the most common reasons patients present to an eyelid specialist. These are inflamed cysts due to blockage of meibomian glands. Initial treatment is warm compress therapy with topical antibiotic ointment with or without corticosteroids. In some instances, corticosteroid injections may be helpful. If medical management fails, incision and drainage through a posterior approach may be indicated.

The area of the chalazion is marked to aid in identification after local anesthesia obliterates the obvious affected portion of the eyelid. Local anesthetic is administered widely across the eyelid to the medial and lateral canthus. The eyelid is everted with a chalazion clamp. If a clamp is not available, the eyelid may be everted over a cotton tip applicator with the aid of a suture passed through the margin. With a #15 or #11 blade, a cruciate incision is

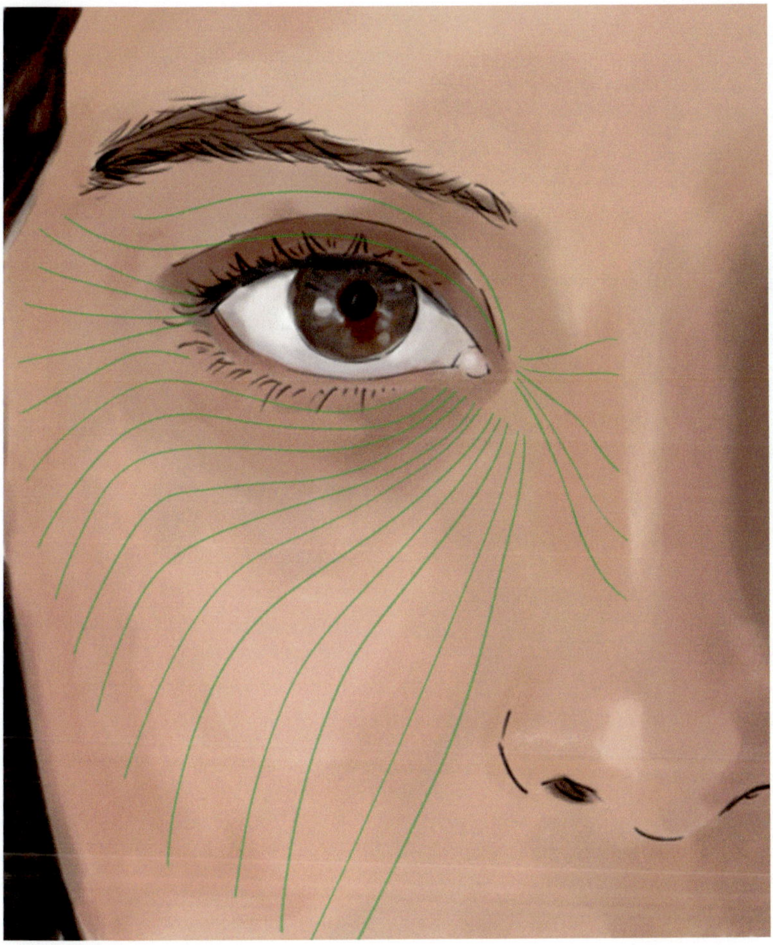

Fig. 1 Relaxed skin tension lines of the lower eyelids and midface *(illustration by Michael Han, MD)*

fashioned on the tarsal side of the chalazion. Intralesional contents are expressed with a blade, scissors, or a curette. Trimming the corners of the cruciate incision may help prevent recurrence and more immediately flatten the eyelid. Electrocautery is helpful to improve hemostasis intraoperatively and especially postoperatively (Video 1).

4 Excisional Techniques for the Removal of Eyelid Lesions

Excision is the exeresis of a tissue fragment. It is performed to remove a benign or malignant lesion, to provide material for histological examination (biopsy) or to correct scars [4]. In many cases of excision of lower eyelid lesions, there is the need for full thickness eyelid resection.

4.1 Shave Excision

Shave excision is recommended for epidermal lesions that do not extend to the dermis. Shave is best for superficial, exophytic, elevated, or pedunculated lesions such as a fibroepithelial papilloma or a seborrheic keratosis. This technique may also be used in tarsal conjunctiva lesions.

A superficial fragment of tissue is removed with a scalpel blade, scissors, or electrosurgical

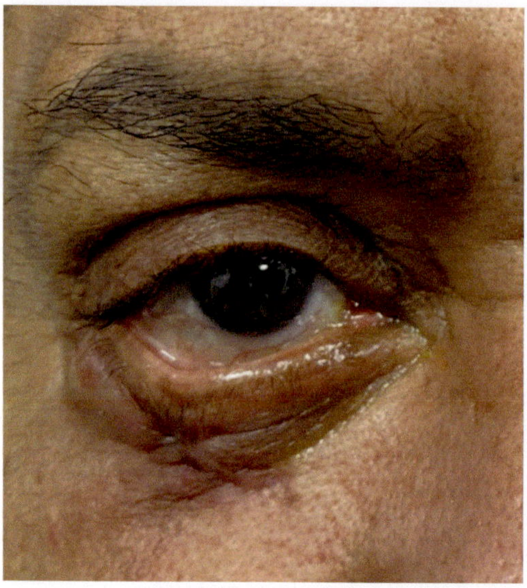

Fig. 2 Lower eyelid scars after incisions traversed relaxed skin tension lines

unit in a plane parallel to the skin. Grasping and elevating the lesion with a toothed forceps aids in the excision. There is no need for subsequent suture, and the technique usually leads to an excellent cosmetic outcome. On the eyelid margin, the shave technique may lead to small hypotrophic scars, trichiasis, or madarosis (local loss of eyelashes).

4.2 Elliptical Excision

Excision in an elliptical pattern may be used for both benign and malignant lesions. It allows for linear closure.

When planning the ellipse, the long axis should ideally run parallel to the relaxed skin tension lines (Figs. 3, 4, 5 and 6) (Video 2). In general, the axis of the ellipse should attempt to follow an inferolateral direction on the lower eyelid, the relaxed skin tension line in this area. To forestall eyelid retraction, closure of the ellipse should cause minimal vertical tension. Ideally, the long axis should be at least three times the width of the lesion to avoid redundant tissue at the ends of the ellipse. This proportion may be smaller when there is extensive skin laxity. Redundant tissue may form a dog ear deformity at the end of the suture closure. This redundant tissue may be excised in small triangles [3].

4.3 Circular Excision

A circular excision is the exeresis of a lesion by demarcating a circumference around it. If the area is small, it may be converted into a fusiform excision, its margins detached and closed primarily; however, in case of larger lesions that do not allow for primary closure, reconstruction may be more complex and may require a graft or flap.

Flaps are discussed in other chapters, but a bilobed is useful for a circular defect. Filling the primary defect with a neighbor flap and creating a second flap to fill the secondary defect can achieve closure and redirect tension appropriately (Figs. 7 and 8).

4.4 Full Thickness Pentagonal Eyelid Excision

A full thickness pentagonal, a.k.a. wedge excision is indicated to remove lesions that affect more than superficial layers of the eyelid. Due to elasticity, up to ¼ to 1/3 of the extent of the lower eyelid may be resected and closed by direct approximation of the free margins. If primary closure is not possible, reconstructive flaps or grafts may be indicated. These are described in Chap. "Repair of Full Thickness Lower Eyelid Defects". Excision of full thickness of the lower eyelid is useful for malignant lesions, owing to a lower probability of leaving behind residual tumor.

Eyelid resection should be in a pentagon to ensure parallel cuts through the tarsus (Fig. 9). Non-parallel incisions risk kinking or non-flush closure. The eyelid is sutured directly, with meticulous alignment of the grey line and eyelash line [5]. Deep sutures to align the tarsus aid in stability [6].

A 6-0 silk suture is used to align the eyelid margin (grey line) (Fig. 10).

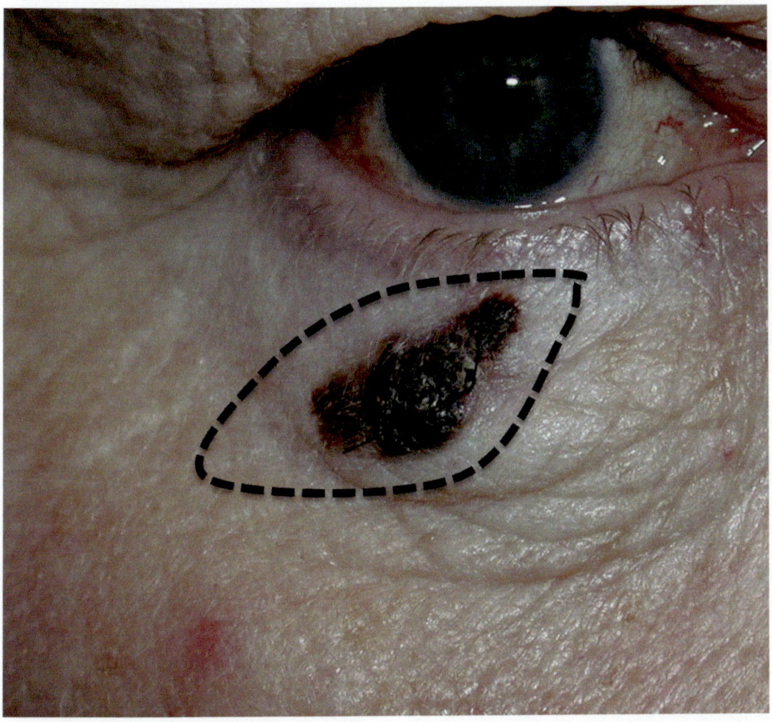

Fig. 3 Ellipse designed surrounding an eyelid melanoma with axis and resultant wound within the inferolateral relaxed skin tension line

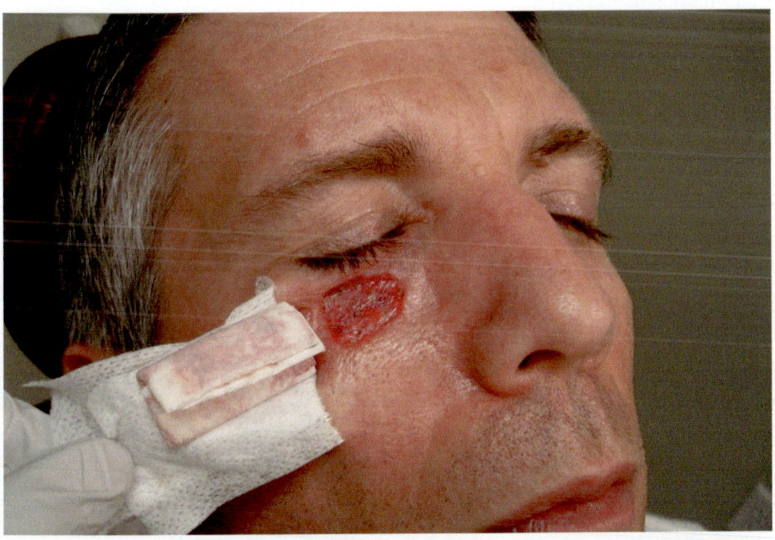

Fig. 4 Large lower eyelid and cheek defect

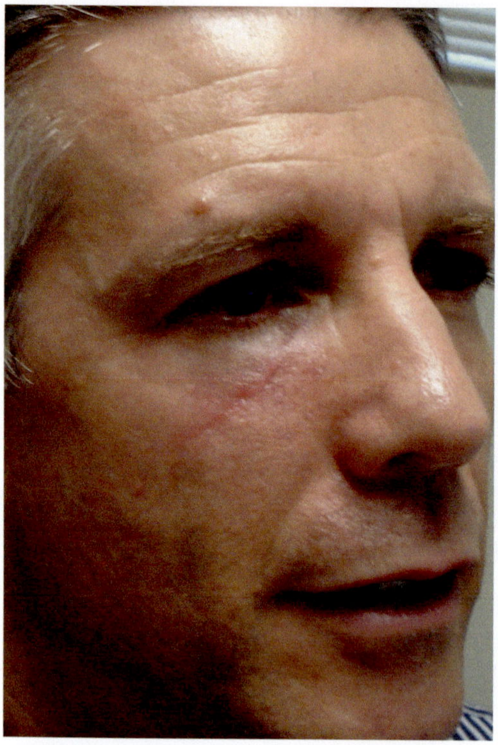

Fig. 5 Patient in Fig. 4 6 weeks post closure via undermining in the superolateral and inferomedial aspect of the wound so that the scar in the inferolateral RSTL and with minimal vertical tension on the eyelid

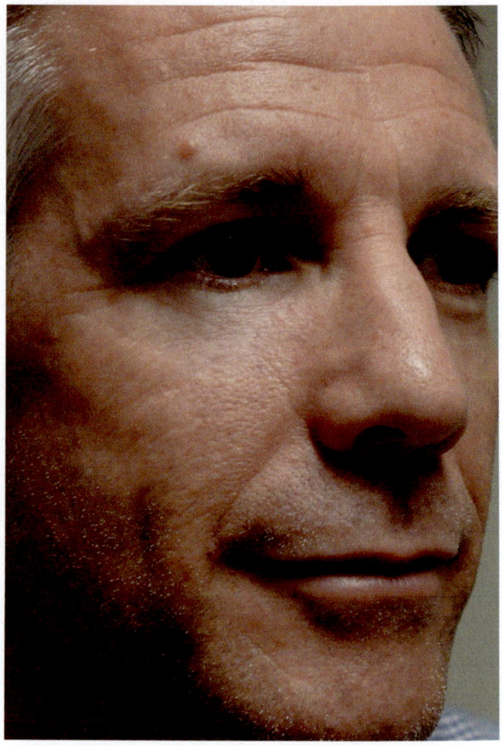

Fig. 6 1 year post repair with scar fully healed with the scar well camouflaged in the RSTL and no eyelid malposition

A second 6-0 silk suture aligns the eyelashes line (a third posterior stitch may be placed to align the mucocutaneous junction but is usually not if necessary). Stitches are knotted and the tails kept long, and are then incorporated into cutaneous sutures to keep the sutures away from the ocular surface (Fig. 11).

The tarsal plate is sutured with one or two absorbable sutures (6-0 polyglactin), with care to take partial thickness passes through tarsus so as to protect the cornea. The orbicularis oculi muscle may be also sutured with 6-0 polyglactin. Skin is closed in its own layer using of 6-0 plain, nylon, or silk (Fig. 12).

After excision and repair, wounds are dressed with antibiotic ointment 2 times per day. Sutures are removed in approximately one week. The initial months are associated with some erythema and trace edema but cosmesis is generally

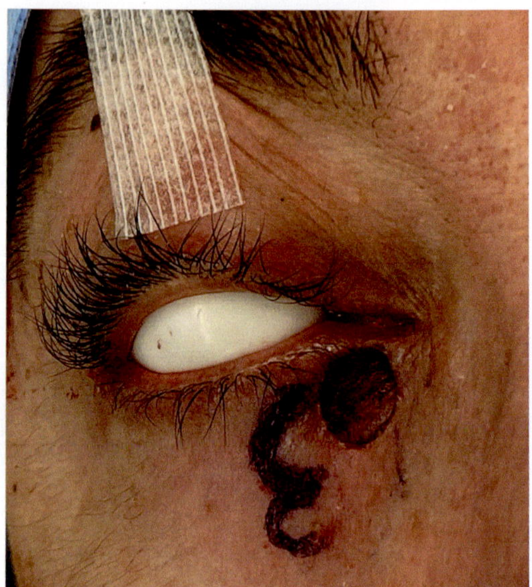

Fig. 7 Circular excision of lower eyelid lesion

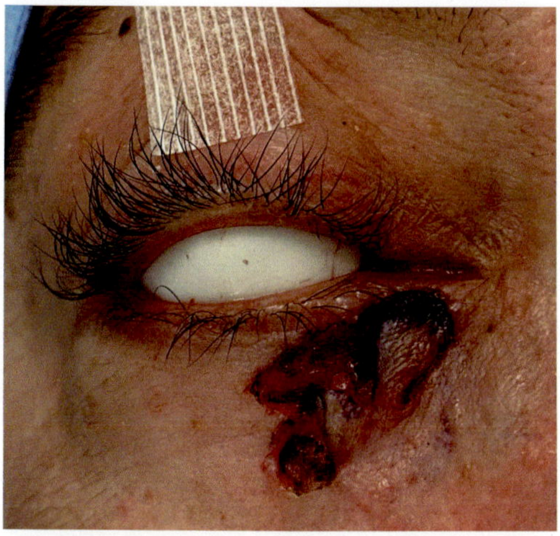

Fig. 8 Bilobed flap transposition

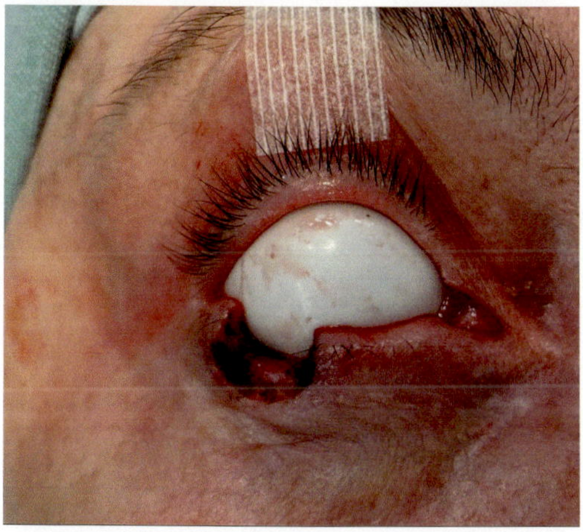

Fig. 9 Excision of a lower eyelid lesion (full-thickness) in pentagonal shape with posterior primary closure of the defect

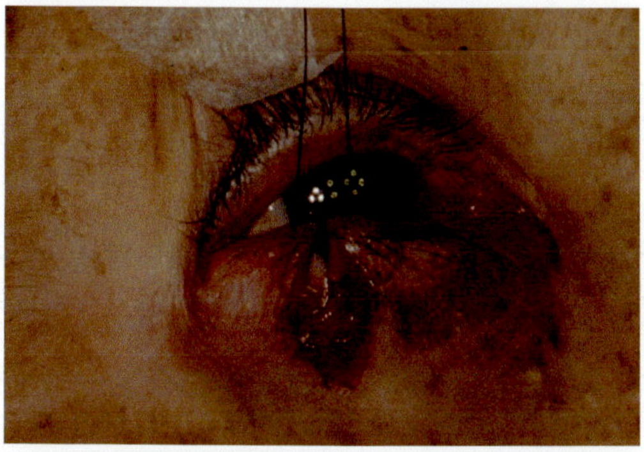

Fig. 10 Repair suture in the eyelid margin (grey line) positioning the structures

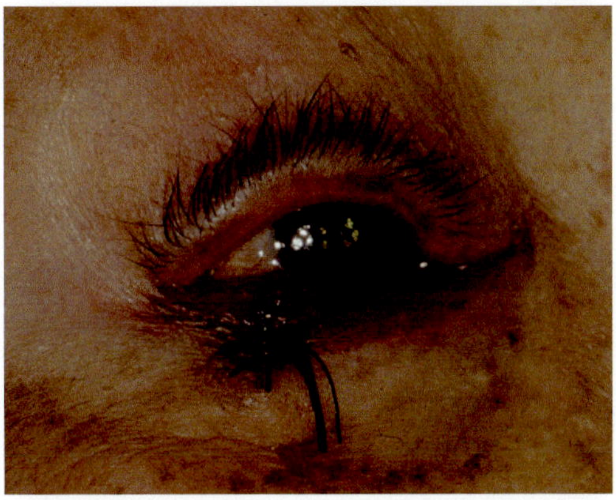

Fig. 11 Immediate postoperative result of primary closure after excision of a lower eyelid full-thickness lesion

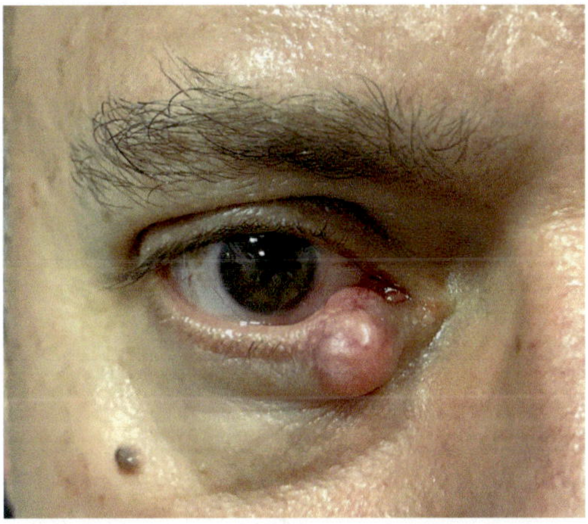

Fig. 12 Preoperative of a full-thickness lesion excision of the lower eyelid with direct closure (with lateral cantholysis)

excellent after full thickness resection, even if a cantholysis is needed (Figs. 12 and 13).

To obviate a conspicuous scar, the wedge resection can be performed posterior to a subciliary incision and anterior lamella flap to avoid facial scars (Figs. 14, 15, 16, 17, 18 and 19) (Video 3).

Larger lower eyelid defects that are not amenable to closure using the above technique may require myocutaneous or tarsoconjunctival flaps or grafts. These are described in other chapters. Spontaneous granulation, a.k.a laissez-faire may be considered for some defects, especially when there exists insufficient tissue for reconstruction

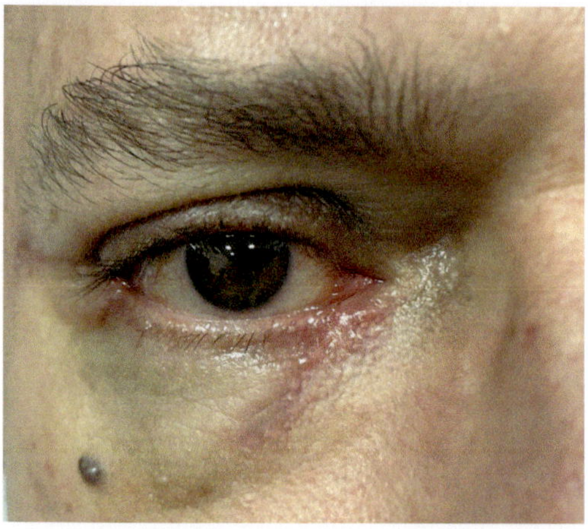

Fig. 13 3 month postoperative appearance of the lower eyelid of the patient in Fig. 12 after full thickness wedge resection

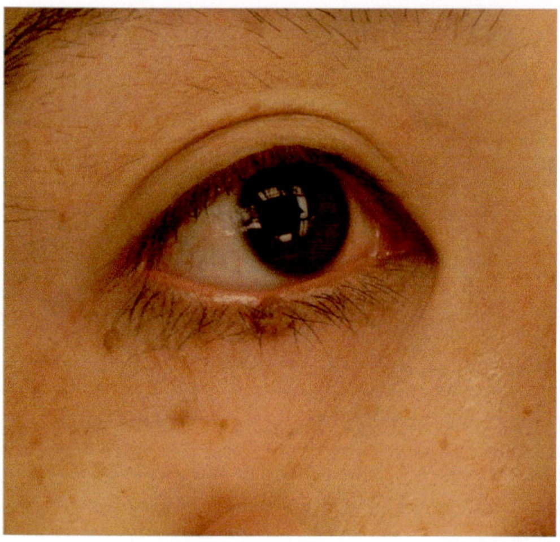

Fig. 14 Lower eyelid margin involving lesion. While a shave may be appropriate, the broad base may result in a conspicuous scar or madarosis

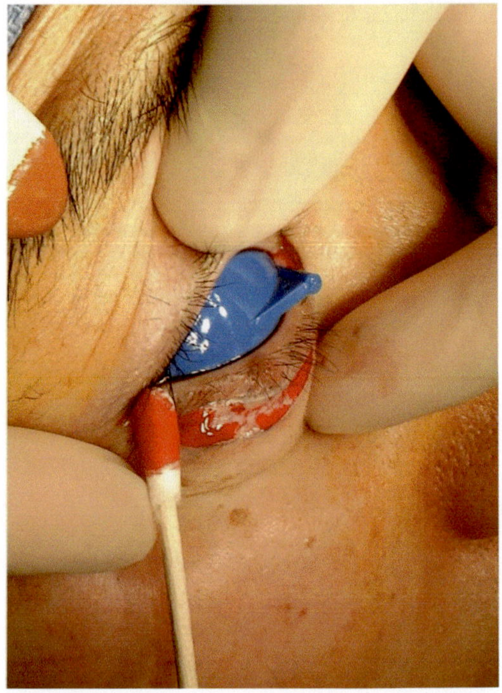

Fig. 15 A subciliary incision is created

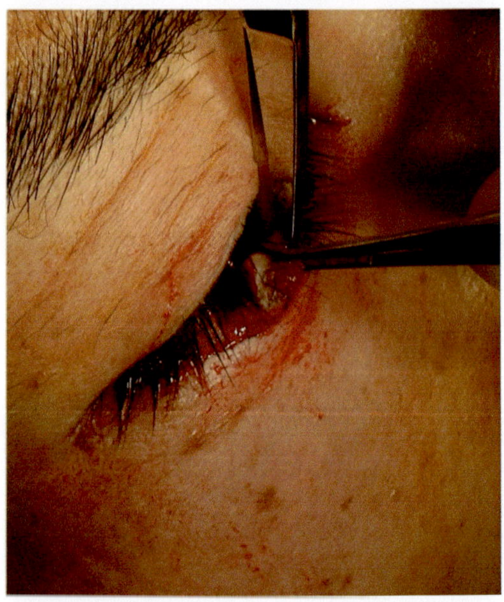

Fig. 16 Pentagonal wedge resection is performed posterior to the anterior lamella flap

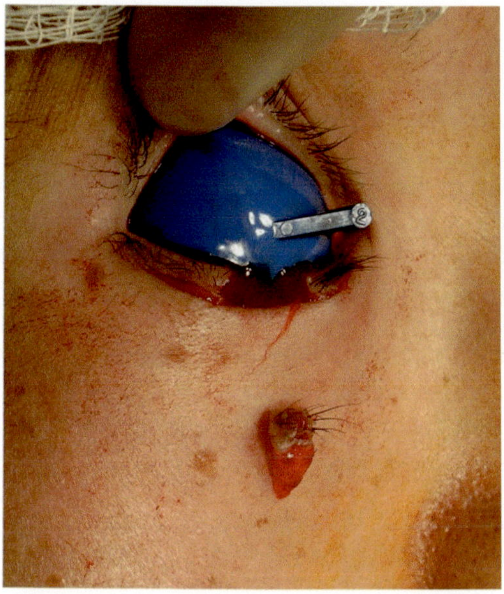

Fig. 17 Segment of the eyelid including the lesion is resected

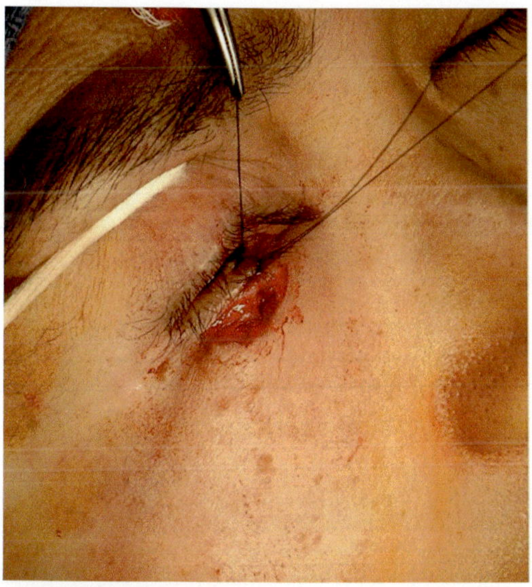

Fig. 18 The eyelid margin is aligned with 6-0 silk sutures to the gray line and lash line, respectively. The tarsus is closed with 6-0 polyglactin suture

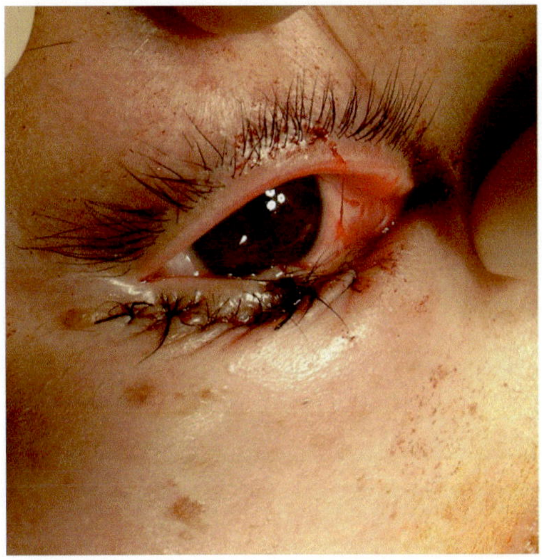

Fig. 19 Anterior lamella flap is redraped over the area of resection to achieve a full thickness eyelid resection without conspicuous scars

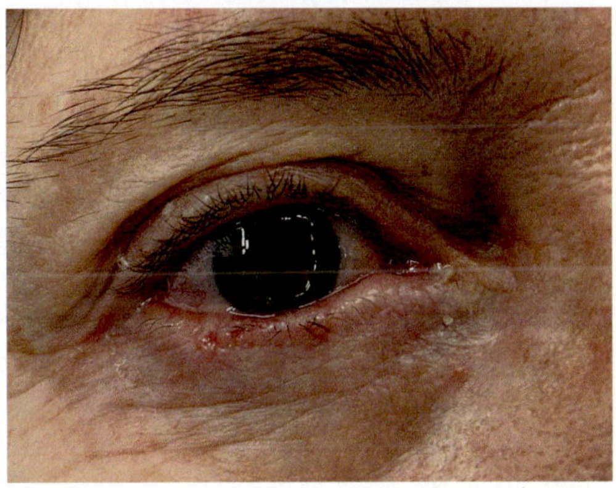

Fig. 20 Basal cell carcinoma. Note madarosis and margin irregularity

such as after extensive burn. With or without recruitment of the adjacent area to reduce the defect size, wound care is performed to allow healing by second intention that takes several months [2].

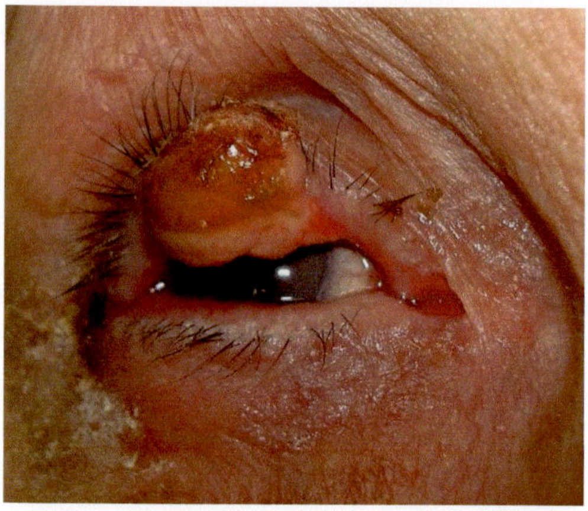

Fig. 21 Example of upper eyelid sebaceous carcinoma

5 Clinical Features of Benign Versus Malignant Eyelid Lesions

Benign eyelid lesions include neoplastic tumors and inflammatory pathologies [7]. Benign lesions typically do not disrupt eyelashes or alter surrounding eyelid architecture. Chronicity often favors a benign process; however recent growth may be seen with both benign and malignant lesions. Common non-inflammatory benign lower eyelid tumors are squamous papillomas, vascular tumors, nevi, cysts, and seborrheic keratosis.

Eyelid malignancies are more common in the lower eyelid and medial canthus. Basal cell carcinoma is most common, followed by squamous-cell carcinoma, melanoma (Fig. 3), sebaceous carcinoma, Merkel cell carcinoma and lymphoma [8–10]. Malignant eyelid tumors are confirmed by histopathology [11]. Progressive increase in size, bleeding, crusting, and lash lass are suspicious behaviors. On clinical assessment, irregularity, madarosis, and ulceration suggest malignancy (Fig. 20). Basal cell carcinoma often has a raised pearly, smooth appearance and under magnification, fine telangiectasia can be seen.

Sebaceous carcinoma is an important malignancy to diagnose because it has aggressive behavior and is potentially lethal. It is a malignancy that originates in a sebaceous gland of the periocular area, usually a Meibomian gland of the tarsal plate, but also of Zeiss gland of the eyelid margin or pilosebaceous gland of the sin, caruncle, or eyebrows. It may present clinically as a chalazion or blepharitis. A classic history is a chalazion that does not respond to usual interventions including incision and drainage [12, 13] (Fig. 21).

6 Conclusion

In summary, eyelid excision is a fundamental lower eyelid surgery. The type of resection depends on features of the lesion including size, location, and level of suspicion for malignancy. Full thickness resection is useful for complete resection of lesions and maintenance of good eyelid structure and function.

References

1. Matayoshi S, Forno EA, Moura EM. Manual de cirurgia plástica ocular. São Paulo: Roca; 2004.
2. Soares EJC, Moura EM, Gonçalves JOR. Cirurgia plástica ocular. São Paulo: Roca; 1997.
3. Volpini M. Técnicas básicas. In: Vital Filho J, Velasco e Cruz AA, Schellini AS, Matayoshi S, Figueiredo ARP, Herzog Neto G, editors. Cultura médica: órbita, sistema lacrimal e oculoplástica. 3rd ed. Rio de Janeiro; 2013. p. 227–241.
4. Hoyama E, Shiratori CA, Stumpft S. Tipos de incisões e excisões. In: Limongi RM, Borba A, editors. Conexão soluções corporativas: oculoplástica e oncologia ocular. Goiânia; 2021. p. 133–138.
5. Souza Júnior AC, Araf D, Matayoshi S. Reconstrução palpebral. In: Vital Filho J, Velasco e Cruz AA, Schellini AS, Matayoshi S, Figueiredo ARP, Herzog Neto G, editors. Cultura médica: órbita, sistema lacrimal e oculoplástica. 3rd ed. Rio de Janeiro; 2013. p. 337–347.

6. Shiratori CA, Stumpft S. Princípios básicos da reconstrução palpebral. pentágono, fechamento direto com ou sem cantólise. Limongi RM, Borba A, editors. Conexão soluções corporativas: oculoplástica e oncologia ocular. Goiânia; 2021. p. 133–138.
7. Abidi U, Maheshwari V, Tyagi N, Tyagi SP, Gogi R. Soft tissue tumours of eyelid. Indian J Pathol Microbiol. 1997;40(4):515–9.
8. Cernea P, Simionescu C, Militaru C. Tumori maligne palpebrale. Consideraţii privind 111 cazuri. Oftalmologia. 1996;40(4):361–7.
9. Abdi U, Tyagi N, Maheshwari V, Gogi R, Tyagi SP. Tumours of eyelid: a clinicopathologic study. J Indian Med Assoc. 1996;94(11):405–9, 416, 418.
10. Margo CE, Mulla ZD. Malignant tumors of the eyelid: a population-based study of non-basal cell and non-squamous cell malignant neoplasms. Arch Ophthalmol. 1998;116(2):195–8. https://doi.org/10.1001/archopht.116.2.195. PMID: 9488271.
11. Kersten RC, Ewing-Chow D, Kulwin DR, Gallon M. Accuracy of clinical diagnosis of cutaneous eyelid lesions. Ophthalmology. 1997;104(3):479–84.
12. Nerad JA. Oculoplastic surgery: the requisites in ophthalmology. St. Louis: Mosby; 2001.
13. Piest K, Lloyd W, Wulc A. Dermatopathology of the ocular adnexa. In: Murphy G, editor. Dermatopathology: a practical guide to common disorders. Philadelphia: WD Saunders; 1995. p. 445–66.

Repair of Full Thickness Lower Eyelid Defects

Lalita Gupta, Mark A. Prendes and Peter J. Timoney

Abstract

A range of techniques exist for the repair of full thickness lower eyelid defects. The aim is to restore structure and function of the eyelid. There are many factors to consider including the width and location of the defect. In this chapter, the authors describe a systematic approach to repair full thickness lower eyelid reconstruction according to size and extent of the defect.

Keywords

Full thickness lower eyelid defects · Tarsoconjunctival flap · Semicircular flap · Skin and muscle flap · Bilobed flap · Glabellar flap

1 Introduction/Background

1.1 Principles

Full thickness lower eyelid defects are chiefly after carcinoma resection but sometimes occur after trauma, and less commonly after infection. The aim of lower eyelid repair is to restore structure and function. Minimizing vertical tension on the eyelid is prioritized to forestall malposition or inadequate eyelid closure that compromise protection of the ocular surface. Whenever possible, incisions should be placed within relaxed facial tension lines that leave better camouflaged scars. Canthal fixation is another important consideration.

The approach to repair depends on various factors including the size and location of the defect. The eyelid is bilamellar and separate flaps or grafts should be utilized for the anterior versus posterior reconstruction. At least one should provide a blood supply, i.e., a graft will not survive upon another graft. The degree of eyelid laxity and quality of the skin will also play a role in the choice of advancement flaps.

Supplementary Information The online version contains supplementary material available at https://doi.org/10.1007/978-3-031-36175-3_4.

L. Gupta · P. J. Timoney (✉)
Department of Ophthalmology, University of Kentucky, Lexington, KY, United States
e-mail: peterjtimoney@gmail.com

M. A. Prendes
Department of Ophthalmology and Visual Sciences, Case Western Reserve University, Cleveland, OH, United States

J. P. Tao (ed.), *Plastic Surgery of the Lower Eyelids*,
https://doi.org/10.1007/978-3-031-36175-3_4

2 Full-Thickness Marginal Defects

The approaches to closure of full thickness marginal defects of the lower eyelid may be organized based on the size of the defect.

2.1 Small Defects (<33–40%)

Small defects, involving less than 33% of the horizontal width of the lower eyelid, may be closed directly (Fig. 1). In older patients, greater skin laxity may allow larger defects involving up to 40% of the lower eyelid to be closed directly. A lateral canthotomy and cantholysis can allow slight additional mobilization of the adjacent tissue and minimize wound tension.

Direct Closure (Video 1; also Described in Chap. "Excision of Lower Eyelid Lesions")

Steps:

1. The margins of the defect should be inspected to ensure that the borders are parallel. Irregular or non-parallel wound edges will not approximate appropriately and risk notch formation at the eyelid margin.
2. If primary closure is not possible and a slight amount of tissue recruitment is needed, a lateral canthotomy and cantholysis may reduce tension. The skin at the lateral canthus is incised with a #15 blade. Sharp dissection is carried down to the lateral orbital rim periosteum. The inferior crus of the lateral canthal tendon is severed with sharp dissection.
3. Attention is then directed to the defect. A 6-0 polyglactin or silk suture is passed through the gray line to close the eyelid margin in a wound everting technique with or without a vertical mattress configuration. An additional 6-0 silk suture is used to approximate the lash line. These margin sutures can be kept long and incorporated into the skin sutures inferior to the eyelash margin to prevent contact with the ocular surface.
4. A 6-0 polyglactin suture is then used to appose the tarsus via partial thickness passes. The deep orbicularis is closed with 6-0 polyglactin. The skin over the defect is closed with 5-0 or 6-0 fast absorbing suture or silk.
5. If a lateral canthotomy and cantholysis was performed, the recruited skin may be secured

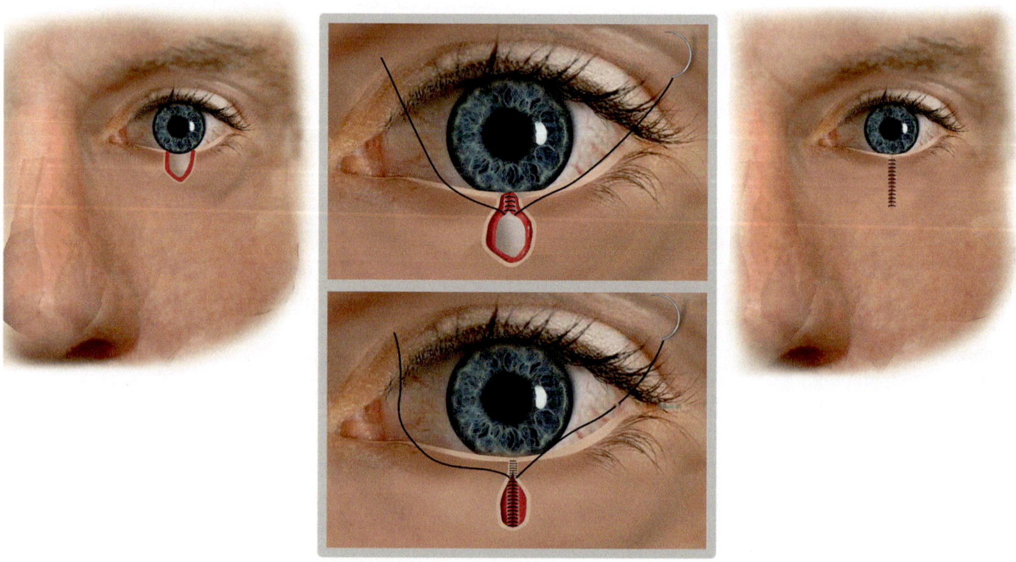

Fig. 1 Direct closure of a full thickness lower eyelid defect

to the lateral rim using 5-0 polyglactin suture to secure the new lateral canthus.

2.2 Moderate Defects (33–50%)

Moderate full thickness lower eyelid defects involving 33–50% of the eyelid margin can be repaired by advancing the lateral portion of eyelid. A semicircular rotational flap is preferred (Fig. 2) [1, 2]. It may also be useful for large defects involving more than 60% of the lower eyelid if orbital rim attachments are released to mobilize the flap [3]. This incision extends laterally and curving upward to the preauricular hair line [4]. A lateral Z plasty at the lateral canthotomy incision is an option that similarly recruits canthal and temple tissues. The chief limitation compared to a semircircular flap is scars that traverse skin tension lines.

3 Semicircular Rotational Flap

Steps

1. An incision is fashioned at the lateral canthus extending first vertically. The arc then extends superotemporally to create a semicircle. A lateral canthotomy and inferior cantholysis are performed. The skin-muscle flap is undermined and elevated allowing the lateral edge of the defect (i.e., the remnant lateral lower eyelid) to be mobilized medially. Attachments down to the inferolateral orbital rim may need to be released to adequately mobilize the flap.
2. The eyelid margin defect is closed directly as described above.
3. At the lateral canthus, the skin and muscle flap is secured to the periosteum at the inner aspect of lateral orbital rim with a 5-0 polyglactin suture.
4. The skin is closed with 5-0 or 6-0 suture.
5. The posterior aspect of the new lateral lower eyelid may be left bare to heal by second intention, however, the authors prefer lining it with a tarsoconjunctival flap from the upper eyelid, as follows.

3.1 Large Defects (>50%)

As above, a semicircular flap is ideal to reconstruct the anterior lamella. Unlike moderate defect that may not require a posterior lamella flap or graft, larger defects generally need posterior support. A tarsoconjunctival flap, is an excellent choice (Fig. 3).

4 Tarsoconjunctival Flap

Tarsoconjunctival flaps have been described since the late 1800s and early 1900s [5–8]. The incision site on the host (upper) eyelid varied in early descriptions, however the general consensus is that a tarsal incision several millimeters superior to the upper eyelid margin best preserves upper eyelid anatomy [9–13].

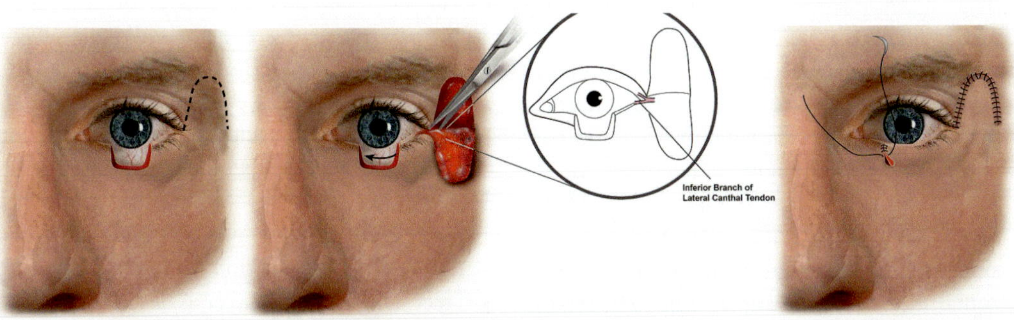

Fig. 2 Closure of a moderate sized lower eyelid defect with recruitment of tissues using a lateral semicircular flap

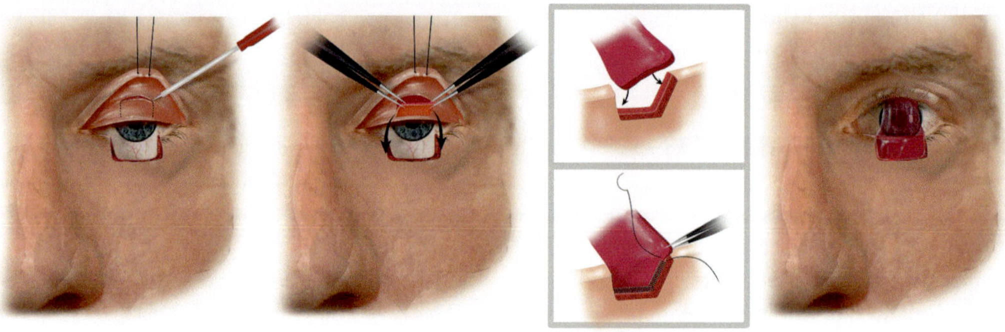

Fig. 3 Traditional repair of a large lower eyelid defect with a tarsoconjunctival flap and skin graft

The flap is created with a horizontal incision 3–4 mm above the margin and then vertical incisions toward the upper fornix. Dissection is carried along the anterior surface of tarsus and then superiorly between the conjunctiva and Muller muscle. Alternatively, Muller muscle may be incorporated into the flap in an attempt to increase flap vascularity [14].

For the anterior lamella, a skin graft or skin flap may be used [9, 14]. The tarsoconjuctival flap is divided weeks later. If it is covered with a well vascularized skin and muscle flap, division can be within 2–3 weeks. In the instance of a skin graft, division is usually postponed to approximately 6 weeks [15–18].

First stage

Steps

1. A traction suture is placed through the upper eyelid margin and the upper eyelid is everted over a Desmarres retractor or cotton tip applicator.
2. The measurement of the lower eyelid defect is used to make a marking of that width on the upper eyelid at least 4 mm from and parallel to the eyelid margin.
3. A #15 blade is used to make a horizontal incision along this marking. Vertical incisions are also made at each end of the horizontal incision to the superior edge of tarsus. Dissection is performed anterior to tarsus to the superior border of tarsus.
4. Dissection is then continued superiorly.
5. The tarsoconjunctival flap is advanced and sutured inferiorly to the remaining lower eyelid tarsus or conjunctiva using 6-0 polyglactin. If there exists insufficient inferior conjunctiva to suture to, the flap may be secured to periorbita at the approximate level of the lower fornix. The tarsoconjunctival flaps may also be secured directly to the posterior aspect of a skin and muscle flap, if applicable.
6. The anterior lamellar defect is repaired with a full thickness skin graft, or preferably an advancement flap.
7. Antibiotic ophthalmic ointment is placed over the surgical site and a pressure patch is placed (if a full thickness skin graft is used).

Second stage

Steps

1. The tarsoconjunctival flap is divided at the site of the newly constructed lower eyelid margin using sharp dissection.
2. The upper eyelid is everted and the host site of the flap is dissected to release adhesions and slightly recess the upper eyelid retractors.
3. At the new lower eyelid margin the mucocutaneous junction is formed so that skin does not come in apposition with the ocular surface. The mucosal layer is secured with 7-0 polyglactin suture or the margin may be left to heal by second intention.

Tarsoconjunctival flap procedures result in good function and cosmesis, with low complication rates [14, 17]. Lower eyelid laxity can be prevented by proper attachment of the tarsoconjunctival flap using small stumps of lower eyelid or other supportive tissue and ensuring that the flap is not too wide [12]. Another concern is upper eyelid entropion which can be prevented by starting the flap at least 3–4 mm from the eyelid margin.

Upper eyelid retraction is more common with host flaps from the central upper eyelid. Lateral tarsoconjunctival flaps, in contrast, are more resistant to retraction since the tissue subtraction is close to the lateral canthal tendon that holds the eyelid in place. A rare complication is tarsal kinking of the upper eyelid immediately after flap division due to fibrosis at the superior edge of tarsus [19]. This can be treated by excision of the fibrotic tissue during the second stage or full thickness excision if persistent. Lower eyelid irregularity, erythema, or scar are common with central tarsoconjunctival flaps covered with a skin graft (Fig. 4). During the second stage, some trim the flap slightly above the margin and then drape the mucosal tissue over the margin to minimize the risk of corneal irritation from keratinized skin [12]. However, this may result in erythema of the eyelid margin. To minimize this, the flap can instead be cut flush with the lower eyelid margin without advancing any excess mucosal tissue and the mucocutaneous junction epithelializes spontaneously without any risk of irritation from keratinized skin [20]. Slight resection or cautery can be used to treat conspicuous overriding, red mucous membrane tissue at the margin.

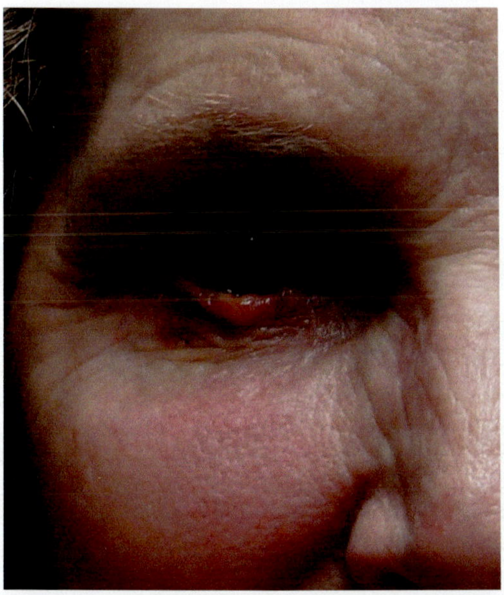

Fig. 4 Lower eyelid irregularity, erythema, and scar after reconstruction of a central lower eyelid defect with a tarsoconjunctival flap and skin graft

5 Tarsoconjunctival Flap Modifications

To avoid ocular occlusion due to eyelid sharing approaches and to obviate a need for a second surgery, Hewes, Sullivan, and Beard described a laterally hinged horizontal designed transconjunctival flap (Fig. 5) [21]. This laterally-based tarsoconjunctival flap from the upper eyelid, is transposed to the lower eyelid to reconstruct the posterior lamella. The anterior lamella is replaced using an advancement flap or a full thickness skin graft [22]. The laterally hinged tarsoconjunctival flap is often used for shallow, lateral defects. If the defect involves the lateral canthus, the technique can be modified by using a higher-based tarsoconjunctival flap not involving the lateral canthal tendon, fixating the flap to the periosteum, reconstructing the superior crus and fixating a tarsal strip to the lateral orbital rim periosteum. If the lateral eyelid is preserved, it can be used for central and medial defects. In that case, the medial defect is closed using a lateral cantholysis and rotational cheek flap and the laterally hinged tarsoconjunctival flap can be transposed into the new lateral defect. Futher stabilization of the posterior lamella laterally can be achieved with a periosteal strip or a free tarsal graft [23]. A myocutaneous advancement flap can be used for the anterior lamella.

The authors' preferred approach is rotation of the remnant lateral lower eyelid with a semicircular flap and a lateral tarsoconjunctival flap (Fig. 6) (Video 2). This method has several

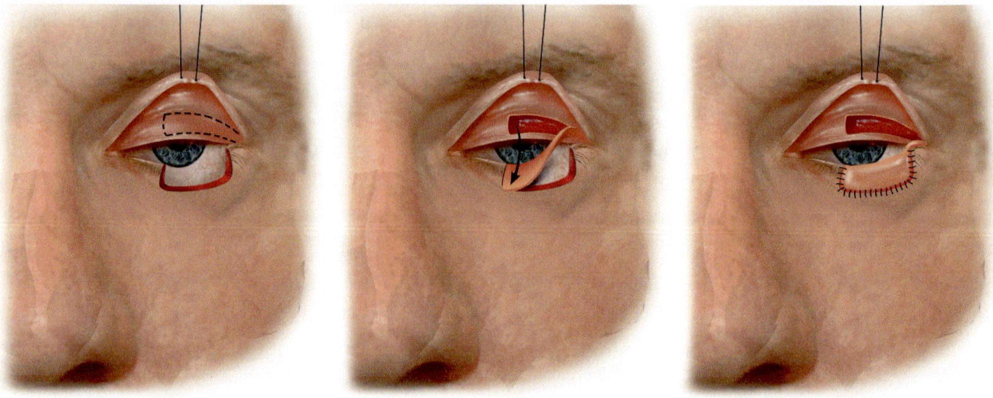

Fig. 5 Laterally hinged tarsoconjunctival flap to repair shallow lateral lower eyelid defects in a single stage

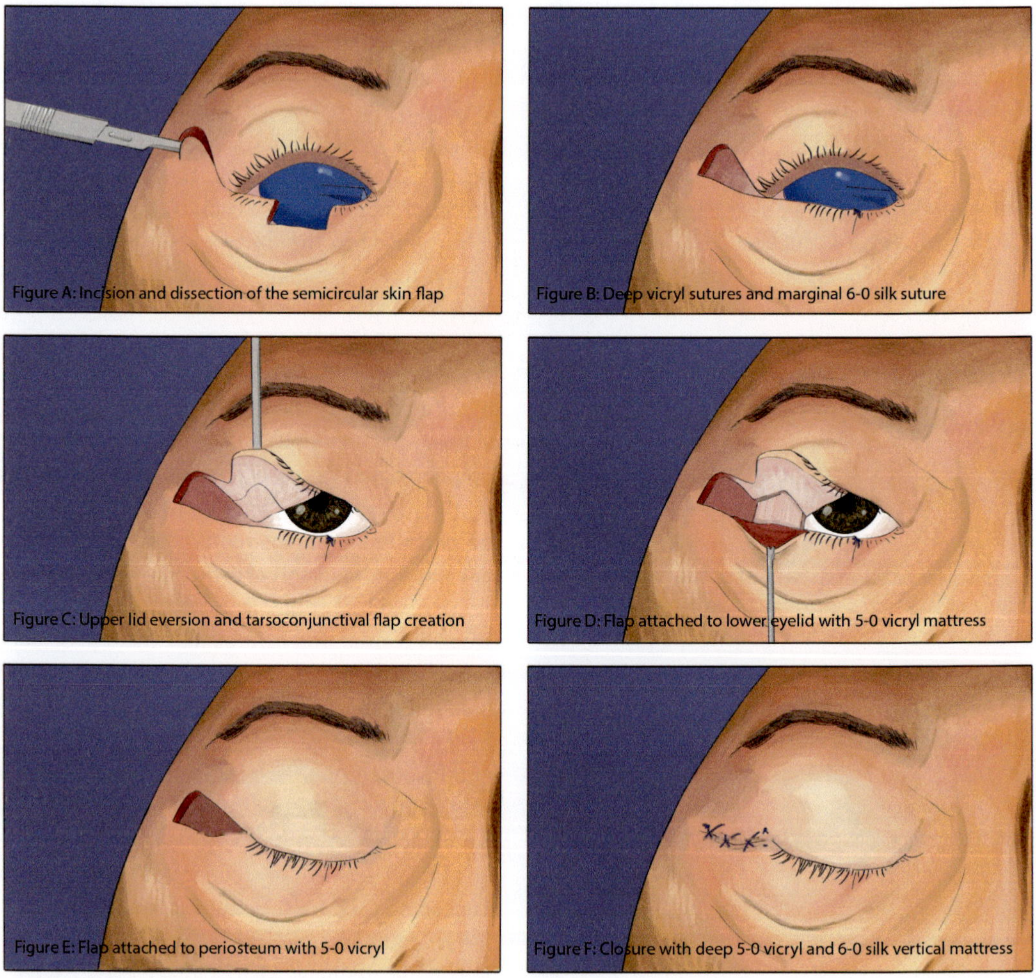

Fig. 6 Reconstruction of large lower eyelid defect with a lateral tarsoconjunctival flap under a semicircular flap (the authors' preferred approach) (illustration by Michael Han)

advantages. First, the flap-on-flap design offers excellent blood supply and excellent healing. The lateral tarsoconjunctival flap obviates a need to occlude the visual axis. Flap division is often not necessary since it is often well camouflaged in the lateral canthus. For larger flaps that do need takedown, the flap-on-flap design heals quicker and separation can commence sooner (several weeks) than with the uses of a skin graft (1–2 months). The lateral tarsoconjunctival flap achieves excellent superolateral traction on the newly constructed lower eyelid. Lastly, this construct leaves resultant wounds and scars that fall mostly within the relaxed skin tension lines.

Sliding tarsal flaps have also been described for the lower eyelid but are limited since the lower fornix is shallow and there exists limited conjunctiva to recruit. Nevertheless, for some shallow tarsal defects with a broad anterior lamellar defect, a sliding tarsal flap can be constructed from the residual tarsus [24]. The anterior lamellar defect can be reconstructed with a full thickness skin graft or advancement flap [24–26]. Other one-stage alternatives including full thickness upper eyelid flaps but these are generally less desirable for their conspicuous scars [26, 36–38].

6 Free Mucosal Grafts (Tarsoconjunctival, Chondromucosa)

An option for reconstruction of the posterior lamella is a free tarsoconjunctival graft [27–30]. This requires an anterior lamella that has good blood supply, ideally a myocutaneous advancement [31, 32]. Another option is an orbicularis flap that is advanced and covered anterioty with a skin graft [33–35]. Free tarsoconjunctival grafts are limited in size. Complications include retraction and scar [27, 29]. Postauricular chondrodermal grafts or acellular dermal matrix implants are an alternative to free tarsal grafts [39, 40]. These are described in other chapters.

For complete lower eyelid loss, a large rotational cervicofacial myocutaneous cheek flap (e.g., Mustarde flap) may be useful (Fig. 7) [41]. A curvilinear incision is made from the lateral canthus as described above except that these larger flaps arch more laterally and superiorly, extending higher than the eyebrow and then turning inferiorly to course in front of the ear 1 to 1.5 cm anterior to the tragus. The inferior crus and attachments to the orbital septum must be incised. The flap is undermined, rotated, and advanced medially. A composite graft of nasal chondromucosa or other mucous membrane (e.g., hard palate, tarsus) is used for the posterior lamella and attached laterally to the lateral canthal tendon or periosteum over the lateral orbital rim and medially to the medial canthal tendon or medial orbital wall. Sutures are used to attach the muscle and fascia of the flap to periosteum above the level of the lateral canthal tendon or the superior crus. Overcorrection is desired. A common concern is sagging of the flap which may lead to lower eyelid retraction and ectropion. This can be prevented by using a high-arched flap so that tissue is brought in from a superolateral position [42]. Other concerns are the quality and laxity of the skin and viability of the flap medially [4]. Complications may also include damage to the facial nerve and facial scarring. In lieu of a graft for the posterior lamella, a tarsoconjunctival flap (the authors' preference) may be used [45–47].

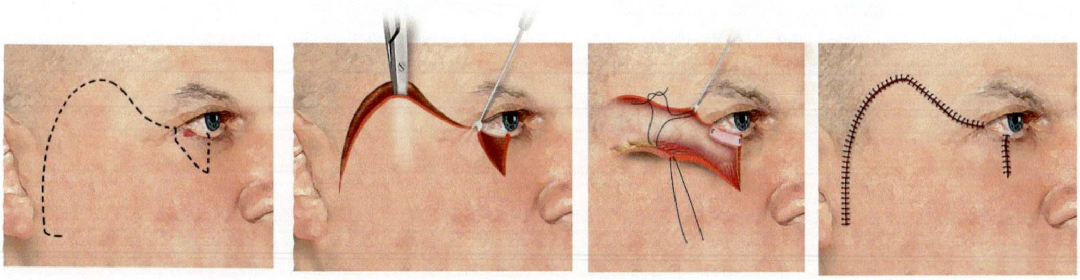

Fig. 7 Large semicircular facial flap for total lower eyelid reconstruction

7 Lateral Canthal Defects

For lower eyelid defects that involve the lateral canthus, the lower eyelid should be fixated to the periosteum of the lateral orbital rim to avoid malposition and ectropion. If additional support is needed, a periosteal flap or temporalis fascia can also be used to attach the residual tarsus of the lateral eyelid margin to the lateral orbital rim [48–52]. They can be used in combination with tarsoconjunctival flaps, free tarsoconjunctival grafts, and tarsal rotational flaps [48].

A rectangular strip of periosteum may be used to achieve posterior and lateral support for a reconstructed eyelid [50] (Fig. 8). The incision is just above the level of the lateral canthal angle with the base at the inner lateral orbital rim. The dimensions of the strip were a width of 5 mm and a length corresponding to the length needed, usually 1 cm [48, 52]. Temporalis fascia may be useful to supplement the periosteal strip. This can be achieved by extending the incision laterally. The strip is elevated, reflected, and attached to the residual tarsus of the eyelid with appropriate tension to allow for apposition of the eyelid to the globe.

If the lateral aspects of both the upper and lower eyelid require reconstruction, two periosteal strips can be created and overlapped [48, 49]. Two parallel incisions are made 1.5 cm apart extending from the temporalis fascia through the periosteum to the inner edge of the lateral rim [49]. The single flap is then elevated with its base at the inner aspect of the lateral orbital rim and split horizontally. Then the two flaps are crossed forming the lateral canthal angle and sutured to tarsus of the upper and lower eyelid. For the anterior lamella, a temporal or cheek myocutaneous flap can be advanced. Complications related to the periosteal strip may include notching, dehiscence, ectropion due to excessive length of the strip, or rounding or blunting of the lateral canthal angle if opposing eyelids heal together [48].

Other materials can be used as slings or patches to provide stronger support at the lateral canthus. Autologous cartilage or tendon can be considered [51, 53, 54]. Acellular dermal matrix grafts are also an option.

8 Medial Canthal Defects

Medial canthus surgery is described in another chapter as well, but the approach to medial canthal defects is based on size and depth of defect. First, direct closure can be attempted.

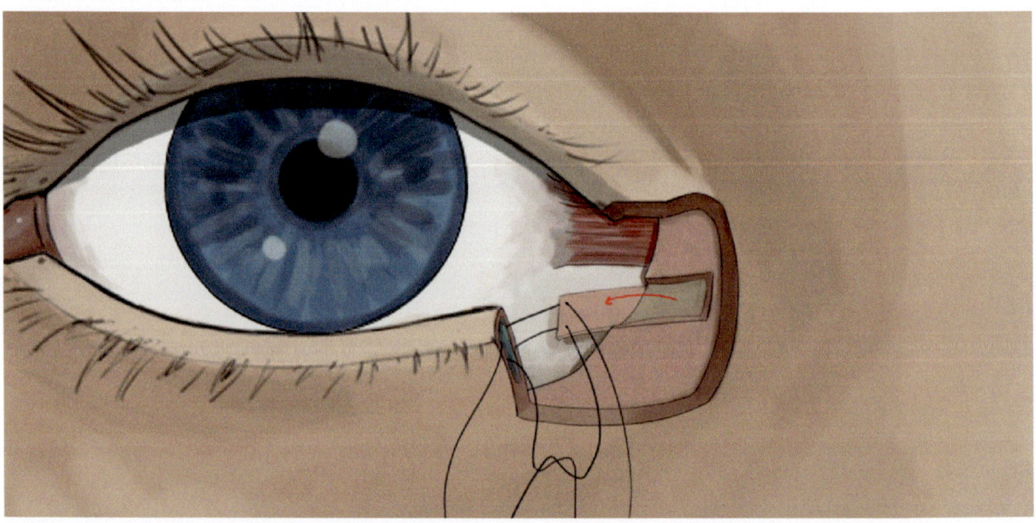

Fig. 8 Periosteal flap to anchor remnant medial eyelid to lateral rim (illustration by Michael, Han, MD)

Spontaneous granulation, a.k.a. laissez faire approach, but it may take a longer time to heal and lead to cicatricial complications including ectropion due to wound contraction [55].

For small shallow defects, a full thickness skin graft can be used from the eyelid, post-auricular area, supraclavicular area, or upper underarm. Advancement and transposition flaps can also be used, sometimes in conjunction with a lateral canthotomy and cantholysis or semi-circular rotational flap to reduce tension. The bilobed flap is described in Chap. "Excision of Lower Eyelid Lesions" and is useful for circular defects and consists of 2 lobes from 1 pedicle [56]. The primary lobe is rotated into the original defect while the secondary lobe is rotated into the secondary defect. The tertiary defect is closed directly. The sizes, angles, and tissues recruited for the lobes have varied [57–59].

A glabellar flap, usually performed as an inverted V–Y, can be useful especially for deep defects (Fig. 9) [60]. There are concerns that it can be aesthetically displeasing due to the skin thickness, prominence of the scar, and narrowing the distance between the brows [61]. Overall, these flaps are advantageous because the superiorly base achieves an appropriate upward vector to maintain good medial lower eyelid position. Also, the incisions can often be camouflaged in the vertical lines evident at the glabella in some patients.

Larger deep defects may require a paramedian forehead flap [62]. In some cases multiple flaps can be combined from various areas including upper or lower eyelid advancement flaps or a cheek advancement flap with the flaps anchored to the medial canthal tendon [63–65] (Video 3).

When the medial canthal tendon is disrupted, posterior fixation of the eyelid medially is important for eyelid position. The eyelid can be reattached directly to the tendon if there are remnants at its origin. If the medial canthal tendon is absent, the approach to fixation depends on whether periosteum is intact. If periosteum is intact, the tendon can be sutured to the periosteum of the posterior lacrimal crest (Video 4). If not, the tendon can be sutured to a titanium miniplate fixated to bone [66]. Transnasal wiring is an older technique to create a tendon fixation point but is usually not necessary with newer miniplate systems that may have less risk of damage to nearby structures especially on the unaffected contralateral side [67]. In cases requiring canalicular repair, the lacrimal stent achieves appropriate medial canthal positioning, with or without sutures to the medial canthal tendon (Video 5).

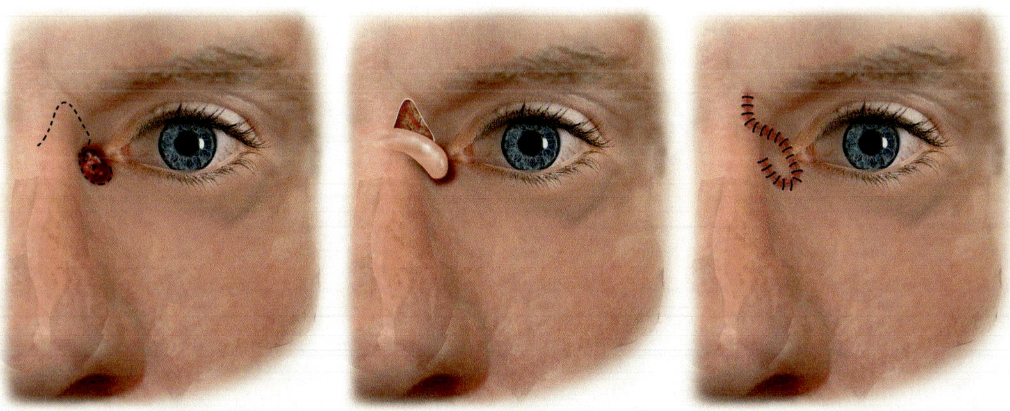

Fig. 9 Small glabella V to Y flap for medial canthal defect

9 Nonmarginal Defects

For nonmarginal defects, if direct closure cannot be performed, various flaps can be used. Flaps provide their own blood supply, contract less, and have better color, contour, texture, durability, and cosmesis than grafts [68]. In the periocular region, most flaps are random pattern skin flaps as opposed to axial pattern skin flaps. Their blood supply is derived from the dermal-subdermal plexus. Viability of a skin flap can be affected by prior surgery, radiation, and impaired perfusion in patients with vasculopathic comorbidities or tobacco use. Delaying the flap may enhance vascularity.

Various periorbital skin flaps are available [68]. For a sliding flap, skin is undermined and moved over to close a skin defect. Examples include the ellipse and its variations. For an advancement flap, a sliding flap with three sides is undermined and advanced to cover an adjacent skin defect. Examples include a single pedicle rectangular advancement flap or V–Y flap. If it is rotated about a pivot point onto an adjacent defect, it is called a rotational flap. Examples include a semicircular (e.g. Tenzel, Mustarde) or glabellar flap. Transposition flaps are when a flap is undermined, elevated, and transposed to a nonadjacent skin defect. Examples include the rhomboid flaps, Z plasty, and bilobed flap.

Full thickness skin grafts can also be used. It is important to match the color, thickness, and texture of the skin. Various locations that can be used include the upper eyelid, preauricular skin, retroauricular area, supraclavicular fossa, and inner upper arm.

10 Conclusion

There are many reconstruction techniques for lower eyelid defects. Procedure selection depends on many factors including the size, location, and depth of the defect. Full thickness defects should generally be approach in a bilamellar fashion. Another key step is strong fixation of flaps at the medial or lateral canthus. Additional thoughtfulness should surround temporary ocular occlusion that while sometimes unavoidable, can be obviated with construction of flaps that are outside the central visual axis.

References

1. Tenzel RR. Reconstruction of the central one half of an eyelid. Arch Ophthalmol. 1975;93:125–6.
2. Tenzel RR, Stewart WB. Eyelid reconstruction by the semicircle flap technique. Ophthalmology. 1978;85:1164–9.
3. Levine MR, Buckman G. Semicircular flap revisited. Arch Ophthalmol. 1986;104:915–7.
4. McGregor IA. Eyelid reconstruction following subtotal resection of upper or lower eyelid. Br J Plast Surg. 1973;26:346–54.
5. Reifler D, editor. The American Society of Ophthalmic Plastic and Reconstructive Surgery (ASOPRS). The First Twenty-Five Years: 1969–1994. History of Ophthalmic Plastic Surgery: 2500 BC-AD 1994. Winter Park, FL: ASOPRS/Norman, 1994.
6. Köllner H. Verfahren für den plastischen Ersatz des Unterlides. Munch Med Wochenschr. 1911;41:2166–8.
7. Dupuy-Dutemps LJBMSFO. Refection d'une paupiere detruite dans toute don epaisseur par greffe cutanee et tarso-donjonctivale prise a l'autre paupiere autoplastie palpebro-palpebrale integrale. 1927;40:262–71.
8. Cirincione GJCO. Sulla blefaroplastica. 1901;2:449–73.
9. Hughes WL. A new method for rebuilding a lower eyelid: report of a case. 1937;17:1008–17.
10. Hargiss JL. Bipedicle tarsoconjunctival flap. Ophthalmic Plast Reconstr Surg. 1989;5:99–103.
11. Moss AL, Cooper MA, Lendrum J, Hiles RW. The sanctity of the upper eyelid in lower eyelid reconstruction questioned. A modification of a eyelid sharing procedure with a long-term follow-up. Br J Plast Surg. 1987;40:246–57.
12. Hughes WL. Total lower eyelid reconstruction: technical details. Trans Am Ophthalmol Soc. 1976;74:321–9.
13. Custer PL, Maamari RN. The Kollner tarsoconjunctival flap for lower eyelid reconstruction: Historical perspective and surgical outcomes of 140 cases. Ophthalmic Plast Reconstr Surg. 2021.
14. Hishmi AM, Koch KR, Matthaei M, Bolke E, Cursiefen C, Heindl LM. Modified Hughes procedure for reconstruction of large full-thickness lower eyelid defects following tumor resection. Eur J Med Res. 2016;21:27.
15. McNab AA. Early division of the conjunctival pedicle in modified Hughes repair of the lower eyelid. Ophthalmic Surg Lasers. 1996;27:422–4.

16. Leibovitch I, Selva D. Modified Hughes flap: division at 7 days. Ophthalmology. 2004;111:2164–7.
17. Bartley GB, Messenger MM. The dehiscent Hughes flap: outcomes and implications. Trans Am Ophthalmol Soc. 2002;100:61–5; discussion 65–6.
18. McNab AA, Martin P, Benger R, O'Donnell B, Kourt G. A prospective randomized study comparing division of the pedicle of modified Hughes flaps at two or four weeks. Ophthalmic Plast Reconstr Surg. 2001;17:317–9.
19. Custer PL. Tarsal kinking after Hughes flap. Ophthalmic Plast Reconstr Surg. 1998;14:349–51.
20. Bartley GB, Putterman AM. A minor modification of the Hughes' operation for lower eyelid reconstruction. Am J Ophthalmol. 1995;119:96–7.
21. Hewes EH, Sullivan JH, Beard C. Lower eyelid reconstruction by tarsal transposition. Am J Ophthalmol. 1976;81:512–4.
22. Leone CR Jr, Van Gemert JV. Lower eyelid reconstruction with upper eyelid transpositional grafts. Ophthalmic Surg. 1980;11:315–8.
23. Perry CB, Allen RC. Repair of 50–75% full-thickness lower eyelid defects: lateral stabilization as a guiding principle. Indian J Ophthalmol. 2016;64:563–7.
24. deSousa JL, Malhotra R, Davis G. Sliding tarsal flap for reconstruction of large, shallow lower eyelid tarsal defects. Ophthalmic Plast Reconstr Surg. 2007;23:46–8.
25. Custer PL, Neimkin M. Lower eyelid reconstruction with combined sliding tarsal and rhomboid skin flaps. Ophthalmic Plast Reconstr Surg. 2016;32:230–2.
26. Skippen B, Hamilton A, Evans S, Benger R. One-stage alternatives to the Hughes procedure for reconstruction of large lower eyelid defects: Surgical techniques and outcomes. Ophthalmic Plast Reconstr Surg. 2016;32:145–9.
27. Hawes MJ, Grove AS Jr, Hink EM. Comparison of free tarsoconjunctival grafts and Hughes tarsoconjunctival grafts for lower eyelid reconstruction. Ophthalmic Plast Reconstr Surg. 2011;27:219–23.
28. Leone CR Jr, Hand SI Jr. Reconstruction of the medial eyelid. Am J Ophthalmol. 1979;87:797–801.
29. Stephenson CM, Brown BZ. The use of tarsus as a free autogenous graft in eyelid surgery. Ophthalmic Plast Reconstr Surg. 1985;1:43–50.
30. Blaskovics LvJO. Über Totalplastik des unteren eyelides. Bildung einer hinteren eyelidplatte durch Transplantation eines Tarsus und Bindehautstreifens aus dem Oberlide. 1918;40:222–7.
31. Katz TL, Pennington TE, Yohendran J, Ghabrial R. One-step reconstruction of large lower eyelid defects: technique and outcomes. Clin Exp Ophthalmol. 2014;42:889–92.
32. Leone CR Jr, Van Gemert JV. Lower eyelid reconstruction using tarsoconjunctival grafts and bipedicle skin-muscle flap. Arch Ophthalmol. 1989;107:758–60.
33. Paridaens D, van den Bosch WA. Orbicularis muscle advancement flap combined with free posterior and anterior lamellar grafts: a 1-stage sandwich technique for eyelid reconstruction. Ophthalmology. 2008;115:189–94.
34. Naugle TC, Levine MR, Carroll GS. Free graft enhancement using orbicularis muscle mobilization. Ophthalmology. 1995;102:493–500.
35. Hawes MJ, Jamell GA. Complications of tarsoconjunctival grafts. Ophthalmic Plast Reconstr Surg. 1996;12:45–50.
36. Jones HW. One stage composite lower eyelid repair. Plast Reconstr Surg. 1966;37:346–8.
37. Anderson RL, Jordan DR, Beard C. Full-thickness unipedicle flap for lower eyelid reconstruction. Arch Ophthalmol. 1988;106:122–5.
38. Anderson RL, Weinstein GS. Full-thickness bipedicle flap for total lower eyelid reconstruction. Arch Ophthalmol. 1987;105:570–6.
39. Porfiris E, Christopoulos A, Sandris P, et al. Upper eyelid orbicularis oculi flap with tarsoconjunctival island for reconstruction of full-thickness lower eyelid defects. Plast Reconstr Surg. 1999;103:186–91.
40. Robbins TH. Chondrodermal graft reconstruction of the lower eyelid. Br J Plast Surg. 1981;34:140–1.
41. Mustarde JC. The use of flaps in the orbital region. Plast Reconstr Surg. 1970;45:146–50.
42. Callahan MA, Callahan A. Mustarde flap lower eyelid reconstruction after malignancy. Ophthalmology. 1980;87:279–86.
43. Manchester WM. A simple method for the repair of full-thickness defects of the lower eyelid with special reference to the treatment of neoplasms. Br J Plast Surg. 1951;3:252–63.
44. Wilcsek G, Leatherbarrow B, Halliwell M, Francis I. The 'RITE' use of the Fricke flap in periorbital reconstruction. Eye (Lond). 2005;19:854–60.
45. Beyer CK, Albert DM. The use and fate of fascia lata and sclera in ophthalmic plastic and reconstructive surgery. Ophthalmology. 1981;88:869–86.
46. Suga H, Ozaki M, Narita K, et al. Comparison of nasal septum and ear cartilage as a graft for lower eyelid reconstruction. J Craniofac Surg. 2016;27:305–7.
47. Jordan DR, Tse DT, Anderson RL, Hansen SO. Irradiated homologous tarsal plate banking: a new alternative in eyelid reconstruction. Part II. Human data. Ophthalmic Plast Reconstr Surg 1990;6:168–76.
48. Weinstein GS, Anderson RL, Tse DT, Kersten RC. The use of a periosteal strip for eyelid reconstruction. Arch Ophthalmol. 1985;103:357–9.
49. Leone CR Jr. Lateral canthal reconstruction. Ophthalmology. 1987;94:238–41.
50. Leone CR Jr. Periosteal flap for lower eyelid reconstruction. Am J Ophthalmol. 1992;114:513–4.
51. Holt JE, Holt GR, van Kirk M. Use of temporalis fascia in eyelid reconstruction. Ophthalmology. 1984;91:89–93.

52. Smith B, English FP. Techniques available in reconstructive surgery of the eyelid. Br J Ophthalmol. 1970;54:450–5.
53. Holt JE, Holt GR, Van Kirk M. Use of temporalis fascia in eyelid reconstruction. Arch Otolaryngol. 1985;111:165–7.
54. Wang W, Meng H, Yu S, Liu T, Shao Y. Reconstruction of giant full-thickness lower eyelid defects using a combination of palmaris longus tendon with superiorly based nasolabial skin flap and palatal mucosal graft. J Plast Surg Hand Surg. 2021;55:147–52.
55. Lowry JC, Bartley GB, Garrity JA. The role of second-intention healing in periocular reconstruction. Ophthalmic Plast Reconstr Surg. 1997;13:174–88.
56. Esser JFS. Gestielte lokale Nasenplastik mit zweizipfligem Lappen, Deckung des sekundären Defektes vom ersten Zipfel durch den zweiten. Deutsche Zeitschrift für Chirurgie. 1918;143:385–90.
57. Meadows AE, Rhatigan M, Manners RM. Bilobed flap in ophthalmic plastic surgery: simple principles for flap construction. Ophthalmic Plast Reconstr Surg. 2005;21:441–4.
58. Sullivan TJ, Bray LC. The bilobed flap in medial canthal reconstruction. Aust N Z J Ophthalmol. 1995;23:42–8.
59. Perry JD, Taban M. Superiorly based bilobed flap for inferior medial canthal and nasojugal fold defect reconstruction. Ophthalmic Plast Reconstr Surg. 2009;25:276–9.
60. Maloof AJ, Leatherbarrow B. The glabellar flap dissected. Eye (Lond). 2000;14(Pt 4):597–605.
61. Meadows AE, Manners RM. A simple modification of the glabellar flap in medial canthal reconstruction. Ophthalmic Plast Reconstr Surg. 2003;19:313–5.
62. Price DL, Sherris DA, Bartley GB, Garrity JA. Forehead flap periorbital reconstruction. Arch Facial Plast Surg. 2004;6:222–7.
63. Harris GJ, Logani SC. Multiple aesthetic unit flaps for medial canthal reconstruction. Ophthalmic Plast Reconstr Surg. 1998;14:352–9.
64. Motomura H, Taniguchi T, Harada T, Muraoka M. A combined flap reconstruction for full-thickness defects of the medial canthal region. J Plast Reconstr Aesthet Surg. 2006;59:747–51.
65. Lee BJ, Elner SG, Douglas RS, Elner VM. Island pedicle and horizontal advancement cheek flaps for medial canthal reconstruction. Ophthalmic Plast Reconstr Surg. 2011;27:376–9.
66. Howard GR, Nerad JA, Kersten RC. Medial canthoplasty with microplate fixation. Arch Ophthalmol. 1992;110:1793–7.
67. Peter H, Freihofer M. Experience with transnasal canthopexy. J Maxillofac Surg. 1980;8:119–24.
68. Patrinely JR, Marines HM, Anderson RL. Skin flaps in periorbital reconstruction. Surv Ophthalmol. 1987;31:249–61.

Canalicular and Tearing Considerations

Cameron B. Nabavi and Andrew J. Mueller

Abstract

Integral to lower eyelid surgery is consideration of tearing and the lacrimal outflow apparatus. Understanding nasolacrimal apparatus anatomy and function allows for the correct treatment of medial eyelid pathology. Medial eyelid malposition can lead to tearing due to poor apposition of the puncta to the tear lake, while punctal stenosis can impair tear entry to the lacrimal outflow system. Proper assessment and management of the tear drainage apparatus is important in any patient undergoing medial lower eyelid surgery with or without epiphora symptoms. This chapter details tear drainage considerations in lower eyelid surgery.

Illustrations by Michael Han

Supplementary Information The online version contains supplementary material available at https://doi.org/10.1007/978-3-031-36175-3_5.

C. B. Nabavi (✉) · A. J. Mueller
Ophthalmic Surgeons and Consultants of Ohio, 262 Neil Ave. Ste 430, Columbus, OH 43201, United States
e-mail: nabavieye@gmail.com

C. B. Nabavi
Department of Ophthalmology and Visual Sciences, The Ohio State University, Columbus, Ohio 43212, United States

Keywords

Tearing · Tear duct · Puncta · Lacrimal outflow · Nasolacrimal duct · Eyelid malposition · Canaliculus · Epiphora

1 Anatomy and Physiology of the Lacrimal Drainage System

The lacrimal drainage system forms embryologically from a cord of ectoderm that becomes the nasolacrimal duct and lacrimal sac, which then extends laterally and superiorly towards the eyelids as the canaliculi and inferiorly into the nasal cavity [1]. Normal anatomy consists of two puncta on each side, one on the medial upper eyelid and one on the medial lower eyelid. The puncta themselves are located on the eyelid margin within a slightly raised area called the papilla. The upper punctum is situated slightly medial to the lower punctum. Both are slightly turned inward posteriorly and are apposed to the tear film. The average punctal size is 0.3 mm, though variation exists [2]. From the punctum, the drainage system continues vertically into the eyelid as the ampulla, a widening of the passageway that allows for collection of tears prior to being pumped through the system into the nose. The ampulla is normally as wide as 1 mm and can dilate to several millimeters in

J. P. Tao (ed.), *Plastic Surgery of the Lower Eyelids*,
https://doi.org/10.1007/978-3-031-36175-3_5

cases of lacrimal stones and canaliculitis. The vertical distance from the punctum to the base of the ampulla is roughly 2 mm. From there, the canaliculus makes a 90 degree turn and travels horizontally, medially, and posteriorly along the eyelid margin for about 8–10 mm. In most patients, the horizontal canaliculi from the upper and lower eyelids join as a common canaliculus just before entering the lacrimal sac. In some patients, however, the two canaliculi enter the sac separately without forming a common canaliculus. Tears then collect in the lacrimal sac before traveling to the nose. The lacrimal sac is an oval-shaped mucosal pocket sitting in the lacrimal sac fossa between the anterior and posterior lacrimal crests on the anterior medial wall of the orbit. The lacrimal sac is roughly 12–15 mm in height and continues inferiorly as the nasolacrimal duct, which empties into the nose in the anterior inferior meatus underneath the inferior turbinate. The course of the nasolacrimal duct is lateral, posterior, and inferior and runs about 12 mm through the bony nasolacrimal canal and 5–6 mm beyond through the nasal mucosa Fig. 1.

The canaliculi are lined by squamous epithelium and are devoid of goblet cells [3]. Although the canaliculi themselves do not contain contractile structures, they run within the medial canthal tendon which is surrounding by the orbicularis oculi muscle. As the eyelids blink, the contraction of the orbicularis oculi muscles pushes tears on the ocular surface towards the puncta. This same contraction propels tears that are already in the lacrimal sac down into the nose through the nasolacrimal duct. The void in the sac then serves as a source of low pressure to pull tears through the punctum and canaliculi into the sac, and the cycle repeats. This coordinated process is the lacrimal pump of the eyelids. Interruptions in this cycle for any reason can lead to decreased lacrimal pump function and decreased clearance of tears from the ocular surface. This can manifest as tearing or epiphora. A common situations in which this is encountered is with senile ectropion, where excess eyelid laxity decreases the ability of the eyelids to funnel tears medially towards the puncta upon orbicularis contraction.

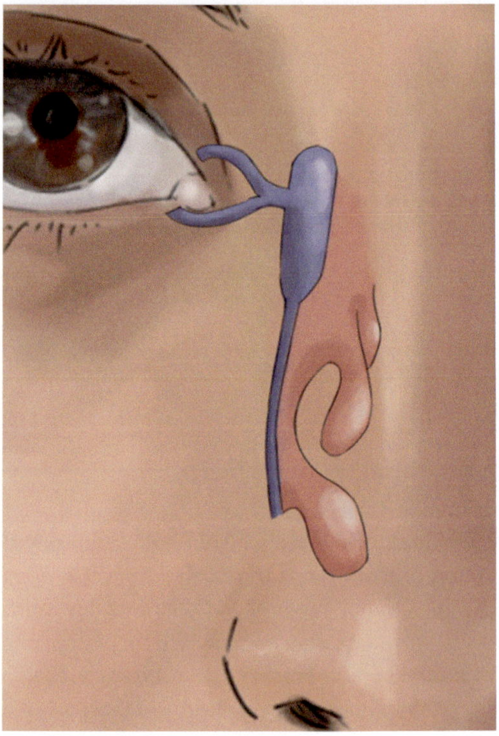

Fig. 1 Lacrimal drainage system

2 Evaluation of Tearing and Epiphora

It is necessary to distinguish between tearing from increased production from tearing due to decreased drainage [4] Tear overproduction can be due to excess lacrimal gland stimulation from several causes. The most common etiology is the spectrum of dry eye disorders, the entirety is beyond the scope of this chapter. Secondly, any other source of ocular irritation can signal for increased tear production. These include misdirected lashes or foreign bodies. Increased tear production can be greater than the amount of normal lacrimal drainage system outflow and lead to the symptom of epiphora.

Decreased lacrimal drainage can occur due to stenosis or blockage at any point in the drainage pathway. Absent, stenotic, or closed puncta can limit passage of tears into the pathway. Stenosed or blocked canaliculi can halt the passage of tears. And an obstructed lacrimal sac or nasolacrimal duct will lead to tear stasis and decreased drainage. In general, symptoms of tears constantly flowing down the cheek or having to wipe incessantly suggest an outflow obstruction rather than an increased secretory state.

To differentiate between the two categories of etiologies, a thorough exam is indicated. Evaluation for dry eye syndrome and other signs of ocular surface disorders and irritation is necessary. This may include a slit lamp examination, fluorescein testing, and Schirmer testing for basal and/or reflex tearing. The examination should also include inspection of the size and position of the lacrimal puncta, the position and laxity of the lower eyelids, and probing and irrigation of the puncta and canaliculus. Probing and irrigation are of utmost importance in cases of tearing due to decreased drainage, as it often localizes the exact level at which there is a stenosis or obstruction. A soft stop during probing can indicate punctal, canalicular, or common canalicular obstruction. In these cases, irrigation results in reflux of fluid back through the same punctum without any passage through the nose or out the other punctum. The exception is in distal common canalicular obstruction, there may be some reflux into the opposite punctum. In cases where there is no soft stop on probing, and a hard stop is felt once the medial wall of the lacrimal sac against the lacrimal fossa bone is contacted, irrigation from one punctum may show reflux through the other punctum, without passage into the nose. This indicates the obstruction is lower than the entrance of the common canaliculus into the lacrimal sac. Most often this is due to obstruction of the nasolacrimal duct, but rarely can be due to pathology within the lacrimal sac that impedes flow into a normal nasolacrimal duct.

3 Excision of Lesions Near Tear Drainage Structures

Often, lesions can present and grow on the medial lower or upper eyelid in proximity to the punctum or canaliculus [5]. A hidrocystoma or papilloma can abut the punctum, and the full spectrum of dermatologic conditions or lesions can be seen on the eyelid skin superficial to the canaliculi. These may not always be symptomatic, but are often removed due to irritation, cosmesis, or for identification via histopathology. Most of these lesions do not directly involve the lacrimal drainage systems and can be separated by meticulous dissection [6]. If there is concern that removal of the lesion will encroach upon the punctum or canaliculus, one can consider placing a probe or stent within the punctum and nasolacrimal system prior to lesion excision. A stent can be left in after the procedure or removed immediately if no concern is present of canalicular violation. Similarly, in cases of suspected malignancy where safety margins are excised around the lesions, it is often helpful to intubate the lacrimal drainage system prior to excision (Video 1) If a large section of medial eyelid and/or medial canthus are to be excised, it may be considered to delay reconstruction of the tear drainage pathway until after the tissue is fully cleared of tumor.

4 Medial Spindle Conjunctivoplasty

In patients who present with poor apposition of the punctum to the ocular surface, the medial spindle procedure [7] can be considered as a method to invert and reposition the punctum to a more anatomical and functional position. The procedure is simple, effective, and can be performed either by itself or in conjunction with other eyelid-inverting or eyelid tightening procedures such as a lateral tarsal strip.

The procedure is started with creating an incision in the medial conjunctival fornix inferior to the tarsus. Visualization can be improved by inserting a lower eyelid traction suture and everting the lower eyelid as necessary. This incision should be placed at least 4 mm inferior to the punctum to avoid the tarsus and the vertical portion of the canaliculus and ampulla. Classically this is a diamond-shaped excision made by tenting and snipping the conjunctiva with small scissors (Fig. 2A). Next, sutures are placed to close the defect. Absorbable buried sutures suffice. Alternatively, sutures may be externalized to the lower eyelid skin (Fig. 2B). The vector of force upon suture closure and tied pulls the posterior lower eyelid to invert the punctum and lower eyelid margin back towards the surface of the eye (Fig. 2C).

This procedure on its own provides modest correction of punctal eversion. In cases where there is severe punctal ectropion, a more extensive inversion may be needed. In these cases, the incision is carried out horizontally over to the caruncle. Dissection with blunt scissors is carried out through the lower eyelid retractors. Next, two 4-0 polyglactin or 4-0 polypropylene sutures are placed like the medial spindle sutures and externalized over a silicone bolster. The medial of the two sutures is also passed through the fibrous tissue of the caruncle to anchor the medial eyelid and prevent it from future eversion, or from lateralizing in cases where the eyelid is tightened or shortened laterally [8]. The bolsters are removed 7–10 days postoperatively. This is typically done in conjunction with horizontal eyelid tightening via a lateral approach.

5 Plastic Repair of Canaliculi

Injuries to the canaliculus can occur via several mechanisms. Most commonly, trauma causes laceration or tearing of the eyelid soft tissue including the lacrimal drainage systems. Notably, dog bites often cause canalicular trauma due to the shearing forces on the lower eyelid, leading to disinsertion of the common canaliculus from the lacrimal sac [9]. Suspicion should be high for a canalicular laceration with any medial lower eyelid trauma. It is important to pull open the wound and probe the canalicular system (Fig. 3).

Trauma to the punctum can be repair with simple approximation of the lacerated edges of the wound. It is beneficial to stent the punctum to preclude stenosis or obstruction secondary to scarring in the following weeks to months. This can be achieved through mono- or bi-canalicular stents, or even with punctal plugs if the laceration is small. Small caliber suture is recommended, such as 7-0 or 8-0 polyglactin to reapproximate lacrimal punctal edges.

Trauma to the canaliculi is repaired with a combination of lacrimal intubation and suturing [10]. Although not an emergency, canalicular

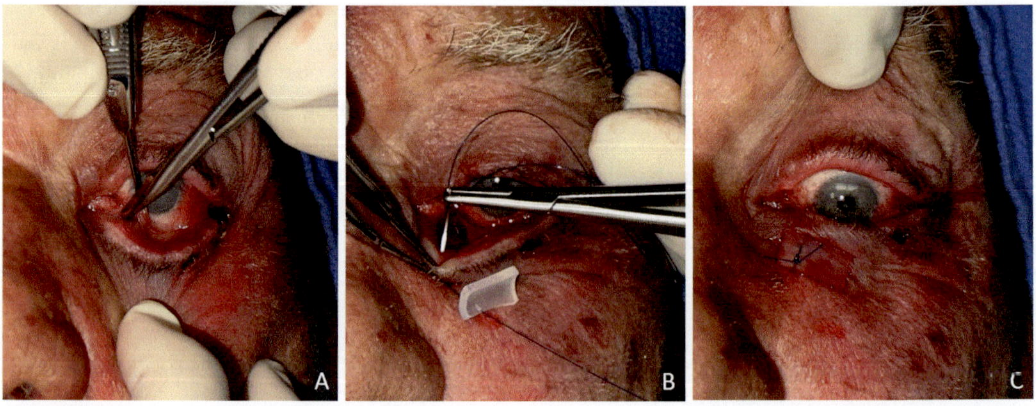

Fig. 2 Key surgical steps of the medial spindle conjunctivoplasty. **A.** A diamond-shaped medial conjunctiva incision is fashioned with scissors inferior to the lower eyelid punctum and lower tarsus. **B.** A 4-0 polypropylene suture is passed through the upper conjunctival edge of the incision and then through the lower conjunctival edge of the incision and externalized over a silicone bolster. (Alternatively, the defect can be closed posteriorly using a buried absorbable suture.) **C.** Tightening of suture provides inward rotation of the medial eyelid margin to reappose the punctum to the ocular surface

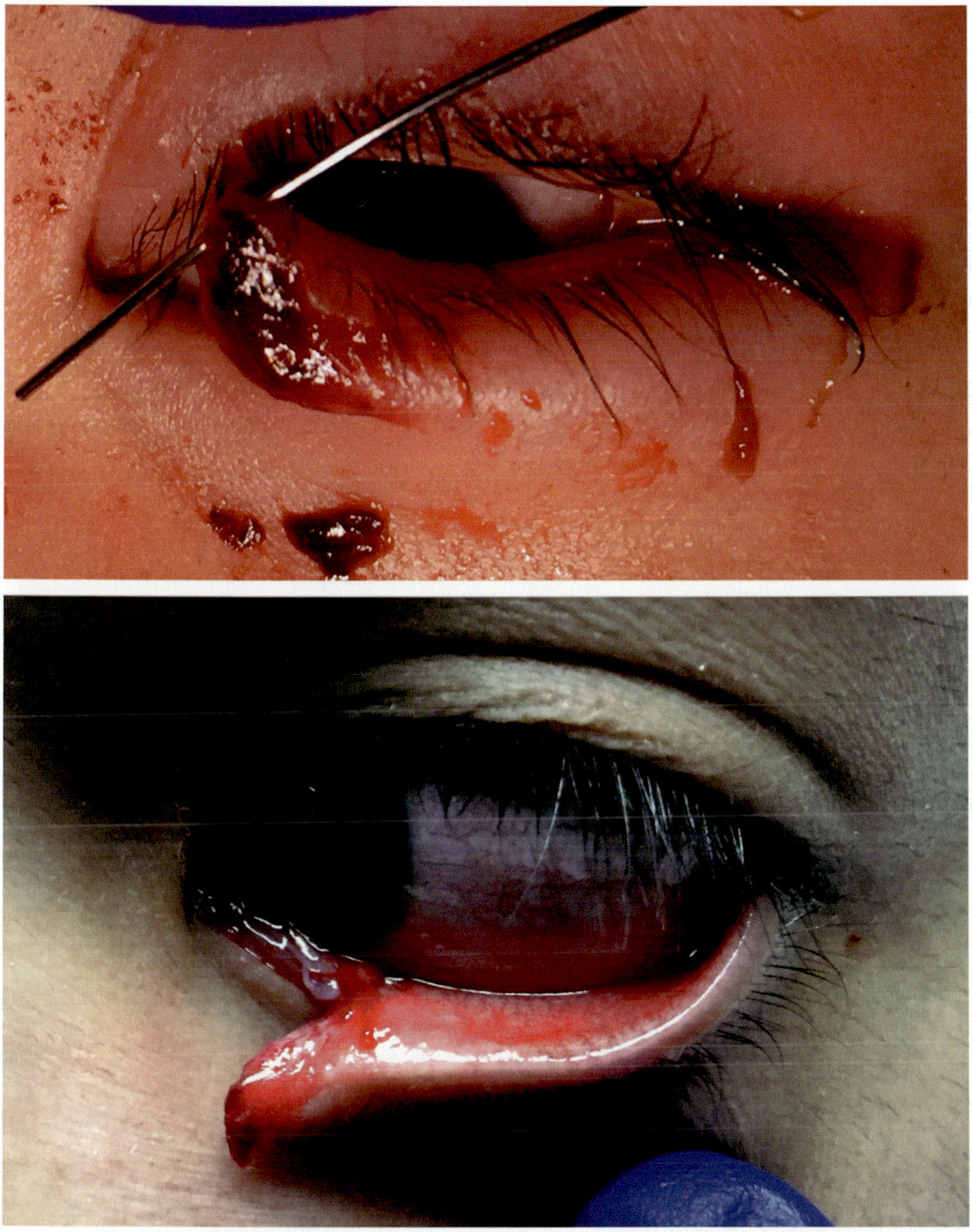

Fig. 3 Medial eyelid laceration involving canaliculus. Probe aids in identification of disrupted canaliculus (image courtesy of Benyam Kinde, and Seana Grob)

repairs should be repaired urgently (within days) before scarring develops which can lead to long term stenosis or obstruction. If a scarred area of canaliculus is encountered, trephination can be attempted to reestablish a patent lumen, or the scarred area can be excised and the fresh edges of the canaliculus re-anastomosed. In acute settings, it is often easier to repair severed canalicular ends early, prior to the onset of significant edema, as the expanding edematous soft tissue can compress the cut edge of the canaliculus and make identification of the lumen difficult.

If there is difficulty finding the medial cut end of a canaliculus there are several aids. The first is to manually manipulate the tissue in opposite directions to open a compressed lumen and see the ring-like cut end of the canaliculus (Fig. 4). Additionally, fluorescein or saline can be injected through the partner punctum/canaliculus (if patent), with digital pressure on the lacrimal sac, to force reflux outflow through the cut end of the canaliculus. Finally, a pig-tail lacrimal probe can be inserted through the partner canaliculus (if patent) to probe in a retrograde fashion the cut end of the canaliculus. However, pigtail probes may risk creation of a false passage.

When probing, it should be confirmed that further passage into the assumed cut canaliculus leads into the lacrimal sac and a hard stop is reached. Monostents that are not passed down the entire duct are an option. The gold standard however is bicanalicular intubation down the nasolacrimal canal and into the nose. This helps to prevent the formation of false passageways which will not prevent scarring and tearing. Additionally, the bicanalicular system may be more stable (Fig. 5).

After intubation, the peri-canalicular tissue should be reapproximated. This can be accomplished with 6-0, 7-0, or 8-0 polyglactin sutures.

Iatrogenic canalicular trauma usually occurs with resection of malignancy, as noted above. Full thickness excisions are treated like trauma cases, where the cut ends of the canaliculus are identified, intubated, and sutured together. In large cases, or cases where it is unclear if residual tumor is present, it may be beneficial to delay canalicular repair until a later date.

6 Canaliculitis

Canaliculitis is a distinct entity from nasolacrimal obstruction/dacryocystitis in pathophysiology, symptoms, and treatment. Canaliculitis occurs when there is obstruction of the canalicular system leading to localized infection and inflammation. Often there is a history of punctal plug administration in the recent or remote past. Patients often report pain or redness of the eyelid, tearing, discharge, and rarely no symptoms at all. Tearing may only be a minor symptom. On examination, there may be localized redness and edema to the medial eyelid or punctum

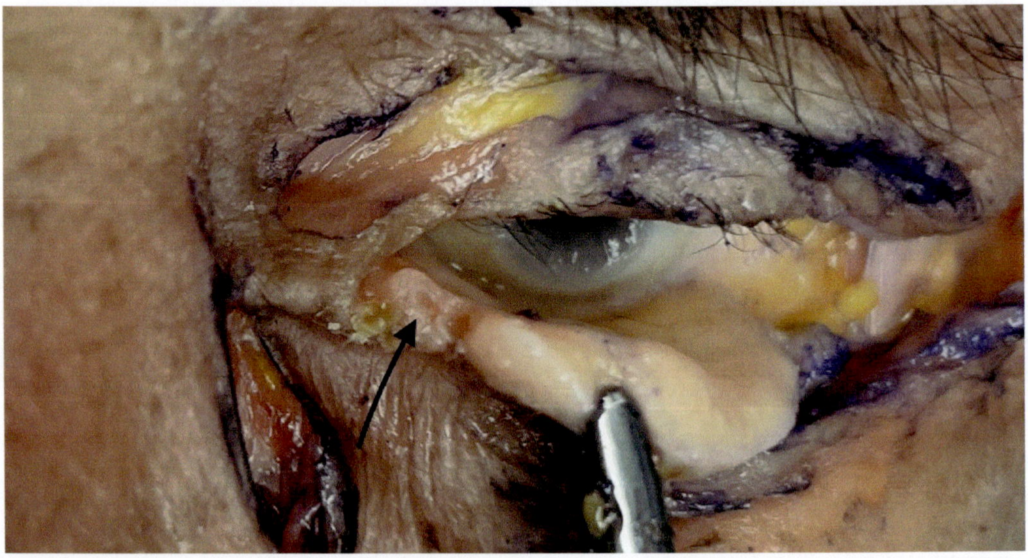

Fig. 4 Distal end of cut canaliculus on a cadaver dissection appearing as circular lumen

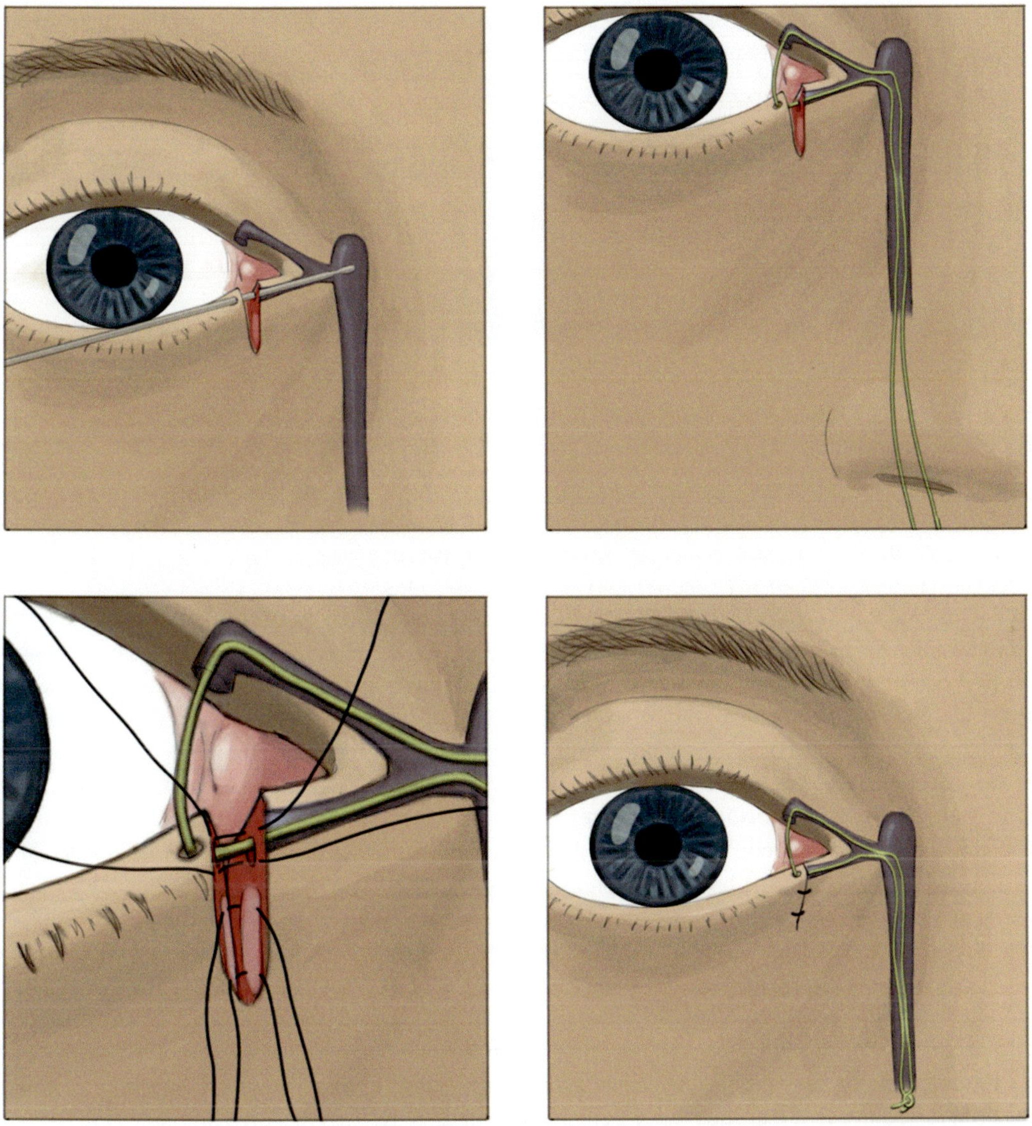

Fig. 5 Bicanalicular intubation of lacrimal systeim including injured lower system *(illustration by Michael Han*

(rather than the medial canthus in dacryocystitis), and the punctum may have a pouty configuration with mucoid material emanating from it (Fig. 6A). Compression of the inflamed area produce further discharge from the punctum, and irrigation usually is not feasible past the obstruction [11].

The inflammation is due to a bacterial infection of a foreign body or lacrimal stone. Lacrimal stones are somewhat misnomers, as the material is often soft, although gritty, the consistency of cheese. The most common organism in canaliculitis is Actinomyces israelii, a normal component of ocular surface flora. Other common infectious agents seen include Streptococcus species, Staphylococcus species, and others.

Treatment involves removing the obstruction in the canaliculus and initiating antibiotic therapy. Incision and curettage of the blocked ampulla or canaliculus is performed with the

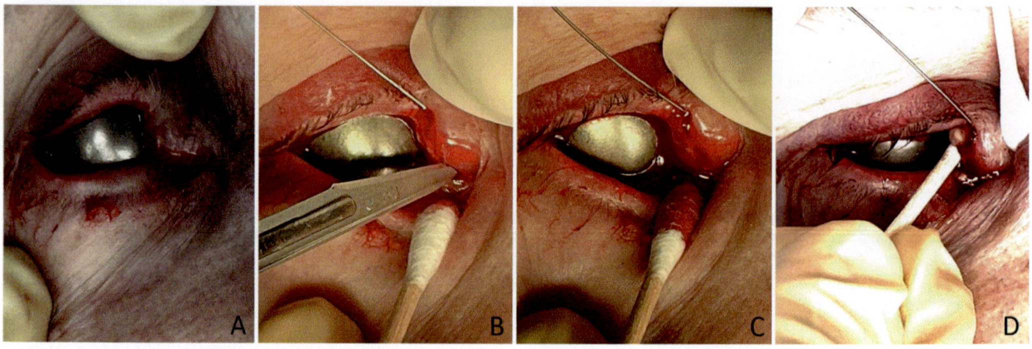

Fig. 6 Key surgical steps of the canaliculotomy procedure for canaliculitis. A. A pre-procedure photo showing the distended upper canaliculus with "pouting" punctum. A small stone is seen on the lower eyelid which was expressed from light digital pressure over the medial upper eyelid. **B.** The horizontal portion of the upper canaliculus is incised with an 11-blade. **C.** Visualization of the incision of the horizontal canaliculus with lacrimal stones present within. **D.** Compression of the distended canaliculus will express the stones through the incision. A curette can also be used to aid in delivery of the stones from the canaliculus

following steps. The incision can either be straight down from the punctum to the ampulla on the posterior side of the punctum, or it could spare the punctum and begin about 1 mm below the punctum on the posterior eyelid surface. If the infection is in the horizontal canaliculus, then the incision can be made directly over the area on the posterior eyelid surface in a horizontal fashion (Fig. 6B and C). Compression or a curette can be used to remove the offending stones or foreign bodies (Fig. 6D) (Video 2) These specimens can be sent for pathological identification and culture to direct antibiotic therapy. The distended canaliculus should be carefully explored to ensure that all infected material is removed. It can then be rinsed with saline or antibiotic solution. Suture closure of the canaliculus is optional. One can also consider silicone intubation if there is concern for canalicular stenosis [12]. The patient should initiate topical antibiotic drops, with oral antibiotics if significant surrounding cellulitis is present.

6.1 Punctoplasty

Punctoplasty is a procedure that can be performed for diagnostic and/or therapeutic reasons. During evaluation of a tearing patient, if the puncta stenotic but dilation is possible, nasolacrimal irrigation can be performed. If the nasolacrimal duct flows freely without resistance, a punctoplasty may be indicated to relieve the bottleneck and input resistance. If dilation is not possible, a punctoplasty can be performed to better assess the remainder of the lacrimal outflow apparatus.

Two main techniques include a snip punctoplasty [13] and Kelly punch punctoplasty [14]. Local anesthetic is injected to area surrounding the puncta. A vertical slit on the posterior aspect of the usually achieves sufficient punctal stenosis relief. A 3 snip punctoplasty involves dilating the puncta and making a vertical cut inferiorly, followed by a horizontal cut medially and then a triangle of tissue is removed, keeping the puncta patent. A Kelly punch punctoplasty is performed by using a standard Kelly Descemet's membrane punch to enlarge the puncta. This can be done in conjunction with silicone intubation.

6.2 Canaliculoplasty

Canaliculoplasty may be indicated if there is stricture or obstruction distal to the punctum. Serial larger Bowmann wire intubation is performed to alleviate blockages. Typically, silicone intubation for several months helps maintain patency. In some instances, double silicone intubation may be useful to further dilate/open the canaliculi. In select cases, a complete and focal canalicular obstruction may be treated by resection of the involved portion of the canaliculus followed by intubation and repair of the cut canalicular ends.

7 Punctal Closure/Cautery

Dry eye syndrome is one of the most common reasons for a visit to an eye specialist. Techniques used to improve dry eye vary from topical lubricants, anti-inflammatory topicals and management of coincident blepharitis. Commonly, punctal plugs can be used to reduce tear drainage, allowing tears to persist for a longer duration. For a patient, when frequent plug loss, difficult plug fitting or plug-related complications occur, permanent punctal closure is an option [15]. This can be performed with varying techniques including punctal cautery [16] and surgical punctal closure. Typically, the lower puncta is addressed, reserving upper punctal closure when severe dryness still persists after treating the lower system. Punctal thermocautery is the commonly employed technique as argon laser closure and suture closure have high rates of recanalization. The drawbacks are that thermal injury may lead to unpredictable scarring that may be resistant to reversal/re-opening sometimes indicated later. For these reasons, a micro wedge resection of the punctum and suture repair may be better. Re-opening can be performed with an eyelid cut down with or without silicone tube intubation.

8 Canalicular Filet Repair

Canalicular filet or cheesewiring can be idiopathic in nature, or it can be secondary to medial traction from silicone intubation. Widening of the puncta along the horizontal portion of the canaliculus can impact the integrity of the canalicular pump and reduce tear outflow, leading to epiphora. Repair of this can improve pump function and restore the integrity of the lacrimal system.

The peri-canalicular tissue is undermined from the surrounding skin and orbicularis muscle. The canaliculus is closed with interrupted 7-0 or 8-0 polyglactin suture. The orbicularis is closed separately from canalicular repair. The skin is closed with interrupted or running 6-0 plain suture. Silicone intubation is typically not recommended at the time of this repair due to concern for creating too much pressure on the closure, putting the repair at risk of dehiscence.

9 Medial Canthopexy (See also Chap. "Medial Canthal Surgery")

Ectropion due to eyelid laxity often can be repaired via horizontal eyelid tightening. However, when laxity of the medial canthal tendon is the predominant contributor, a medial canthopexy may be preferable as a standalone technique or in conjunction with lateral eyelid tightening. Repair of medial laxity can help narrow the widened palpebral fissure in cases of 7th nerve palsy. Further, trauma involving the posterior limb of the medial canthal tendon may require reconstruction of the medial canthus to prevent traumatic telecanthus.

During medial canthopexy, care must be taken preserve the canalicular system integrity. This can be done with lacrimal probes that can also be used to retract the upper and lower eyelids. An approach can be done at the mucocutaneous junction or just anterior to the caruncle on the conjunctival surface.

9.1 Anterior Approach Technique

An incision is made at the mucocutaneous junction 1–2 mm medial to the upper and lower puncta and extended to the medial canthal angle, where the incisions are united. Skin flaps are elevated. While carefully avoiding canalicular damage, the upper and lower medial canthal limbs are secured together with interrupted 6-0 or 7-0 polyglactin sutures [17].

9.2 Posterior Approach Technique

A precaruncluar incision is made through the conjunctiva and dissection is carried medially along the posterior limb of the medial canthal tendon, guiding the dissection towards the posterior lacrimal crest. A screw is placed at the posterosuperior lacrimal crest. A suture is tied around the screw and anchored deeply to the medial end of the tarsal plate as close to the eyelid margin as possible [18].

10 Conclusion

The lacrimal drainage apparatus is key in eyelid and ocular surface physiology. Adequate tear outflow depends on not only a patent lacrimal system, but also good medial lower eyelid positioning and tone. Probing the canaliculi may be useful during surgery and silicone stent placement into the lacrimal outflow system is useful when there exists a concern for occlusion.

References

1. Sevel D. Development and congenital abnormalities of the nasolacrimal apparatus. J Pediatr Ophthalmol Strabismus. 1981;18(5):13–9.
2. Saude T. Ocular anatomy and physiology. Oxford, UK: Blackwell Scientific Publications; 1993.
3. Kominami R, Yasutaka S, Taniguchi Y, Shinohara H. Anatomy and histology of the lacrimal fluid drainage system. Okajimas Folia Anat Jpn. 2000;77(5):155–60.
4. Hartstein ME. The Complete Guide to the Evaluation and Management of the Tearing Patient. American Academy of Ophthalmology Annual Meeting. Dallas, TX. October 2000
5. Eagle R. The eyelid and lacrimal drainage system. In Eye Pathology: An Atlas and Text. Philadelphia: LWW; 2011. p. 241–242.
6. Singh AD, McCloskey L, Parsons MA, Slater DN. Eccrine hidrocystoma of the eyelid. Eye (Lond). 2005;19:77–9.
7. Nowinski TS, Anderson RL. The medial spindle procedure for involutional medial ectropion. Arch Ophthalmol. 1985;103(11):1750–3.
8. Czyz CN, Wulc AE, Ryu CL, Foster JA, Edmonson BC. Caruncular fixation in medial canthal tendon repair: the minimally invasive purse string suture for tendinous laxity and medial ectropion. Ophthalmic Plast Reconstr Surg. 2015;31(1):34–7.
9. Prendes MA, Jian-Amadi A, Chang SH, Shaftel SS. Ocular trauma from dog bites: characterization, associations, and treatment patterns at a regional level I trauma center over 11 years. Ophthalmic Plast Reconstr Surg. 2016;32(4):279–83.
10. Baylis HI, Axelrod R. Repair of the lacerated canaliculus. Ophthalmology. 1978;85(12):1271–6.
11. Rumelt S, Remulla H, Rubin PA. Silicone punctal plug migration resulting in dacryocystitis and canaliculitis. Cornea. 1997;16(3):377–9.
12. Wang M, Cong R, Yu B. Outcomes of canaliculotomy with and without silicone tube intubation in management of primary canaliculitis. Curr Eye Res. 2021;46(12):1812–5.
13. Caesar RH, McNab AA. A brief history of punctoplasty: the 3-snip revisited. Eye (Lond). 2005;19(1):16–8.
14. Carrim ZI, Liolios VI, Vize CJ. Punctoplasty with a Kelly punch. Ophthalmic Plast Reconstr Surg. 2011;27(5):397–8.
15. Dohlman CH. Punctal occlusion in keratoconjunctivitis sicca. Ophthalmology. 1978;85(12):1277–81.
16. Ohba E, Dogru M, Hosaka E, Yamazaki A, Asaga R, Tatematsu Y, Ogawa Y, Tsubota K, Goto E. Surgical punctal occlusion with a high heat-energy releasing cautery device for severe dry eye with recurrent punctal plug extrusion. Am J Ophthalmol. 2011;151(3):483-7.e1.
17. Maamari RN, Custer PL, Neimkin MG, Couch SM. Medial canthoplasty for the management of exposure keratopathy. Eye (Lond). 2019;33(6):925–9. https://doi.org/10.1038/s41433-019-0347-9.
18. Fante RG, Elner VM. Transcaruncular approach to medial canthal tendon plication for lower eyelid laxity. Ophthalmic Plast Reconstr Surg. 2001;17(1):16–27.

Extraocular Muscle Considerations in Lower Eyelid Surgery

Vivek R. Patel

Abstract

Important relationships exist between the lower eyelid and the inferior extraocular muscles. Lower eyelid surgery can impact ocular motility. In turn, strabismus surgery can influence the position of the lower eyelids. Knowledge of these interactions are important to avoid complications as well as anticipate the need for future interventions. This chapter describes common interactions between the extraocular muscles and the lower eyelid, important for the oculofacial surgeon.

Keywords

Retraction · Thyroid eye disease · Restrictive strabismus · Ectropion · Entropion · Brown syndrome · Diplopia

1 Introduction

The lower eyelids and inferior extraocular muscles are intimately associated. They are linked directly through the capsulopalpebral fascia. Moreover, surgery on one, can affect the other. Chiefly, the inferior oblique, if not recognized, is at risk for damage during many lower eyelid surgeries, especially blepharoplasty. Lastly, in the absence of eyelid pathology, strabismus may induce relative positional changes in the eyelid. For example, hypertropia induces a relative increase in the lower eyelid margin to light reflex distance (MRD2).

Several anatomical, clinical and surgical factors are important in lower eyelid-eye muscle relationships. This chapter will review two broad categories: (1) scenarios where lower eyelid surgery can affect ocular motility; (2) eye muscle surgery and considerations that may influence lower eyelid position.

1. Eyelid surgeries and their impact on ocular motility:

Canthoplasty surgery such as a lateral tarsal strip are commonly employed to address horizontal laxity of the lower eyelid [1]. Overtightening the lower eyelid or excessive supraplacement of the periosteal fixation suture can result in restriction of inferior oblique excursion. Clinically, this can result in vertical and torsional diplopia, similar in pattern to an acquired Brown Syndrome. New onset postoperative diplopia and degree of vertical misalignment may be greatest when the affected eye is adducted, and excyclotorsion can be appreciated on double Maddox rod testing or direct

V. R. Patel (✉)
Chief, Neuro-Ophthalmology, Gavin Herbert Eye Institute, University of California, Irvine, USA
e-mail: vivekrp@hs.uci.edu

J. P. Tao (ed.), *Plastic Surgery of the Lower Eyelids*,
https://doi.org/10.1007/978-3-031-36175-3_6

evaluation of the fundus. There is generally a degree of limitation of supraduction of the eye in adduction.

The same Brown syndrome-type strabismus pattern can be seen following lower eyelid blepharoplasty [2]. Care should be taken when removing fat from the inferior compartments to avoid direct injury (Fig. 1). In the absence of direct injury, excessive cautery in the region can cicatrize the connective tissues surrounding the inferior oblique muscle (capsulopalpebral fascia and Lockwood ligament), and restrict ocular movement. The inferior oblique muscle originates at the anterior lacrimal crest, inserts on the posterior globe, just inferior to the posterior aspect of the lateral rectus muscle, and travels below the inferior rectus muscle. The proximal inferior oblique muscle is in very close proximity to the lower eyelid tissues. Both anterior and posterior lower eyelid blepharoplasty approaches require careful attention to path of the inferior oblique muscle and its surrounding connective tissues to maintain its anatomical and functional integrity. Some surgeons advocate blunt dissection to identify the inferior oblique muscle during blepharoplasty. Direct visualization is not mandatory, but the eyelid surgeon should be mindful to not injure the muscle during fat manipulation.

In these scenarios of diplopia following eyelid surgery, ocular motility and alignment often gradually improve during the post-operative course, typically over weeks but occasionally requires several months. Strabismus surgery is rarely required to improve alignment, and should generally not be considered for at least 6 months after eyelid surgery. Consultation with a strabismus specialist familiar with acquired cyclo-vertical

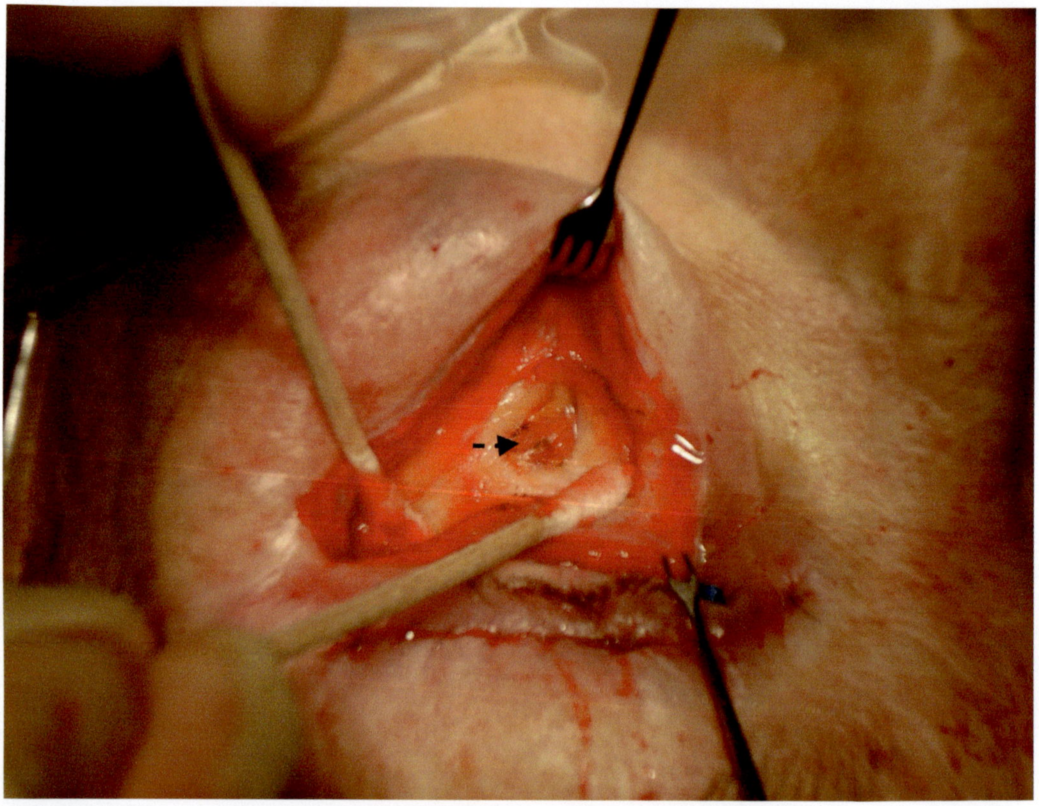

Fig. 1 Intraoperative external lower eyelid blepharoplasty image demonstrating the proximal inferior oblique muscle (arrow) evident between the medial and central fat compartments

deviations may be indicated. Medical management includes spectacle correction with prisms. If these fail, strabismus surgery may be required.

2. Eye muscle considerations that may influence lower eyelid position:

The posterior aspect of the inferior eyelid and orbital surface of the inferior rectus (IR) are directly connected by the capsulopalpebral fascia (a.k.a retractor band) (see Figs. 2 and 3). This continuous musculo-tendinous system originates near the region of intersection between the inferior rectus and inferior oblique muscles, then extends anteriorly to surround the inferior oblique, and inserts into the inferior border of the tarsal plate [3]. There is considerable variability in how anteriorly the fascia inserts along the longitudinal axis of the muscle. Careful blunt technique is used to separate these from the inferior rectus belly without extending the dissection beyond Tenon capsule

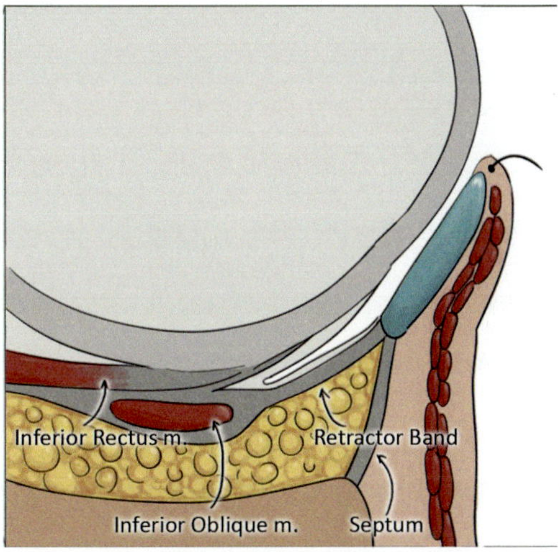

Fig. 2 Sagittal section diagram demonstrating relationship between the retractor band (a.k.a capsulopalpebral fascia) and the inferior extraocular muscles. *Image by Michael Han*

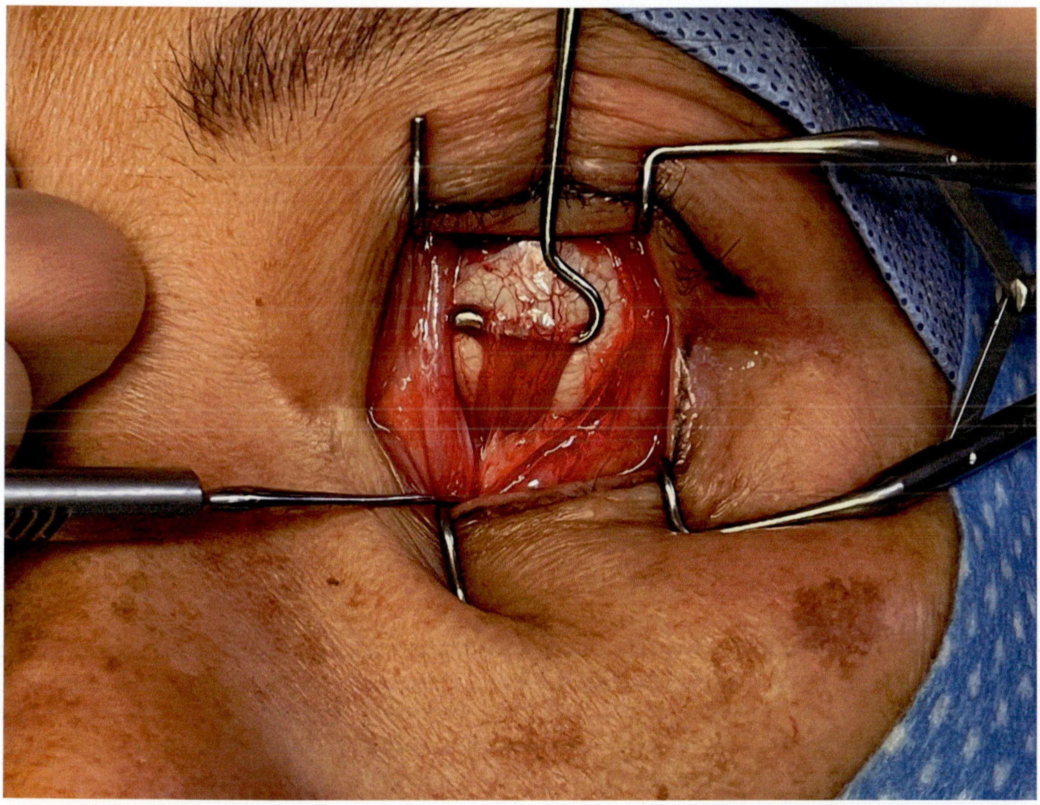

Fig. 3 Intra-operative photo of the inferior rectus and capsulopalpebral fascia which is identified as the white bands attached to the orbital surface of the inferior rectus muscle. Careful blunt technique is used to separate these from the inferior rectus belly without extending the dissection beyond Tenon capsule

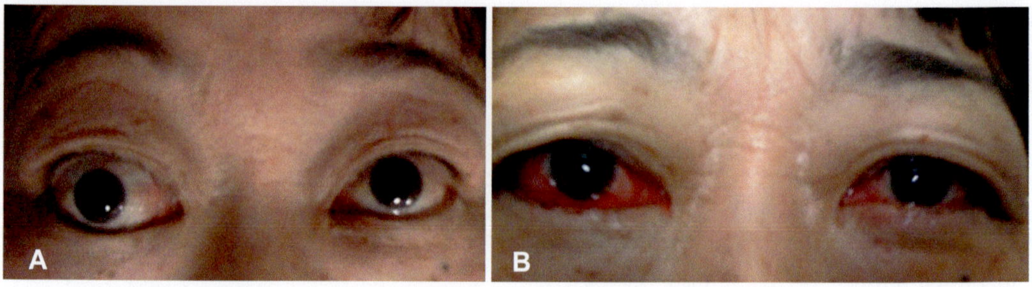

Fig. 4 A) Pre-operative photo of a TED patient with bilateral orbitopathy. Note the inferior scleral show in both eyes with greater upper eyelid retraction the right eye. The large angle right hypotropia required right inferior rectus recession (6 mm) and left superior rectus recession (6 mm) to neutralize the deviation. B). Immediate post operative appearance

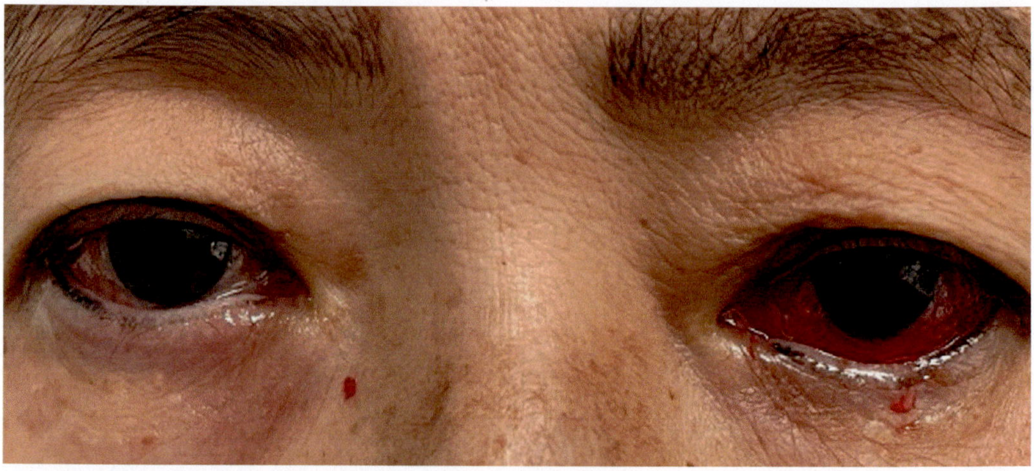

Fig. 5 Same day post-operative after inferior rectus recession photo shows mild worsening of pre-existing left lower eyelid retraction which improved over the next few weeks, and did not require surgical intervention

IR. As expected, younger patients tend to have more firm attachments. This anatomical connection between the lower eyelid and IR allows the lower eyelid to be pulled inferiorly on infraduction, keeping the pupil and visual axis from being obscured.

In patients with thyroid eye disease (TED), fibrosis within the lower eyelid tissues, proptosis and contraction of the sympathetically innervated inferior tarsal muscle can each contribute the development of inferior eyelid retraction (see Fig. 4). The angle of vertical strabismus can be large in patients with TED given the propensity for IR involvement, producing a marked restrictive vertical strabismus. Since the eye is typically pulled down by a fibrotic IR, the primary approach to improve alignment is performing a recession of this muscle, with or without a contralateral superior rectus recession for cases with larger deviations. Reducing IR restriction is an essential component of relieving this type of strabismus. Given the direct attachment between the IR and inferior eyelid via the capsulopalpebral fascia, recession of the IR accordingly pulls the eyelid inferiorly (Fig. 5). In anticipation of this, the capsulopalpebral fascia needs to be released by carefully creating separation between the fascia and surface of the IR muscle belly. This can usually be accomplished by blunt technique alone (cotton-tip gently yet firmly used to separate the fascia from the muscle's surface), but in cases where the fascia is

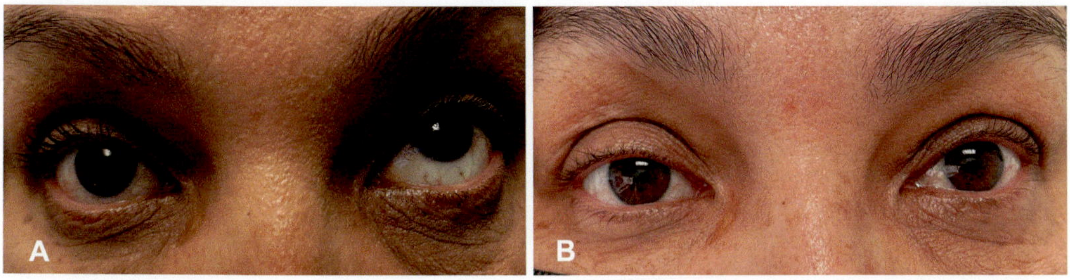

Fig. 6 A) TED patient with greater than 50 Prism Diopter (PD) left hypertropia due to right IR restriction and secondary overaction of the left superior rectus (SR). Large left SR recession (8 mm) and right IR recession (8 mm) were required to effectively neutralize the deviation. B) 6 weeks post-operatively, note the desirable right lower eyelid position despite large amplitude IR recession, achieved by effective disinsertion of the lower eyelid retractors from the IR muscle belly

quite adherent, the desired anatomical plane can be established by initial sharp dissection, taking care not to injure the muscle itself or violate tenon's capsule. If orbital fat is allowed to encroach upon the IR surface, fat adherence can occur. In the author's experience, any IR recession greater than 5 mm requires a generous release of this attachment, but in some patients even smaller amplitude recessions can result in post-operative lower eyelid retraction. Although this concept is described in this chapter in relation to IR recessions in TED, the principle of attentive dissection of the capsulopalpebral fascia off the orbital surface of the IR applies to all cases of IR recession, in particular larger amplitude ones. Some strabismus surgeons recommend disinserting the lower eyelid retractors from the inferior border of the tarsal plate for larger IR recessions, where post-surgical eyelid retraction is expected (Fig. 6). Lower eyelid spacers using a variety of techniques may be considered in cases where eyelid retraction cannot be avoided despite attention to these factors [4].

2 Conclusion

The lower eyelids and inferior extraocular muscles are intimately associated and surgery on one can impact each other. Knowledge of these relationships are important to achieve optimal results.

References

1. Jordan DR, Anderson RL. The lateral tarsal strip revisited. The enhanced tarsal strip. Arch Ophthalmol. 1989;107(4):604–6.
2. Syniuta LA, Goldberg RA, Thacker NM, Rosenbaum AL. Acquired strabismus following cosmetic blepharoplasty. Plast Reconstr Surg. 2003;111(6):2053–9.
3. Basic and Clinical Science Course, Orbit, Eyelids and Lacrimal System (Section 7), American Academy of Ophthalmology, 2002–2003, pp 124–8.
4. Cypen SG, Conger JR, Chen LE, Tao JP. Treatment options for lower eyelid retraction in thyroid eye disease. Int Ophthalmol Clin. 2021;61(2):145–59.

Inflammatory Symblepharon

Cinthia Kim and Sanjay Kedhar

Abstract

Symblephara are adhesions between the palpebral and bulbar conjunctiva and may occur as a complication of infectious, inflammatory, or neoplastic diseases. They may also be due to trauma or surgery. A loss of epithelial cells on both the palpebral and bulbar conjunctival surfaces results in adhesion formation that may be asymptomatic or, in more severe forms, obliterate the fornix resulting in an insufficient tear reservoir and secondary ocular surface keratinization. Symptoms of symblepharon can include eye redness, tearing, pain, photophobia, diplopia, restricted extraocular motility, lagophthalmos, entropion and reduced visual acuity. This chapter will provide a brief overview of the differential diagnosis, evaluation, and medical management of eyes with inflammatory symblephara.

Keywords

Symblepharon · Ocular inflammatory disease · Stevens-Johnson Syndrome · Mucous membrane pemphigoid

C. Kim · S. Kedhar (✉)
Gavin Herbert Eye Institute, University of California, Irvine, Irvine, CA, USA
e-mail: skedhar@hs.uci.edu

1 Introduction

Symblepharon is a partial or complete adhesion of the palpebral conjunctiva of the eyelid to the bulbar conjunctiva of the eye [1]. While most symblepharon are acquired, congenital cases may rarely occur. Symblephara occur as a complication of various infectious, inflammatory, and neoplastic diseases or due to trauma or surgery. It is incumbent on the treating physician to carefully investigate for an etiology in cases of symblephara, including taking a complete history and performing any diagnostic procedures such as conjunctival biopsy or serologies. A thorough history is a key part of evaluating these patients as findings will guide the workup and may avoid unnecessary diagnostic procedures. A history of exposure to sulfonamides prior to the development of ocular inflammation can suggest a diagnosis of Stevens-Johnson syndrome for example. Likewise, examination of extraocular tissues, especially the skin and oral mucosa may aid in elucidating the underlying etiology. Patients with mucous membrane pemphigoid may also oral mucosa disease and ulcerative gingivitis may be present on examination. Conjunctival biopsy should be considered in most patients without a pre-existing definitive diagnosis or in those patients whose course is atypical or progressive despite conventional therapy.

J. P. Tao (ed.), *Plastic Surgery of the Lower Eyelids*,
https://doi.org/10.1007/978-3-031-36175-3_7

Regardless of etiology, patients with symblepharon may experience a multitude of symptoms. Some, such as redness, pain, tearing, photophobia and reduced visual acuity may be related to the inflammatory effect on the ocular surface and secondary dry eye. These are typically managed with topical anti-inflammatories, lubricants and possibly barrier methods to protect the ocular surface such as bandage contact lenses or amniotic membrane transplant. Others, such as diplopia, restricted extraocular motility, lagophthalmos, and entropion may be a direct effect of the adhesion itself which are generally managed with surgical interventions [2]. Of note, control of any underlying inflammation for at least 3 to 6 months, is paramount before undertaking any surgical corrections unless the intervention is urgent.

2 Physical Examination

Because symblephara are a complication of conjunctival inflammation, exam findings distinguishing one etiology from another are often not apparent. Examination of the periocular area may reveal additional clues as to the diagnosis; central facial erythema, papulopustular lesions or extensive facial telangiectasias may suggest a diagnosis of acne rosacea. As another example, examination of the skin may show purple-red papules with irregular white streaks consistent with a diagnosis of lichen planus. Symblepharon has variable severity and tissue involvement. On physical exam, there may be only a small adhesion between the two layers of conjunctiva with no obvious symptoms. However, in more severe cases, the fornix of the eye may become obliterated, cicatricial entropion may form, or there may be permanent lagophthalmos with exposure of the cornea [3]. Obliteration of the fornix can cause insufficient tear reservoir and blinking leading to eventual keratinization of the ocular surface. Entropion can cause ocular trauma to the surface of the eye as the eyelashes rub on the outer surface. With greater tissue involvement, restrictions in extraocular movements may be seen [4]. Depending on the severity, the symblepharon may or may not involve the cornea.

3 Differential Diagnosis

There are many causes of symblepharon, which is typically a response to trauma or inflammation [2]. Immune mediated inflammatory conditions include:

- Stevens-Johnson Syndrome /Toxic Epidermal Necrolysis
- Mucous membrane pemphigoid
- Atopic keratoconjunctivitis
- Rosacea
- Sarcoid
- Granulomatosis with Polyangiitis
- Chronic Ocular Graft-versus-host disease
- Sjogren's Syndrome
- Lichen Planus
- Paraneoplastic Mucous Membrane Pemphigoid
- Recessive Dystrophic Epidermolysis Bullosa

A complete discussion of each disease entity is beyond the scope of this book, however Stevens-Johnson syndrome and mucous membrane pemphigoid, the two major causes of symblephara are described in this chapter.

4 Stevens-Johnson Syndrome/ Toxic Epidermal Necrolysis

Stevens-Johnson syndrome (SJS) and toxic epidermal necrolysis (TEN) are hypersensitivity reactions to drugs or infectious diseases (e.g., those due to herpes simplex virus, streptococcus, adenovirus). Approximately 80% of TEN and 50–80% of SJS cases are thought to be drug induced; the ocular conjunctiva and oropharynx are the tissues most frequently affected. Sulfonamides, anticonvulsants, NSAIDs, and allopurinol are most frequently involved. Although the pathogenesis of the disease is not completely understood, several genetic factors are implicated in the onset of SJS/TEN with ocular complications [7, 8].

It is characterized by an acute inflammatory vesiculobullous reaction of the skin and mucous membranes. The distinctive pathologic changes of SJS are subepithelial bullae and subsequent scarring. When these hypersensitivity disorders involve only the skin, the term erythema multiforme minor is used; when the skin and mucous membranes are involved, the condition is SJS, or erythema multiforme major. The most severe form of this condition is TEN [8]. SJS occurs most commonly in female children and young adults. Fever, arthralgia, malaise, and upper or lower respiratory symptoms are usually sudden in onset. Skin eruption follows within a few days, with a classic target lesion consisting of a red center surrounded by a pale ring and then a red ring, however maculopapular or bullous lesions are also common. The mucous membranes of the eyes, mouth, and genitalia may be affected by bullous lesions with membrane or pseudomembrane formation. The primary ocular finding is a mucopurulent conjunctivitis and episcleritis [9, 10]. Conjunctival and corneal epithelial sloughing and necrosis with severe inflammation and scarring may develop. Long-term ocular complications result from ocular surface cicatrization, resulting in conjunctival shrinkage, keratinization of the eyelid margins, trichiasis, and tear deficiency. Management of acute SJS is like that of extensive thermal burns; patients are often treated in burn units at major tertiary care centers. Immediate discontinuation of the offending agent has been associated with reduced mortality and improved outcome. Systemic therapy is mainly supportive and is aimed at managing dehydration and superinfection. Acute ocular therapy includes lubrication with preservative-free artificial tears and ointments; topical antibiotics are occasionally used as prophylaxis. More recently, significant long-term benefit has been demonstrated from the early transplantation of amniotic membrane over the entire ocular surface, including the eyelid margins for severe epithelial defects of the cornea and/or conjunctiva. This is one of the few potentially beneficial therapeutic interventions for this devastating disease. Corticosteroids may decrease surface inflammation and corneal angiogenesis but the efficacy of topical corticosteroids for the ocular manifestations of this condition has not been established and remains controversial. Additionally, therapeutic contact lenses may be used as a temporizing measure. Scleral contact lenses can play a critical role in the long-term rehabilitation of these patients. Systemic immunosuppression is often required to suppress the severe inflammatory response in these cases [9–12].

Symblepharon may form during the acute phase because the raw, necrotic palpebral and bulbar conjunctival surfaces can adhere to one another. Late eyelid sequelae, such as entropion, trichiasis, and keratinization, result in chronic ocular surface inflammation that can be difficult to manage [8, 12].

5 Mucous Membrane Pemphigoid

Mucous membrane pemphigoid (also known as ocular cicatricial pemphigoid or OCP) is an autoimmune disease characterize by mucous membrane fibrosis and skin changes resulting in scarring. It is characterized by a chronic bilateral conjunctivitis with relapsing–remitting periods. With a worldwide distribution and no racial predilection, mucous membrane pemphigoid predominantly affects women aged around 60 years. The pathogenic mechanisms of mucous membrane pemphigoid remain unknown probably linked to an autoimmune type II hypersensitivity response in patients with a genetic predisposition and exposure to different environmental triggers [13, 14].

Without therapy up to 75% of patients develop vision loss due to major ocular complications. Conjunctival fibrosis may cause severe dry eye syndrome, corneal epithelial erosions or ulceration, corneal keratinization, entropion, trichiasis and symblepharon. Secondary glaucoma is one of the most frequent complications. Conjunctival biopsy with direct immunofluorescence is the gold standard in diagnosis confirmation, but up to 40% of the patients can have a negative biopsy result that does not rule out the diagnosis. Conjunctival biopsy should be performed in cases of persistent conjunctival inflammation. Perilesional biopsy specimens may have the highest yield for direct immunofluorescence. If involvement is diffuse, the biopsy may be taken from the inferior conjunctival fornix. The skin and many other mucous membranes (e.g., oral, trachea, esophagus, pharynx, larynx, urethra, vagina, and anus) may also be involved. Oral mucosal biopsies may be useful, especially in the presence of an active lesion [13–15]. Once the diagnosis is established, a multidisciplinary approach to management is of utmost importance. Any nose or throat symptoms should prompt an immediate referral to otolaryngology as these complications may be life-threatening.

Local treatment of mucous membrane pemphigoid is adjunctive and will not halt progression of the disease. Treatment can include topical drops or ointments including lubricants, corticosteroids, antibiotics, and glaucoma medications as indicated.

Because progression is often slow, careful clinical staging of the disease and photo documentation in differing positions of gaze is generally recommended in evaluating the disease course and response to therapy. Severity of pemphigoid can be judged by measuring the shortening of the inferior fornix depth and degree of cicatrix formation [14, 15].

The main goals of treatment are to stop disease progression, relieve symptoms and prevent complications. With long-term systemic therapy 90% of the cases can be effectively controlled. Patients may be divided into low and high-risk categories. Low-risk patients include those with disease occurring only in the oral mucosa or oral mucosa and skin may have a much lower incidence of scarring; thus, they can be treated more conservatively. High-risk patients are characterized by ocular, genital, nasopharyngeal, esophageal, and/or laryngeal mucosa involvement, requiring more aggressive treatment. Treatment regimens vary, but the prevailing wisdom is to be as aggressive as necessary to prevent progression of the disease. Oral dapsone and corticosteroids may control the activity of the disease in mild disease without rapid progression. While dapsone is the first-line treatment in mild to moderate disease in patients without G6PD deficiency, more severe cases may require immunosuppressant therapy with azathioprine, mycophenolate mofetil, methotrexate or cyclophosphamide. Cyclophosphamide can produce a durable drug-free remission but carries with it significant risks. The anti-CD20 biologic rituximab and intravenous immunoglobulin therapy are often reserved for recalcitrant disease or those with unsatisfactory results to conventional therapy. Dry eye syndrome requires constant lubricating medication and can also involve topical steroids, cyclosporine or lifitegrast and tacrolimus ointment. Surgery should be planned only in the quiescent phase as minor conjunctival trauma can significantly worsen the disease [13, 14, 16].

6 Medical Management

Medical management of symblepharon consists of treatment of the underlying disease to prevent or decrease additional symblepharon. In inflammatory conditions, immune modulating therapy to suppress inflammation can improve outcomes, such as rituximab for Severe Refractory Paraneoplastic Mucous Membrane Pemphigoid [17]. Systemic steroids and other immunosuppressive drugs such as azathioprine, methotrexate, mycophenolate mofetil or cyclophosphamide may also be used depending on the severity of the disease. In some instances, use of a particular immunosuppressive drug will be dictated by the underlying condition (i.e. granulomatosis with polyangiitis) while in others it will be dictated by the ocular severity itself. The symptoms of dry eye caused by symblepharon can be managed using preservative free artificial tears, lubricating ointments, and topical anti-inflammatory medications [18, 19]. A symblepharon ring may forestall further

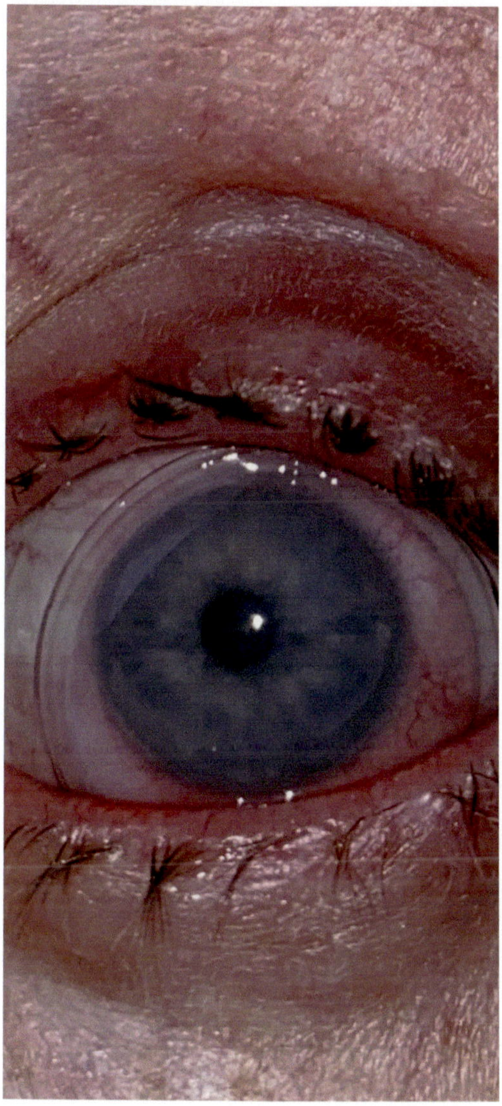

Fig. 1 Self-retaining amniotic membrane mounted on a symblepharon ring. (*Photo courtesy of Olivia Lee*

adhesions between the bulbar and palpebral conjunctiva (Fig. 1).

Various surgical interventions may also be used to treat symptomatic symblepharon. The conventional surgical approach is reconstruction of the ocular surface by symblepharon lysis and buccal mucosal graft or amniotic membrane transplantation [5, 6]. These are described in Chap. Symblepharon and Conjunctival Scarring.

7 Conclusion

Symblepharon is characterized by an adhesion that forms between the palpebral and bulbar conjunctiva. Immune mediated inflammatory causes of symblepharon include Stevens-Johnson syndrome /toxic epidermal necrolysis, mucous membrane pemphigoid, atopic keratoconjunctivitis, and acne rosacea, among others. Conjunctival biopsy is the gold standard for diagnosing the underlying etiology of symblephara and should be considered in most patients without a definitive diagnosis or in those patients whose course is atypical or progressive despite conventional therapy. Treatment aims include arrest of disease progression, prevention of complications and relief of symptoms. Medical management must include treatment of the underlying inflammatory disease process and coordination with physicians who are familiar with systemic anti-inflammatory therapy including oral steroids and immunosuppressants. Symptomatic management often involves therapies such as frequent use of preservative-free artificial tears and lubricating ointments, as well as punctal occlusion. Additional treatments such as topical anti-inflammatories (including courses of topical steroids or tacrolimus ointment, and long-term use of topical cyclosporine or lifitegrast), therapeutic bandage contact lenses and amniotic membrane transplantation may also be used to optimize the ocular surface. Various surgical interventions may also be used to treat symptomatic symblepharon and are described in Chap. Symblepharon and Conjunctival Scarring.

References

1. Basic and Clinical Science Course, Section 8: External Disease and Cornea. American Academy of Ophthalmology, 2017–2018 edition.
2. Li T, Shao Y, Lin Q, Zhang D. Reversed skin graft combining with lip mucosa transplantation in treating recurrent severe symblepharon: a case report. Medicine (Baltimore). 2018;97(35): e12168. https://doi.org/10.1097/MD.0000000000012168.

3. DeVoe AG. System of ophthalmology, diseases of the outer eye; part 1: Conjunctiva, part 2: Cornea and Sclera. Arch Ophthalmol. 1965;74(6):884–5. https://doi.org/10.1001/archopht.1965.00970040886033.
4. Catt CJ, Hamilton GM, Fish J, Mireskandari K, Ali A. Ocular manifestations of Stevens-Johnson syndrome and toxic epidermal necrolysis in children. Am J Ophthalmol. 2016;166:68–75. https://doi.org/10.1016/j.ajo.2016.03.020.
5. Kheirkhah A, Blanco G, Casas V, et al. Surgical strategies for fornix reconstruction based on symblepharon severity. Am J Ophthalmol. 2008;146:266–75.
6. Jonathan E, Harminder S, Albert B, et al. Ocular surface reconstruction in LOGIC syndrome by amniotic membrane transplantation. Cornea. 2001;20:753–6.
7. Araki Y, Sotozono C, Inatomi T, et al. Successful treatment of Stevens-Johnson syndrome with steroid pulse therapy at disease onset. Am J Ophthalmol. 2009;147(6):1004–1011.
8. Borchers AT, Lee JL, Naguwa SM, Cheema GS, Gershwin ME. Stevens-Johnson syndrome and toxic epidermal necrolysis. Autoimmun Rev. 2008;7(8):598–605.
9. Gerull R, Nelle M, Schaible T. Toxic epidermal necrolysis and Stevens-Johnson syndrome: a review. Crit Care Med. 2011;39(6):1521–32.
10. Gregory DG. Treatment of acute Stevens-Johnson syndrome and toxic epidermal necrolysis using amniotic membrane: a review of 10 consecutive cases. Ophthalmology. 2011;118(5):908–14.
11. Frantz R, Huang S, Are A, Motaparthi K. Stevens-Johnson syndrome and toxic epidermal necrolysis: a review of diagnosis and management. Medicina (Kaunas). 2021;57(9):895. https://doi.org/10.3390/medicina57090895. PMID:34577817;PMCID: PMC8472007
12. Ueta M. Stevens-Johnson syndrome/toxic epidermal necrolysis with severe ocular complications. Expert Rev Clin Immunol. 2020;16(3):285–91. https://doi.org/10.1080/1744666X.2020.1729128. Epub 2020 Feb 28 PMID: 32045311.
13. Branisteanu DC, Stoleriu G, Branisteanu DE, Boda D, Branisteanu CI, Maranduca MA, Moraru A, Stanca HT, Zemba M, Balta F. Ocular cicatricial pemphigoid (Review). Exp Ther Med. 2020;20(4):3379–3382. https://doi.org/10.3892/etm.2020.8972. Epub 2020 Jul 7. PMID: 32905166; PMCID: PMC7465597.
14. Thorne JE, Anhalt GJ, Jabs DA. Mucous membrane pemphigoid and pseudopemphigoid. Ophthalmology. 2004;111(1):45–52; Williams GP, Radford C, Nightingale P, Dart JK, Rauz S. Evaluation of early and late presentation of patients with ocular mucous membrane pemphigoid to two major tertiary referral hospitals in the United Kingdom. Eye (Land). 2011;25(9):1207–1218.
15. Saw VP, Dart JK, Rauz S, et al. Immunosuppressive therapy for ocular mucous membrane pemphigoid: strategies and outcomes. Ophthalmology. 2008;115(2):253–261; Srikumaran D, Tzu JH, Akpek EK. Cicatrizing conjunctivitis. Focal Points: Clinical Modules for Ophthalmologists. San Francisco: American Academy of Ophthalmology; 2011, module 1.
16. Foster CS, Chang PY, Ahmed AR. Combination of rituximab and intravenous immunoglobulin for recalcitrant ocular cicatricial pemphigoid: a preliminary report. Ophthalmology. 2010;117(5):861–9.
17. Wittenberg M, Worm M. Severe refractory paraneoplastic mucous membrane pemphigoid successfully treated with rituximab. Front Med (Lausanne). 2019;6:8. Published 2019 Jan 29. https://doi.org/10.3389/fmed.2019.00008.
18. Kaufman HE, Thomas EL. Prevention and treatment of symblepharon. Am J Ophthalmol. 1979;88(3 Pt 1):419–23. https://doi.org/10.1016/0002-9394(79)90642-1.
19. Brydak-Godowska J, Moneta-Wielgoś J, Pauk-Domańska M, Dróbecka-Brydak E, Samsel A, Kecik M, Kowalewski C, Mackiewicz W, Kecik D. Diagnostyka i leczenie zachowawcze ocznego pemfigoidu bliznowaciejacego [Diagnostics and pharmacological treatment of ocular cicatrical pemphigoid]. Klin Oczna. 2005;107(10–12):725–7. Polish. PMID: 16619831.

Symblepharon and Conjunctival Scarring

Non-inflammatory Symblepharon

Eric J. Shiuey and Marjan Farid

Abstract

Symblepharon is an abnormal adhesion between the bulbar and palpebral conjunctiva. It can cause ocular surface disease, restriction of eye motility, obstruction of the visual axis, or irregular astigmatism, among other problems. Numerous etiologies exist and treatment in the inflammatory phase is largely medical and includes lubrication, corticosteroids, and ring spacer. Surgical intervention with active inflammation is not advised because it may exacerbate the condition and increase morbidity. When the conjunctiva is quiescent, surgical interventions include mucous memberane grafts, amniotic membrane transplantation, and adjuvant therapies such as mitomycin C, or 5 fluorouracil, and post-operative beta irradiation. Keratolimbal allograft (KLAL) segments are a novel tissue alternative for treatment of symblepharon that mechanically deter symblepharon reformation and provide conjunctival stem cells. This chapter will review surgical management of non-inflammatory symblephara.

Keywords

Symblepharon · Keratolimbal allograft transplantation · Ocular surface reconstruction · Amniotic membrane transplantation

1 Introduction

Symblephara involve abnormal partial or complete adhesions of palpebral conjunctiva to bulbar conjunctiva following conjunctival injury (Figs. 1A, 2A, 3A, 4A and 5A). They may damage the corneal surface via reduction of tear reservoir, interruption of tear flow and spread, and microtrauma from an irregular tarsal surface, and cause symptoms such as dry eye, burning, photophobia, and decreased vision [1–4]. In severe cases, cicatrix formation may result in entropion and lagophthalmos, which can eventually result in keratinization and neovascularization. These adhesions can limit extraocular movement, which can ultimately lead to causing diplopia in side gaze. Aside from inflammatory causes covered in Chap. Inflammatory Symblepharon (e.g. autoimmune disease such as Stevens-Johnson syndrome, ocular cicatricial

E. J. Shiuey
Sidney Kimmel Medical College, Thomas Jefferson University, Philadelphia, PA, USA

M. Farid (✉)
Gavin Herbert Eye Institute, University of California, Irvine, CA, USA
e-mail: mfarid@hs.uci.edu

J. P. Tao (ed.), *Plastic Surgery of the Lower Eyelids*,
https://doi.org/10.1007/978-3-031-36175-3_8

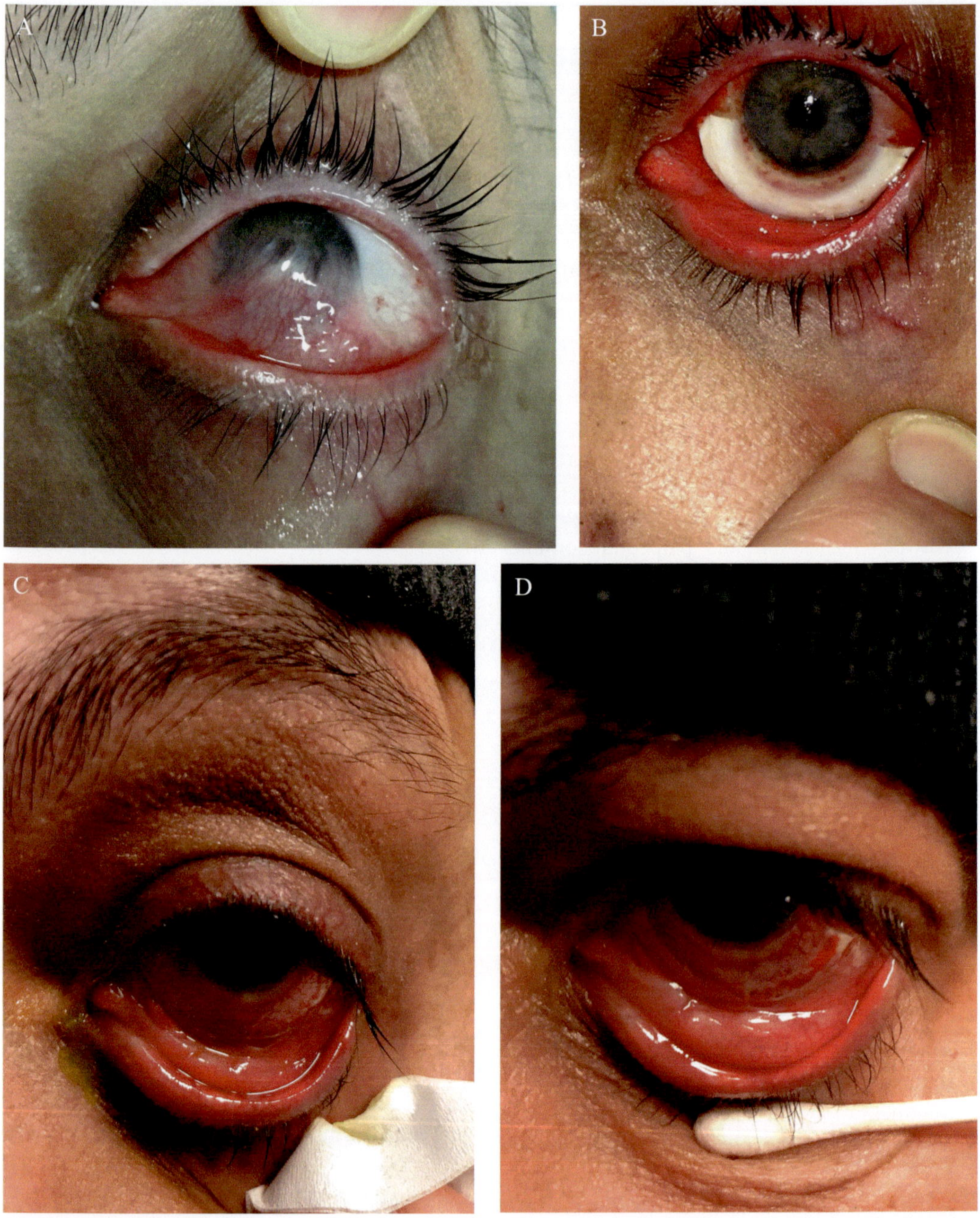

Fig. 1 (A) Symblepharon adhering the palpebral conjunctiva of the left lower eyelid to the inferior bulbar conjunctiva due to previous pterygium excision with reactivation of inflammation and fibrosis. (B) One day after keratolimbal allograft surgery (KLAL) in the left eye. (C) Two weeks after KLAL. (D) Two months after KLAL

pemphigoid, atopy, infection, and other chronic conjunctivitis), non-inflammatory etiologies of symblephara include trauma, iatrogenic (e.g. post pterygium excision, radiation, drug use), and chemical injury.

While medical therapy for mildly symptomatic symblepharon may include artificial tears and other eye lubrications or immune modulation in inflammatory cases, surgical techniques for more debilitating disease includes ocular

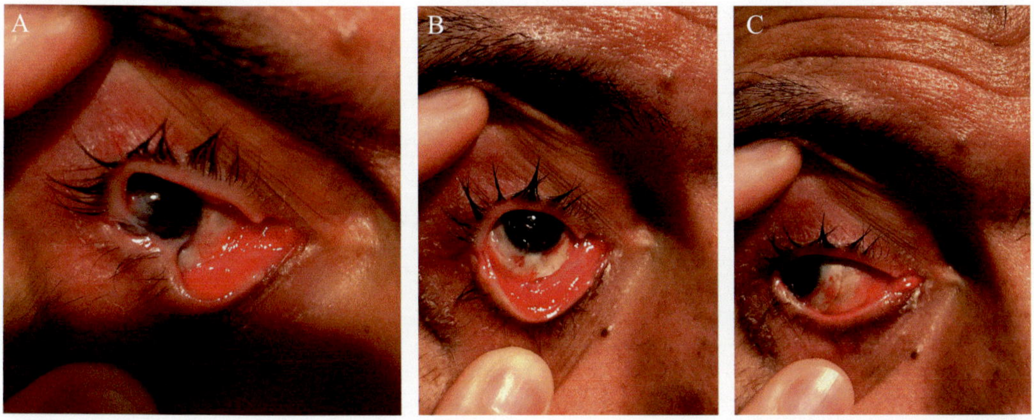

Fig. 2 (A) Symblepharon of the right eye secondary to pterygium surgery. (B) One week postoperative images after keratolimbal allograft surgery, with demonstration of successful symblepharolysis in upgaze. (C) The patient exhibits good range of motion in abduction

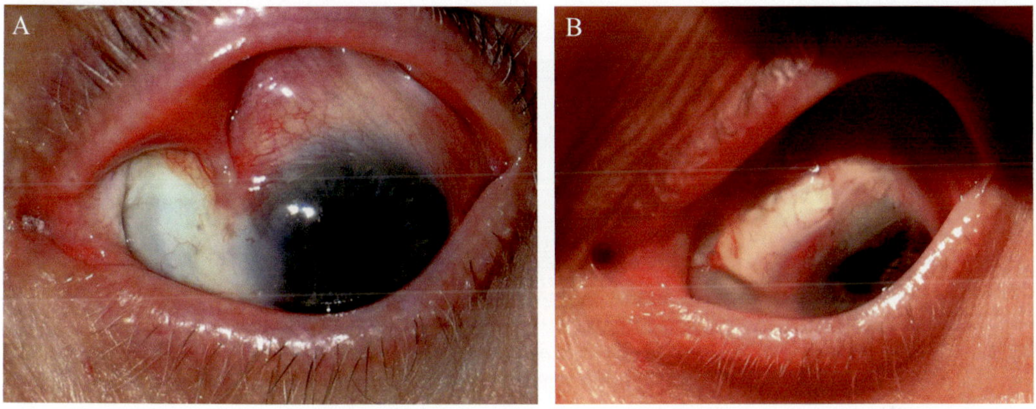

Fig. 3 (A) Formation of a dense symblepharon causing restriction to downward gaze after a reactive inflammatory response post-pterygium surgery. (B) Postoperative month 4

surface reconstruction with tissue substitutes such as conjunctival, oral, and nasal mucousal membranes and/or amniotic membrane grafts (Table 1) [3, 5–8]. Adjuvant techniques, not limited to mitomycin C, use of ring spacers, and subconjunctival steroid injections, reduce the likelihood of fibrovascular regrowth and are commonly used to ameliorate re-scarring [1, 2, 9]. However, many symblephara are refractory to these traditional therapies and recur.

More recently, keratolimbal allograft (KLAL) tissue has been used refractory symblephara. Traditionally, KLAL tissue has been used in the treatment of limbal stem cell deficiency to replace defective corneal/limbal stem cells [10], KLAL may be more robust than other graft tissue and may provide a physical barrier to scar extension. The supply of limbal stem cells may explain its efficacy, although the longevity of the stem cells and their role in long term survival has not been shown. This tissue alternative may prevent recurrence of symblepharon and corneal conjunctivalization [10, 11]. Presently the authors favor the use of KLAL to treat symptomatic recurrent or severe primary symblepharon, with symptomatic diplopia in primary gaze.

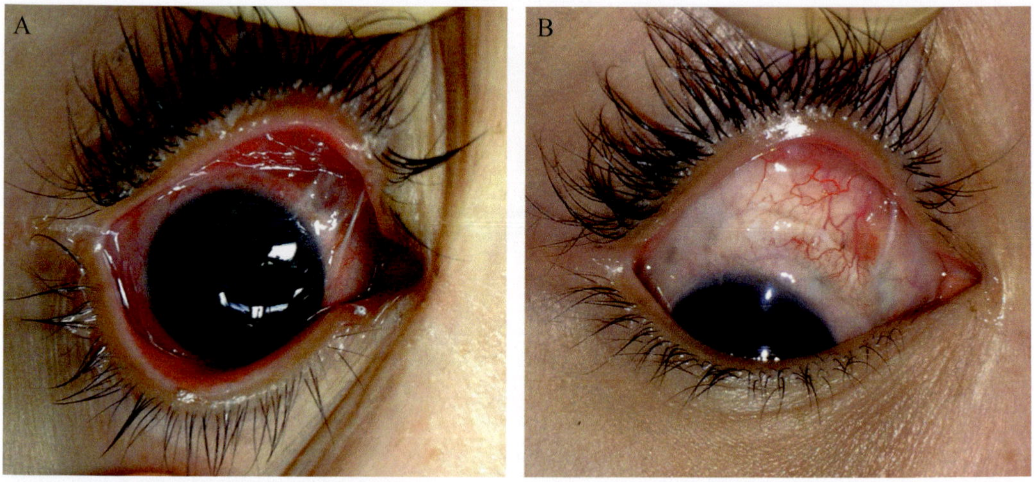

Fig. 4 (A) A patient who developed secondary symblepharon formation after eyelid reconstruction necessitated following a motor vehicle accident. (B) Postoperative month 4

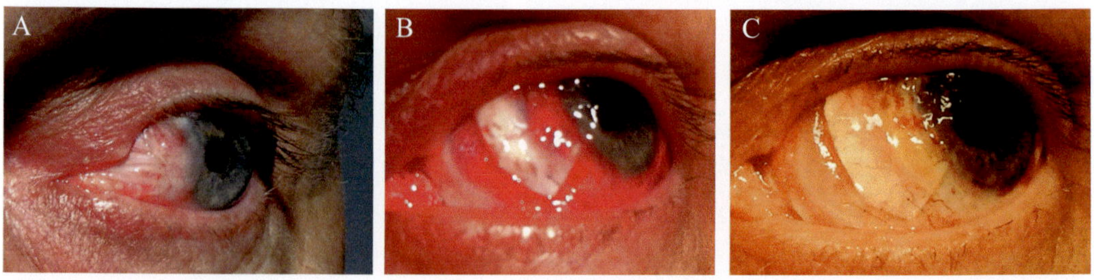

Fig. 5 (A) Following pterygium surgery, development of severe symblepharon is often mistaken for recurrent pterygium. This patient required two keratolimbal allograft segments. (B) Postoperative day 1. (C) Postoperative week 2

Table 1 Management of recurrent non-inflammatory symblephara

Medical/procedural	Surgical techniques	Adjuvant therapy
• Artificial tears and other eye lubrication • Mechanical lysis with glass rods (in acute phase) • Immunomodulation (topical/systemic)	Release and ocular surface reconstruction with: • Conjunctival graft • Oral mucosal graft • Nasal mucosal graft • Amniotic membrane transplantation • Split-thickness skin graft[a] • Vaginal/labial mucosal graft[b] Keratolimbal allograft	• Intraoperative mitomycin C • Symblepharon ring spacers • Subconjunctival corticosteroid injection • Post-operative beta irradiation

[a] Skin grafts are largely a historical surgical option; epithelial desquamation is poorly-tolerated by the cornea and the graft becomes edematous and pale post-operatively [20]
[b] Also historical [21]

2 Indications and Evaluation

While there are no major absolute or relative contraindications for surgery to treat non-inflamed symblepharon, indications for surgical management of symblephara may include:

- Severe ocular irritation
- Restricted extraocular motility with symptomatic diplopia
- Lagophthalmos
- Entropion or trichiasis

We review various surgical techniques below, of which most involve tissue grafting and forniceal reconstruction.

3 Conjunctival Grafts

More commonly used in smaller conjunctival defects, autologous conjunctival transplantation after severe alkali burn was proposed by Thoft in 1977 [12]. In a prospective study of conjunctival allograft transplantation by Kwitko et al. in 12 eyes of 10 patients with predominantly inflammatory bilateral surface disorders were predominantly positive, but this study did not include patients with symblephara and follow-up was limited [5].

The procedure described by Kwitko et al. is as follows: 5×8 mm flaps are prepared from donor conjunctiva adjacent to the limbus (excluding the corneal limbus) and kept moist with balanced salt solution. In the recipient eye, a 360° peritomy and a superficial keratectomy are performed, after which the donor flaps are sutured at the cornea and conjunctiva, with the limbal flap edge abutting the recipient limbus. Patching is performed, and cycloplegic and neomycin-dexamethasone drops are administered postoperatively [5].

4 Amniotic Membrane Grafts

Amniotic membrane, the innermost layer of the placenta and a more traditional substrate for replacing damaged conjunctival membranes, has been demonstrated to effectively rehabilitate the ocular surface from various processes that have caused conjunctival stem cell deficiency [13, 14]. Though numerous reports have studied amniotic membrane transplantation (AMT) in inflammatory conditions [8, 15], Solomon et al. reported results from 17 eyes of 15 patients with symblepharon due to a variety of causes over 37 ± 24 months (range, 9–84 months) [16]. They achieved complete fornix reconstruction in 12 of 17 eyes, while 2 eyes had partial success, and 3 eyes had recurrence of symblepharon with restricted motility. The most successful outcome was observed in eyes with symblepharon associated with trauma. However, eyes with partial success or failure originally had an autoimmune disorder or a recurrent pterygium and fibrosis. The authors contend that an epithelial component in addition to AMT (e.g. conjunctival autograft or ex vivo expanded epithelial stem cells) may improve outcomes.

The procedure [8, 16] involved dissection of subconjunctival scar tissue from the episclera, with the freed conjunctival flap recessed to the fornix. A layer of amniotic membrane was applied to cover the exposed episclera, and the fornical edge of the membrane was anchored with sutures passing through the full thickness of the eyelid. Topical steroid and ofloxacin were prescribed postoperatively, and subconjunctival steroid was administered if proliferative or congested vessels were noted at the graft edge. More recently, Kheirkhah et al. described three to five minutes of adjuvant 0.04% mitomycin C with glued AMT and anchoring sutures in 30 eyes with symblepharon, observing higher success rates in patients with less extensive disease [2].

Patients who fail AMT may have diseased conjunctiva incapable of proper ocular surface reepithelialization. Thus, they may be especially prone to surface breakdown and consequently symblepharon recurrences. Rehabilitation techniques using grafts that provide barriers to adhesion formation, such as the keratolimbal allografts, may have a role in these situations.

5 Oral Mucosal Graft

Kheirkhah et al. in a prospective study of 32 eyes with severe symblepharon due to chemical or thermal burns achieved restoration of a deep fornix without scar or motility restriction in 84.4% of patients at 16.4 ± 7.6 months (range, 6–22 months) follow-up using oral mucosal transplantation and sutureless amniotic membrane [3]. Complications included entropion in 2 eyes, ocular surface keratinization in 1 eye, and pyogenic granuloma in 4 eyes. Notably, cases with severe dry eye were excluded from this study.

The surgical technique is as follows: after dissecting adherent conjunctiva to expose bare sclera, subconjunctival fibrovascular tissue is removed, bleeding vessels are cauterized, and 0.04% mitomycin C is applied for 5 min then washed out with balanced salt solution. An oral mucosal graft 30% larger than the tarsal conjunctival defect is harvested from the lower lip, thinned, and then sutured to the residual conjunctival edge or the eyelid margin and deep into the fornix. Then, a single layer of cryopreserved amniotic membrane, stromal side down, is glued to cover exposed sclera and create an anatomically-deep fornix. Topical antibiotics and steroids are administered for 3 weeks and 3 months, respectively. For eyes with severe conjunctival inflammation site at 1 month after surgery, subconjunctival steroids are injected. Additional surgical procedures for visual rehabilitation may be performed at least 3 to 4 months after the reconstruction.

Shore et al. described oral mucosal grafting alone in 42 eyelids (23 eyes) of 17 patients with ocular cicatricial pemphigoid with mixed outcomes [17]. Complications included breakthrough trichiasis, surface keratinization of the graft, blepharoptosis, phimosis, depressed eyelid blink, incomplete eyelid closure, submucosal abscess formation, and persistent nonhealing epithelial defects of the cornea.

6 Nasal Mucosal Graft

Naumann et al. described nasal mucosal grafting in 24 patients with massive symblephara (including eyelid fusion) and mucus deficiency after chemical and thermal burns predominantly [6]. Over a follow-up period ranging from 1 to 63 months, visual outcomes were modest at best, and complications included glaucoma, recurrence, and cataract. However, 17 patients were pain-free postoperatively. After eyelid separation, dissection of scar tissue, and fixation of the rectus muscles, the surgical procedure involved partial resection of the middle or inferior turbinates, trimming bone and cavernous tissue to achieve a 2 × 4 × 0.1 to 0.2 cm graft, and fixation to the conjunctiva from the limbus to the rectus muscles. Local antibiotics and steroids were applied for at least 3 weeks.

A similar study and procedure were published by Kuckelkorn et al. featuring reconstruction in 17 patients followed-up for between 6 to 31 months [18]. Similarly, they report improved Schirmer testing and mucus production by goblet cells on pathology but still modest visual outcome when using only the inferior concha. They also concede that such cases are performed unilaterally given the limited tissue available for grafting, though counter that this procedure is better than buccal mucosal grafts for patients with burns due to the presence of intraepithelial goblet cells.

7 Keratolimbal Allografts

In 5 eyes from 5 patients with symptomatic diplopia in primary gaze because of marked symblepharon formation, the authors reported that KLAL successfully resolved diplopia in all cases, offering near complete eye motility (two patients had residual diplopia on severe lateral gaze but none in primary) [4]. Over the range of follow-up (12 to 28 months), no symblepharon recurrences onto the KLAL tissue itself were observed. Subsequently, unpublished data from over 30 eyes that have undergone ocular surface reconstruction with KLAL for recurrent or severe symblepharon exhibited no recurrence of fibrosis past the area of the KLAL segments.

The authors believe that this method offers distinct benefits from traditional management of symblephara. For example, (1) in severe or bilateral disease, there may be insufficient conjunctival tissue for autografting; (2) buccal grafts have been reported to shrink; (3) mitomycin C carries risks of ischemia, necrosis, and ocular perforation; (4) subconjunctival steroids are limited by their half-lives, and may require repeated injections; and (5) silicone spacers and symblepharon rings may provide temporary barriers to symblepharon formation, which may recur when the devices are removed. KLAL tissue achieves functional and anatomic successes in patients with recurrent or severe symblepharon (Figs. 1, 2, 3, 4 and 5). The main steps of this procedure are as follows:

1. Lysis and excision of the symblepharon with careful excision of surrounding fibrosis and scarred Tenons. Isolation and hooking of the extraocular muscles may be needed if the scarring is extensive and includes the muscles. (Fig. 6A)
2. Custom trimming of the keratolimbal allograft segments. (Fig. 6B) (detailed below)
3. Lamellar thinning of the keratolimbal allograft segments by 50%.
4. Tapering the corneal side of the keratolimbal allograft segment for smooth transitioning onto the recipient ocular surface. (Fig. 6C)
5. Positioning each keratolimbal allograft segment on to the ocular surface to fully cover the area of defects and to ensure no gaps on the ocular surface. (Fig. 6D)

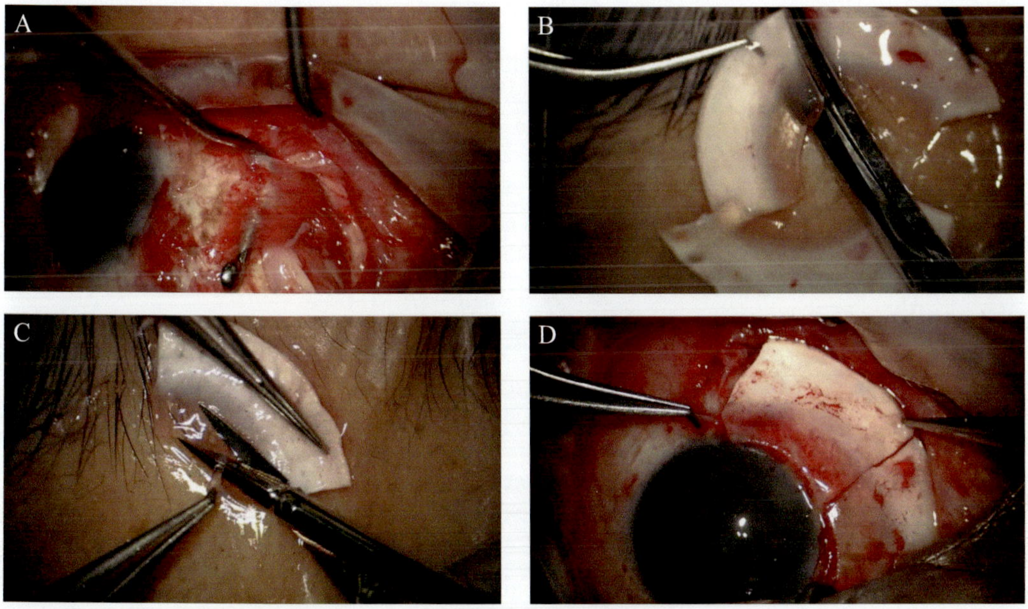

Fig. 6 The keratolimbal allograft procedure in an eye with symblepharon. (A) After lysis and excision of the symblepharon, isolation and hooking of the extraocular muscles may be required. (B) Custom trimming of the keratolimbal allograft segments; afterwards, the allograft lamella is thinned by 50%. (C) Tapering the corneal edge for smooth transitioning onto the recipient ocular surface. (D) Positioning each segment to fully cover the defective area and ensure no gaps on the ocular surface

It is important to request a donor cornea with a large scleral rim that has the conjunctiva attached, and care must be taken during tissue preparation to ensure preservation of the donor conjunctiva. The KLAL segments are prepared as previously described (Fig. 7) [19].

- A 7.5-mm corneal button is trephined from the donor tissue and discarded.
- The corneoscleral rim is custom sectioned to cover bare sclera.
- The segments are thinned (about 50%) in lamellar fashion and the corneal edges tapered.

Each segment is positioned concentrically from the host limbus to cover the exposed bare sclera without overlap or gaps (Fig. 8).

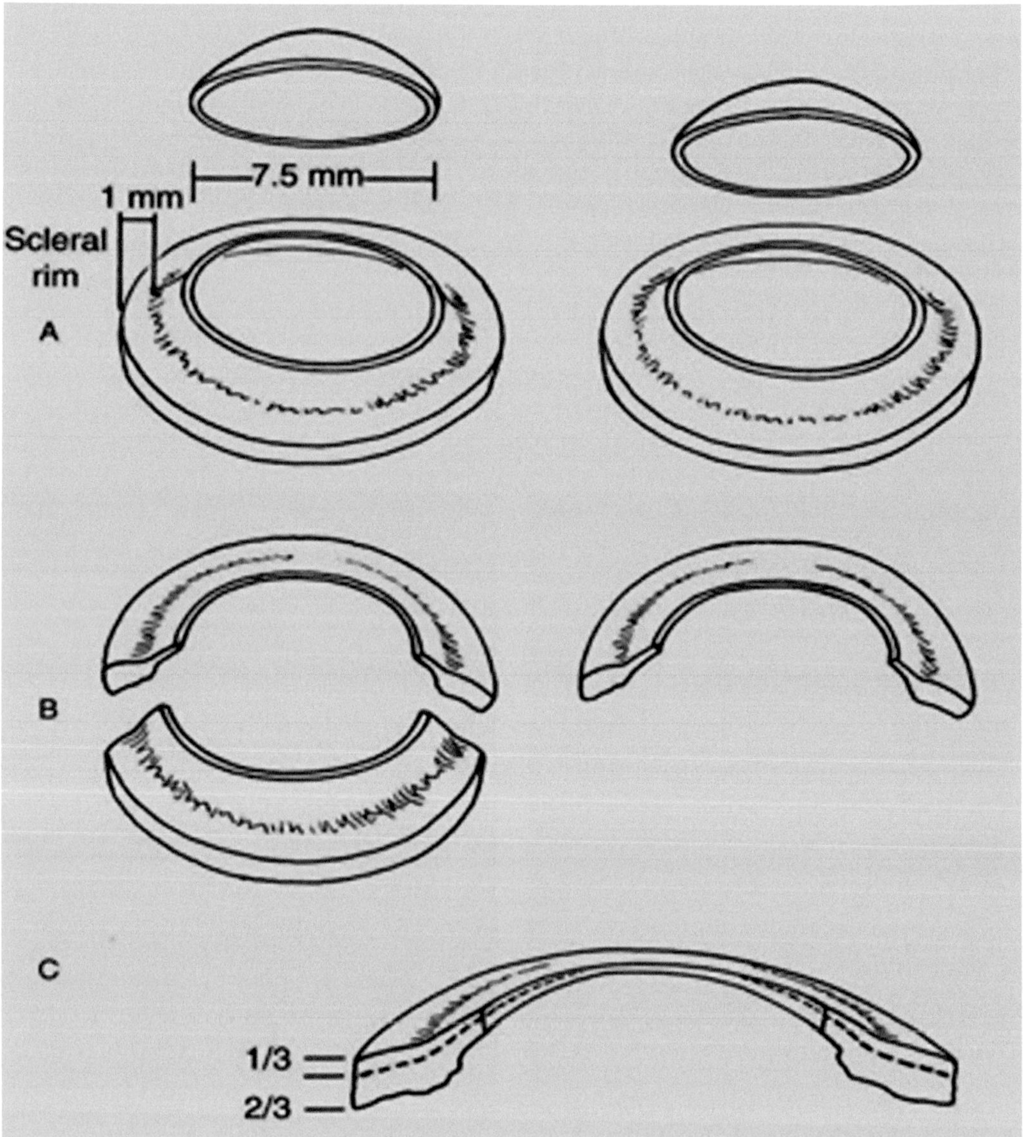

Fig. 7 Keratolimbal allograft segment preparation. (A) A 7.5-mm corneal button is trephined from the donor tissue and discarded. (B) The corneoscleral rim is custom sectioned to cover bare sclera. (B) The segments are thinned by two-thirds in lamellar fashion and the corneal edges tapered

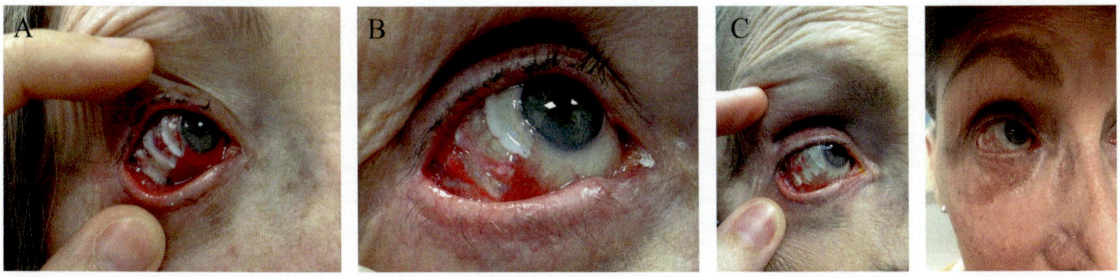

Fig. 8 Postoperative keratolimbal allograft (KLAL) images for a patient with symblepharon after orbital floor fracture repair. The patient had undergone three previous attempts at repair using conjunctival autograft, amniotic membrane transplantation with mitomycin C, and a symblepharon spacer. The symblepharon continued to recur over the spacer. (A) Postoperative day one. (B) Postoperative week 3. Near post-operative month two, the patient developed slight recurrence abutting the third KLAL segment. Placement of a fourth segment resolved the globe restriction. (C) Postoperative month 3. (D) Postoperative year 2. The patient exhibited full range of motion. (E) Postoperative year 7

Peripheral segments are placed deep into the fornix for simultaneous use as a spacer to prevent restrictive adhesions. Each segment is glued and sutured to episclera and surrounding conjunctiva. Antibiotic and steroids are injected subconjunctivally.

Postoperatively, topical steroids and a fourth-generation fluoroquinolone are prescribed four times a day, with the antibiotic discontinued after seven days and the steroid tapered based on recurrence or inflammation.

KLAL provides a healthy supply of epithelial stem cells that may serve as a barrier to conjunctivalization of the cornea and a mechanical barrier to scar extension. The role of the cadaveric stem cells that are transferred through the KLAL graft in the prevention of symblepharon recurrence and previous use of mitomycin C, as well as efficacy in larger randomized studies or autoimmune cicatrization are unknown.

8 Conclusion

Symblephara and conjunctrival scarring present many problems including ocular irritation, restricted eye motility, and tearing. Mucous membrane or amniotic membrane grafts are generally required to treat cicatricial bands after surgical release. Keratolimbal autografts may offer another option that may obviate recurrent scar formation.

References

1. Yao YF, Qiu WY, Zhang YM, Tseng SC. Mitomycin C, amniotic membrane transplantation and limbal conjunctival autograft for treating multirecurrent pterygia with symblepharon and motility restriction. Graefes Arch Clin Exp Ophthalmol. 2006;244:232–6.
2. Kheirkhah A, Blanco G, Casas V, Hayashida Y, Raju VK, Tseng SC. Surgical strategies for fornix reconstruction based on symblepharon severity. Am J Ophthalmol. 2008;146:266–75.
3. Kheirkhah A, Ghaffari R, Kaghazkanani R, Hashemi H, Behrouz MJ, Raju VK. A combined approach of amniotic membrane and oral mucosa transplantation for fornix reconstruction in severe symblepharon. Cornea. 2013;32:155–60.
4. Farid M, Lee N. Ocular surface reconstruction with keratolimbal allograft for the treatment of severe or recurrent symblepharon. Cornea. 2015;34:632–6.
5. Kwitko S, Marinho D, Barcaro S, et al. Allograft conjunctival transplantation for bilateral ocular surface disorders. Ophthalmology. 1995;102:1020–5.
6. Naumann GO, Lang GK, Rummelt V, Wigand ME. Autologous nasal mucosa transplantation in severe bilateral conjunctival mucus deficiency syndrome. Ophthalmology. 1990;97:1011–7.
7. Azuara-Blanco A, Pillai CT, Dua HS. Amniotic membrane transplantation for ocular surface reconstruction. Br J Ophthalmol. 1999;83:399–402.
8. Tseng SC, Prabhasawat P, Barton K, Gray T, Meller D. Amniotic membrane transplantation with or without limbal allografts for corneal surface reconstruction in patients with limbal stem cell deficiency. Arch Ophthalmol. 1998;116:431–41.
9. Patel BC, Sapp NA, Collin R. Standardized range of conformers and symblepharon rings. Ophthalmic Plast Reconstr Surg. 1998;14:144–5.

10. Biber JM, Skeens HM, Neff KD, Holland EJ. The Cincinnati procedure: technique and outcomes of combined living-related conjunctival limbal allografts and keratolimbal allografts in severe ocular surface failure. Cornea. 2011;30:765–71.
11. Liang L, Sheha H, Tseng SC. Long-term outcomes of keratolimbal allograft for total limbal stem cell deficiency using combined immunosuppressive agents and correction of ocular surface deficits. Arch Ophthalmol. 2009;127:1428–34.
12. Thoft RA. Conjunctival transplantation. Arch Ophthalmol. 1977;95:1425–7.
13. Koizumi N, Fullwood NJ, Bairaktaris G, Inatomi T, Kinoshita S, Quantock AJ. Cultivation of corneal epithelial cells on intact and denuded human amniotic membrane. Invest Ophthalmol Vis Sci. 2000;41:2506–13.
14. Meller D, Tseng SC. Conjunctival epithelial cell differentiation on amniotic membrane. Invest Ophthalmol Vis Sci. 1999;40:878–86.
15. Tsubota K, Satake Y, Ohyama M, et al. Surgical reconstruction of the ocular surface in advanced ocular cicatricial pemphigoid and Stevens-Johnson syndrome. Am J Ophthalmol. 1996;122:38–52.
16. Solomon A, Espana EM, Tseng SC. Amniotic membrane transplantation for reconstruction of the conjunctival fornices. Ophthalmology. 2003;110:93–100.
17. Shore JW, Foster CS, Westfall CT, Rubin PA. Results of buccal mucosal grafting for patients with medically controlled ocular cicatricial pemphigoid. Ophthalmology. 1992;99:383–95.
18. Kuckelkorn R, Schrage N, Redbrake C, Kottek A, Reim M. Autologous transplantation of nasal mucosa after severe chemical and thermal eye burns. Acta Ophthalmol Scand. 1996;74:442–8.
19. Chan CC, Holland EJ. *Ocular Surface Disease: Cornea, Conjunctiva, and Tear Film*. London, UK: Elsevier Saunders; 2013.
20. Hartman DC. Use of free grafts in correction of recurrent pterygia, pseudopterygia and symblepharon. Calif Med. 1951;75:279–80.
21. Castroviejo R. Plastic and reconstructive surgery of the conjunctiva. Plast Reconstr Surg Transplant Bull. 1959;24:1–12.

Prominent Eye Considerations in Lower Eyelid Surgery

Raneem D. Rajjoub and Andrew R. Harrison

Abstract

The risk of postoperative lower eyelid malposition is amplified in patients with prominent eyes. Thyroid eye disease, midface hypoplasia, or long axial eye length are common causes of a prominent eye, but it also may be a normal variant. This chapter highlights clinical assessment lower eyelids in the setting of a prominent eye.

Keywords

Prominent eyes · Midface hypoplasia · Negative malar vector · Postoperative lower eyelid malposition · Thyroid eye disease · Proptosis

Illustrations by Michael Han

Supplementary Information The online version contains supplementary material available at https://doi.org/10.1007/978-3-031-36175-3_9.

R. D. Rajjoub · A. R. Harrison (✉)
Department of Ophthalmology—Oculoplastic and Orbital Surgery, University of Minnesota, 516 Delaware St SE, 9th Floor, Minneapolis, MN 55455, USA
e-mail: harri060@umn.edu

1 Anatomy

The lower eyelid consists of an anterior, middle, and posterior lamellae. The anterior lamella is comprised of skin and orbicularis oculi muscle, the middle lamella consists of the orbital septum, preaponeurotic fat, and lower eyelid retractors, and the posterior lamella is comprised of the tarsal plate and palpebral conjunctiva (Fig. 1).

A normal lower eyelid margin rests at the inferior corneal limbus and has a slight upward curve towards the lateral canthus where it attaches to the lateral orbital tubercle. The lateral canthus is positioned 1 to 2 mm higher than the medial canthus. The position of the lower eyelid, measured as the margin-to-reflex distance 2 (MRD2), is measured as the distance in millimeters from the corneal light reflex to the lower eyelid margin. A normal MRD2 is 5 mm. Lower eyelids resting below the lower limbus are defined as having eyelid retraction and can be further described by the amount of inferior sclera visible between the inferior limbus and the eyelid margin.

2 Preoperative Assessment

Several factors affect the position of the lower eyelid, including the degree of horizontal tension of the lower eyelid, the anterior projection of the

J. P. Tao (ed.), *Plastic Surgery of the Lower Eyelids*,
https://doi.org/10.1007/978-3-031-36175-3_9

inferior orbital rim, and the relative lengths of the anterior, middle, and posterior lamellae [4]. A feared complication following lower eyelid surgery is eyelid retraction. Lower eyelid retraction may occur due to aging, thyroid eye disease, cicatricial skin disease, anterior lamellar shortening, or postoperatively. A prominent eye may be a normal variation. High myopia (i.e., high axial length) is another common cause. Space occupying lesions in the orbit can certainly cause proptosis. If an underlying cause is present, treatment of this proceeds before eyelid surgery. In cases in which orbital interventions are not indicated, eyelid surgery may be necessary to treat ocular surface exposure or an unsatisfactory appearance or both, Patients with prominent eyes often have increased inferior scleral show at baseline, which predisposes them to the development of postoperative ectropion or worsened eyelid retraction.

3 Diagnostic Tests to Evaluate Lower Eyelid Laxity

- Eyelid distraction test
- Eyelid snap-back test
- Finger test

The eyelid distraction test measures the distance that the lower eyelid can be anteriorly displaced from the globe (Fig. 2). Eyelid distraction greater than 6–8 mm indicates significant lower eyelid laxity. The eyelid snap-back test evaluates the time required for the eyelid to return to its native location after inferiorly displacing the eyelid towards the inferior orbital rim. An eyelid without laxity will return to normal position without blinking. If eyelid laxity is present, the lower eyelid has measurable lag that requires one or more blinks for the eyelid to return to its native position.

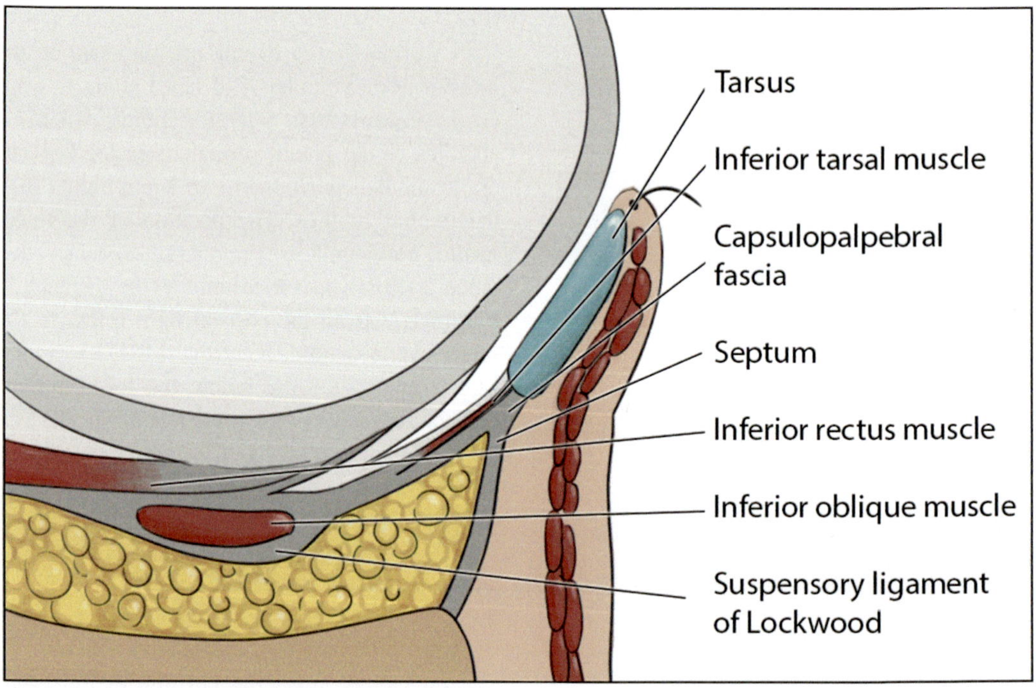

Fig. 1 Lower eyelid anatomy

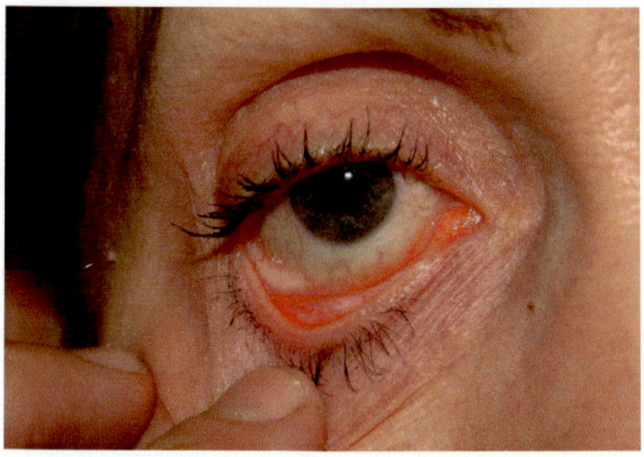

Fig. 2 Eyelid distraction test. The eyelid is manually pulled away from the globe. Eyelid distraction greater than 6–8 mm indicates significant lower eyelid laxity

To determine the extent of surgical correction needed to treat a malpositioned lower eyelid, the lateral canthus is manually lifted until adequate eyelid support is achieved. If minimal manual support is required and the eyelid distraction test measures less than 6 mm, a canthopexy may be performed. An eyelid distraction test measuring greater than 6 mm may be better addressed with a canthoplasty. When performing lateral canthal surgery in patients with prominent eyes, the lateral canthus must be fixated superior to the lateral orbital tubercle. Fixating the lateral canthus at too low or too posteriorly in prominent eyes may lead to worsened lower eyelid retraction as the lower eyelid becomes further displaced under the inferior globe.

In the finger test, if the central lower eyelid remains retracted despite manual/digital support of the lateral canthus, recession of the lower eyelid retractors or the placement of a spacer graft may be required to enhance lower eyelid support. The finger tests mimic the effects of surgical horizontal tightening to assess for slippage of the central margin inferiorly, toward the equator (Fig. 3). Recession of the lower eyelid retractors provides 1 to 2 mm of lower eyelid elevation. Spacer grafts such as acellular dermal matrix grafts, donor sclera, autologous hard palate, or autologous tarsus, or autologous ear cartilage provide additional eyelid elevation [1].

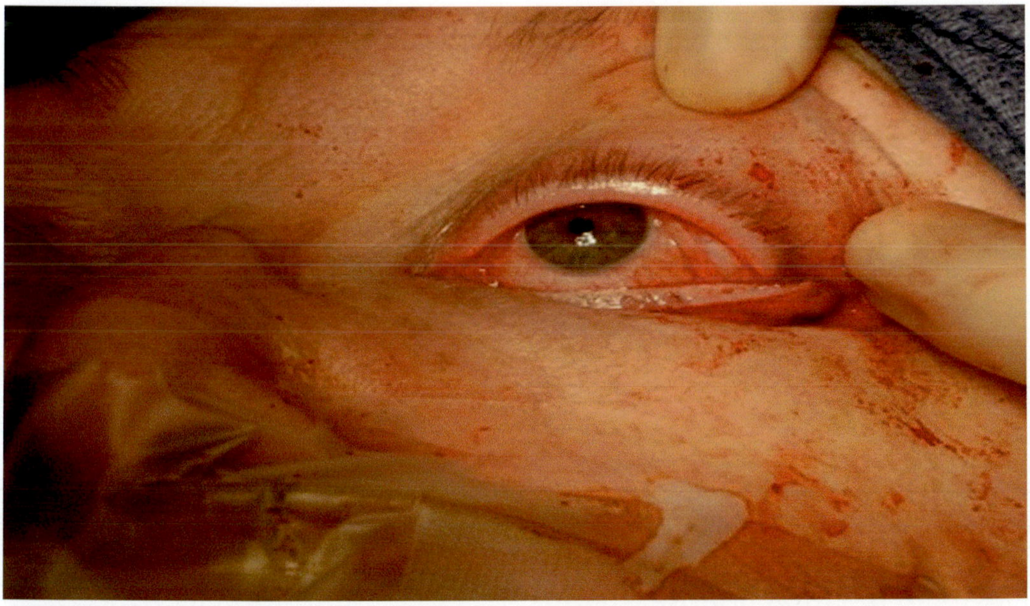

Fig. 3 Inferior scleral show due to horizontal tightening in the presence of a prominent eye. A finger test preoperatively can assess for this to indicate if lateral canthal tightening alone may be insufficient or may cause retraction

4 Evaluating the Inferior Orbital Rim

The degree of anterior projection of the malar eminence creates a vector that affects the lower eyelid position. Evaluating the relationship between the inferior orbital rim and the globe is used to determine whether the patient has a positive or negative malar vector. A positive malar vector is created when the inferior orbital rim is located anterior to the surface of the cornea, while a negative malar vector occurs when the inferior orbital rim is oriented posterior to the cornea (Fig. 4). A negative malar vector results in less support of the lower eyelid, and further amplifies lower eyelid retraction in patients with prominent eyes. Correcting lower eyelid laxity using horizontal shortening techniques predisposes patients to eyelid retraction, ectropion, and dry eye when a negative malar vector is present.

Eye prominence may result from a deficiency in skeletal support of the lower eyelid and midface and is associated with a negative malar vector. The presence of midface hypoplasia provides decreased mechanical support of the lower eyelid and leads to a higher incidence of lower eyelid retraction and inferior scleral show preoperatively. Hypoplasia of the midface further amplifies the appearance of prominent or proptotic eyes in which the inferior globe is particularly pronounced. Rounding of the eyes is also seen in midface hypoplasia due to medial displacement of the lateral canthus.

Especially in thyroid eye disease, but in other cases of proptosis, orbit decompression is indicated to alleviate the negative vector (Figs. 5 and 6). In marked globe prominence, most eyelid surgeries are destined to fail owing to the globe physically pushing the lower eyelid down. Orbital decompression is beyond the scope of this chapter, but in general, should be considered

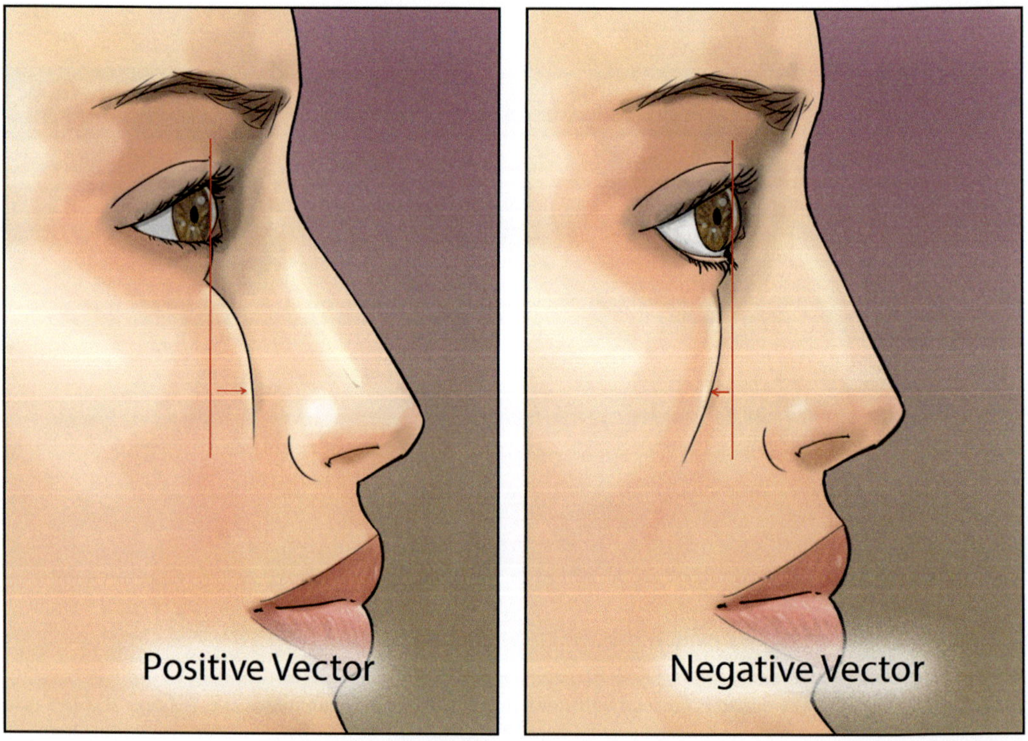

Fig. 4 Positive and negative malar vectors. In a positive vector, the globe remains at or behind the plane of the malar eminence. In a negative vector, the globe projects anterior to this plane

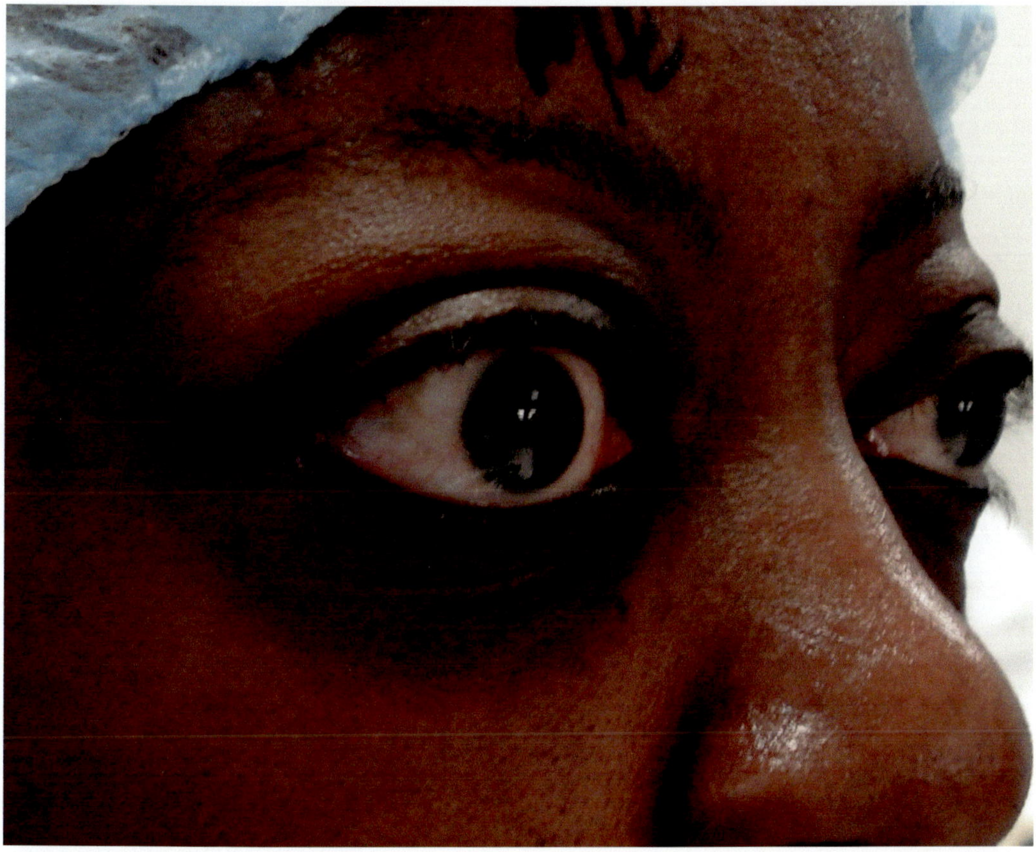

Fig. 5 Prominent eye and negative vector due to thyroid eye disease

in patients with marked proptosis and especially those with thyroid eye disease.

In lieu of orbit decompression that aims to retroplace or inferiorly displace or both the globe, augmentation of the inferior orbital rim with the placement of an implant can be considered. In addition, a midface lift may add support to the lower eyelid to offset the negative malar vector [4]. The placement of an implant provides support for the cheek and the lower eyelid by increasing the sagittal projection of the inferior orbital rim. A subperiosteal midface lift elevates the cheek and the suborbicularis oculi fat inferiorly, which further supports the lower eyelid and counteracts lower eyelid descent.

5 Anterior Lamellar Surgical Considerations

Surgical manipulation of the anterior lamella must be approached conservatively in all patients, especially in cases of eye prominence. Cicatricial disease of the skin as well as excessive surgical excision of the skin and orbicularis oculi muscle leads to lower eyelid retraction

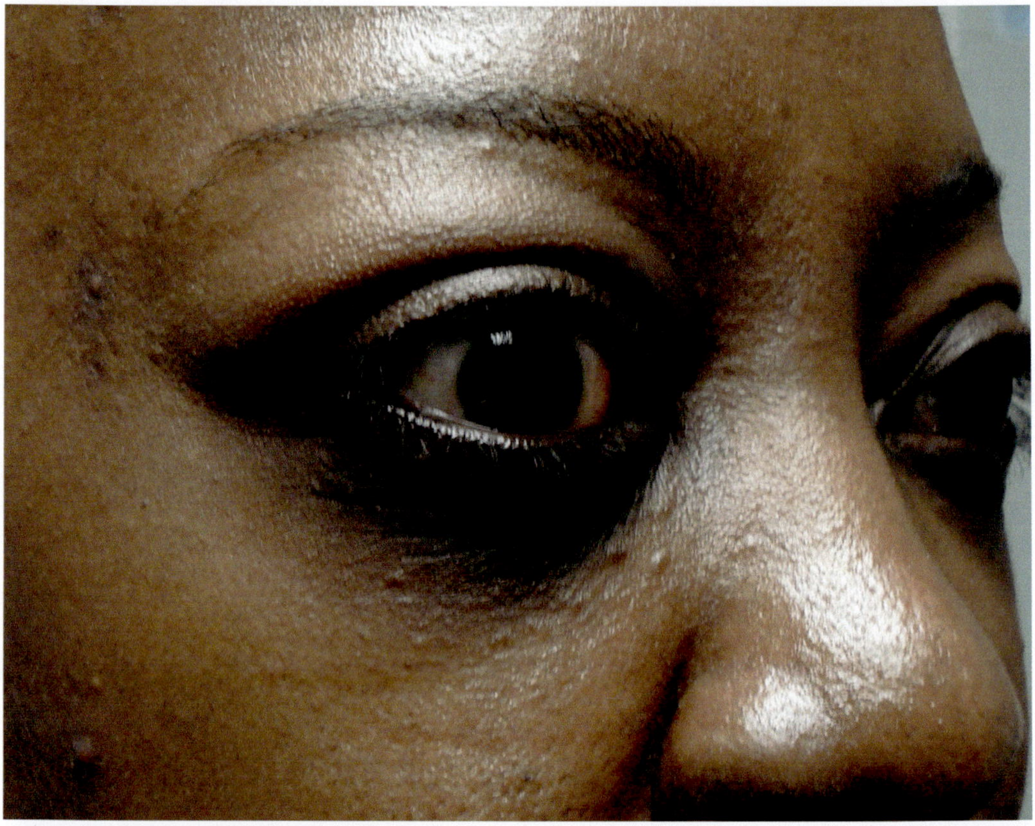

Fig. 6 Patient in Fig. 5 after orbital decompression surgery that alone improved the eyelid retraction

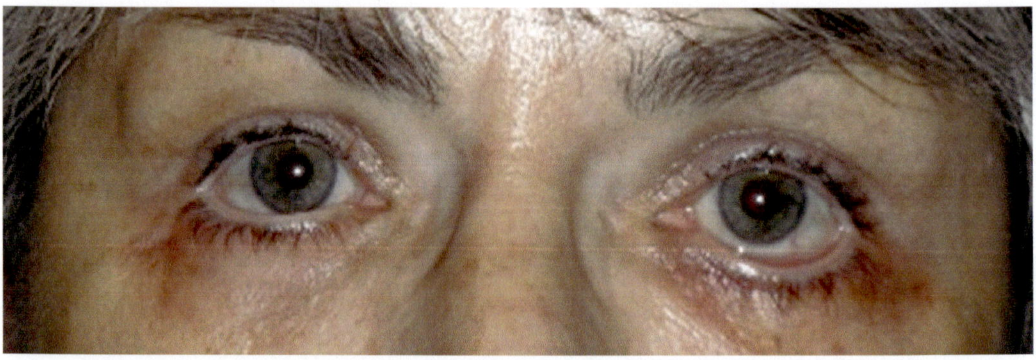

Fig. 7 Anterior lamellar shortening causing lower eyelid retraction and ectropion

(Fig. 7). Postoperative lower eyelid malposition has been reported as high as 30% following lower eyelid blepharoplasty [1, 4, 5], thus simultaneous lateral canthal support should be considered when performing a lower eyelid blepharoplasty. When anterior lamellar shortening is present, releasing the cicatrix and placing a full thickness skin graft aids in lengthening the anterior lamella and thus decreases eyelid retraction [4].

6 Conclusion

The presence of eye prominence may exacerbate postoperative complications following lower eyelid surgery. Understanding eyelid anatomy, and identifiying preoperative risk factors that increase the likelihood of lower eyelid malposition is integral to creating an appropriately tailored surgical plan that is often multimodal (Figs. 8 and 9; Video 1).

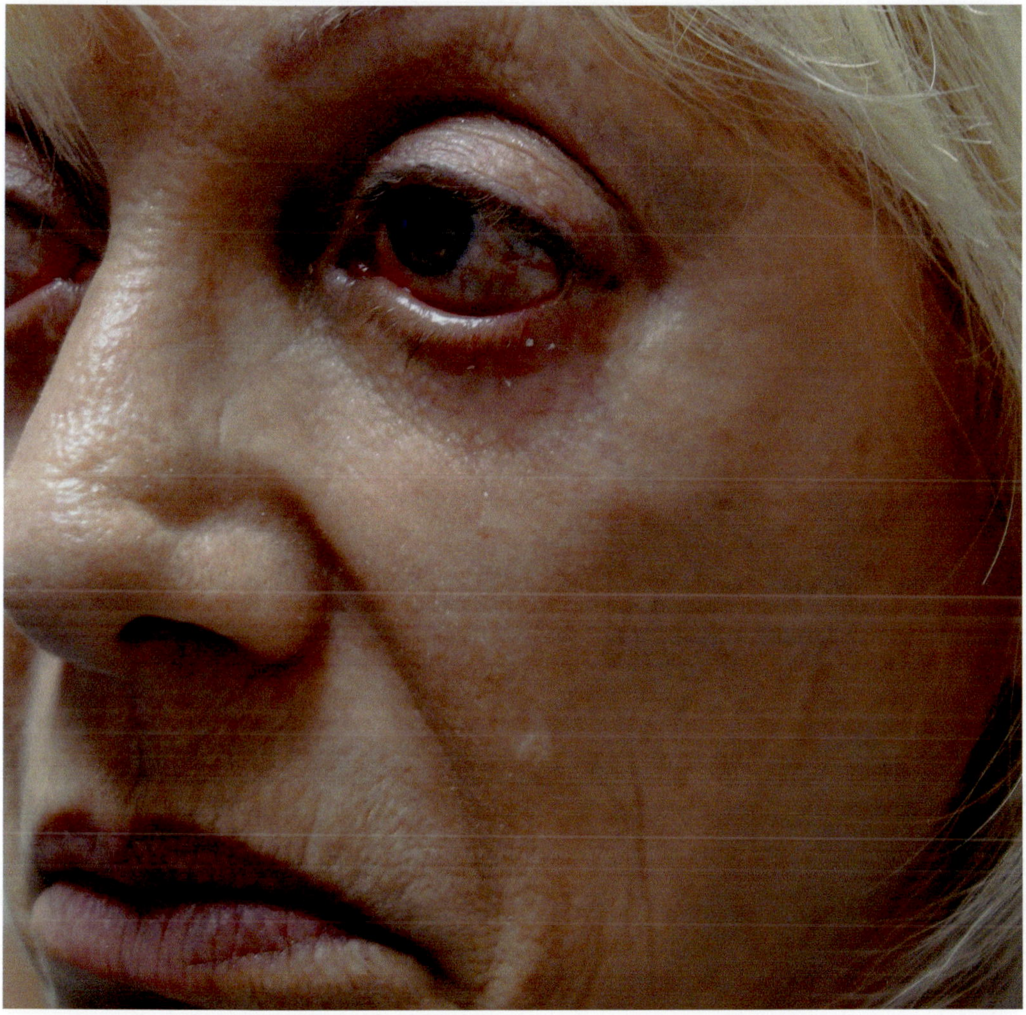

Fig. 8 Lower eyelid retraction after blepharoplasty. In addition to cicatricial vectors that were iatrogenic, a prominent globe and profound negative vector predisposed to this complication

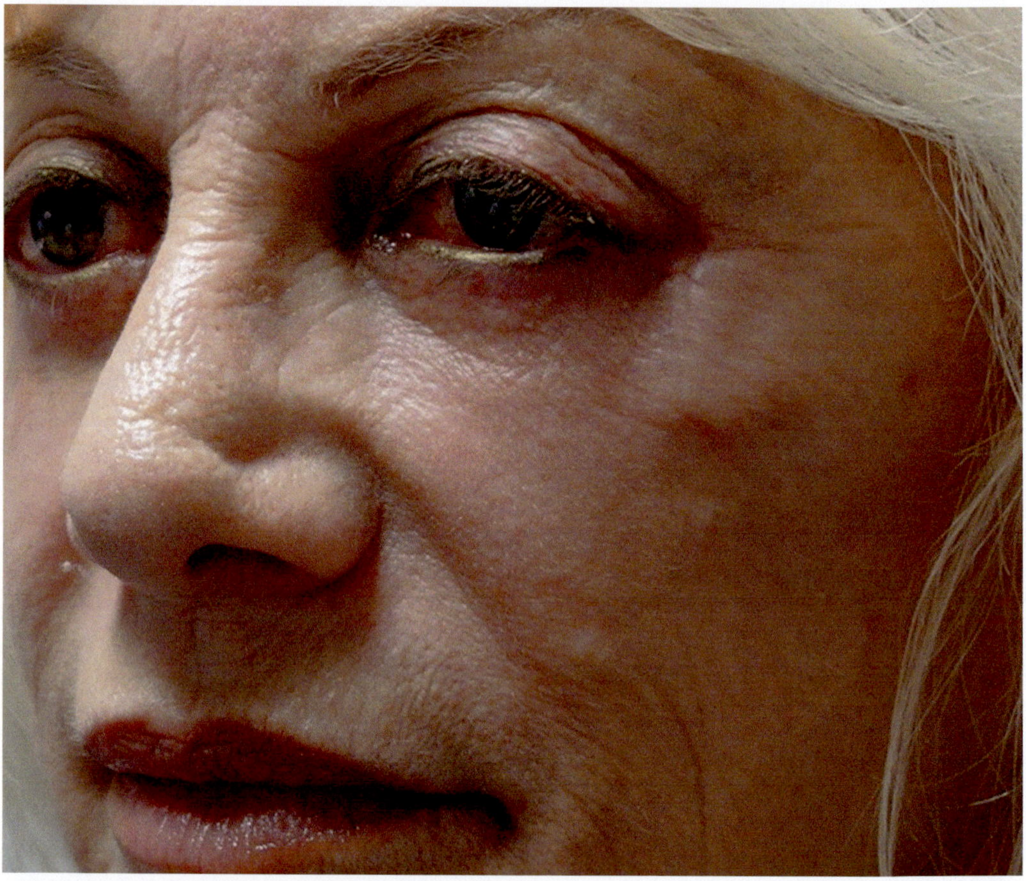

Fig. 9 Patient in Fig. 8 3 months status post lower eyelid retraction repair that included midface lift, posterior lamella spacer, canthal anchoring and a lateral tarsoconjunctival suspension flap

References

1. Carraway JH, Mellow CG. The prevention and treatment of lower eyelid ectropion following blepharoplasty. Plast Reconstr Surg. 1990;85:971–81.
2. Codner MA, Kikkawa DO, Korn BS, Pacella SJ. Blepharoplasty and brow lift. Plast Reconstr Surg. 2010;126:1e–17e.
3. Codner MA, Wolfli JN, Anzarut A. Primary transcutaneous lower blepharoplasty with routine lateral canthal support: a comprehensive 10-year review. Plast Reconstr Surg. 2008;121:241–50.
4. Nerad J. Techniques in ophthalmic plastic surgery: a personal tutorial. 2nd ed. Philadelphia, PA: Elsevier; 2021.
5. Rohrich RJ, Ghavami A, Mojallal A. The five-step lower blepharoplasty: Blending the eyelid-cheek junction. Plast Reconstr Surg. 2011;128:775–83.

Repair of Tarsal Ectropion Using a Putterman Ptosis Clamp

Katherine M. Lucarelli, Sruti S. Akella and Pete Setabutr

Abstract

Tarsal ectropion represents a severe variant of involutional ectropion. It is caused by disinsertion of the lower eyelid retractors at the tarsal border with or without significant horizontal eyelid laxity. Clinically, this manifests as complete eversion of the lower eyelid limited to the region of the tarsal plate. This chapter describes repair of tarsal ectropion using a Putterman ptosis clamp that is analogous to a upper eyelid Müller's muscle-conjunctiva resection for blepharoptosis.

Keywords

Tarsal ectropion · Putterman ptosis clamp · Eyelid laxity · Marginal ectropion · Eyelid eversion

1 Introduction

Tarsal (marginal) ectropion is a severe form of involutional ectropion described by Fox in 1960 and characterized by complete eversion of the tarsal plate and overlying conjunctiva [1]. In comparison to typical involutional ectropion, eyelid eversion is limited to the portion of the eyelid containing the tarsus with an absence of tissue laxity below the tarsus. Tarsal ectropion requires moderate digital pressure to re-invert and immediately everts when the eyelid is released, whereas classic involutional ectropion demonstrates a lower eyelid that is more easily manually pulled into position.

2 Pathophysiology

Tarsal ectropion, initially called chronic spastic ectropion, was originally thought to be the result of orbicularis oculi spasm [2]. Fox discredited this theory and attributed the condition to horizontal tarsoligamentous relaxation [1]. White later postulated that the primary etiology of tarsal ectropion is disinsertion or dehiscence of the lower eyelid retractors at the tarsal border, although horizontal eyelid laxity may also be present [3, 4].

K. M. Lucarelli · S. S. Akella · P. Setabutr (✉)
Department of Ophthalmology, University of Illinois at Chicago, Chicago, IL 60623, USA
e-mail: Psetabutr@yahoo.com

J. P. Tao (ed.), *Plastic Surgery of the Lower Eyelids*,
https://doi.org/10.1007/978-3-031-36175-3_10

3 Anatomy

The eyelids are comprised of seven structural layers: skin and subcutaneous connective tissue, muscles of protraction, orbital septum, orbital fat, muscles of retraction, tarsus, and conjunctiva [5]. Below the tarsus, the lower eyelid can be divided into anterior and posterior lamellae. The anterior lamella includes the skin and orbicularis oculi muscle. The posterior lamella contains the lower eyelid retractors, tarsal plate, and conjunctiva [6]. Some sources also characterize the orbital septum, fat, and suborbicularis fibroadipose tissue dividing the anterior and posterior layers as the middle lamella [7].

The lower eyelid retractors are the capsulopalpebral fascia (analogous to the levator aponeurosis in the upper eyelid and the inferior tarsal muscle (analogous to the superior tarsal muscle, i.e., Müller muscle) [5]. The capsulopalpebral fascia (CPF) extends from the terminal muscle fibers of the inferior rectus muscle as the capsulopalpebral head (CPH). The CPH divides to encircle the inferior oblique muscle and rejoins to form the Lockwood suspensory ligament. Extending anteriorly from the suspensory ligament, the CPF sends attachments to the inferior conjunctival fornix, inferior tarsal border and septum, and lower eyelid skin. The inferior tarsal muscle runs posterior to the CPF [8]. Some cadaveric studies have delineated the retractors into distinct anterior and posterior layers, and suggest that a posterior layer containing the denser fibers of the CPF and smooth inferior tarsal muscle fibers provides the main tractional force on the lower eyelid [9, 10]. The traction generated by the lower eyelid retractors is the basis for surgical procedures aimed at treating vertical laxity in tarsal ectropion.

4 Management

Treatment for tarsal ectropion may be medical and focused on maintaining lubrication of the ocular surface with artificial tears, gels or ointments. When chronic exposure of the inferior sclera or cornea results in symptomatic irritation or keratopathy, surgical correction is indicated. Putterman first to described correction of both horizontal and vertical components of laxity in a patient who developed tarsal ectropion after blepharoptosis repair and lateral canthal tightening [11]. Via a transcutaneous approach, the inferior tarsal muscle and capsulopapelbral fascia were identified and found to be detached from the tarsus. Reattachment to the inferior tarsus resulted in complete resolution of the lower eyelid eversion. A posterior approach with conjunctival resection was later proposed by Wesley to avoid an external scar [12].

5 Repair of Tarsal Ectropion Using the Putterman Ptosis Clamp

This technique uses the Putterman clamp to resect conjunctiva and the inferior tarsal muscle in adjunct with a lateral canthal tendon tuck for patients with severe tarsal ectropion. The procedure is analogous to the Müller muscle-conjunctival resection ptosis repair of the upper eyelid.

The surgical technique is described as follows:

A lateral canthotomy and cantholysis are performed under local anesthesia, with or without sedation. A lateral tarsal strip is created but left free for the time being.

A 4–0 silk traction suture is placed anteriorly through the lower-eyelid margin, and the lower eyelid is everted over a Desmarres retractor to expose the inferior tarsus and overlying inferior palpebral conjunctiva.

A caliper is used to measure 2 to 3 mm below the inferior tarsal border nasally, centrally, and temporally. For marking, three 6–0 silk traction sutures are placed through the conjunctiva and tied at these positions.

With an assistant placing gentle but sustained tension on the nasal and temporal silk traction sutures, the surgeon grasps the central traction suture. The Desmarres retractor is removed, and a Putterman ptosis clamp is placed to imbricate the conjunctiva and the inferior tarsal muscle between the inferior tarsal border and the marking sutures.

A 6–0 double-armed plain gut suture is placed temporally to nasally in a running horizontal mattress fashion approximately 1 mm below the clamp.

The tissue incarcerated within the ptosis clamp is excised using a #15 blade, with the blade hugging the clamp to avoid cutting the suture. This results in 4 to 6 mm resection, or double the amount measured in Step 3.

The conjunctiva and inferior tarsal muscle and capsulopalpebral fascia are then closed by running the 6–0 plain gut suture nasally to temporally, with the knots buried to prevent corneal irritation in the postoperative period. Alternatively, each arm of the suture may be externalized and tied together over skin.

The lateral tarsal strip is reattached to the lateral orbital rim periosteum using a 5–0 monofilament polypropylene suture. A 6–0 plain gut suture is used to reform the canthal angle, the orbicularis is closed with 6–0 polyglactin and the skin is closed with 6–0 polyglylene suture (Fig. 1).

The Putterman clamp technique avoids tedious lower eyelid retractor dissection and reinsertion [13]. A cadaveric model confirmed that this technique results in advancement of the CPF and the inferior tarsal muscle by the clamp [14]. This technique is advantageous because it is quick and efficient, allows for resection of redundant conjunctiva, and eliminates the need for extensive posterior dissection.

6 Surgical Outcomes

In a retrospective case series, 75% of patients undergoing tarsal ectropion repair via the aforementioned technique had complete resolution of ectropion. Twenty-five percent had mild residual ectropion, but no patient required re-operation. One hundred percent of patients reported symptomatic improvement. In patients who had inferior scleral show, an average of 1.875 mm of improvement was measured post-operatively. There were no adverse events [13].

7 Conclusion

Tarsal ectropion is a severe variant of involutional ectropion in which the entire tarsal plate and conjunctiva of the lower eyelid are everted. The pathophysiology of this disorder can be primarily attributed to disinsertion of the lower

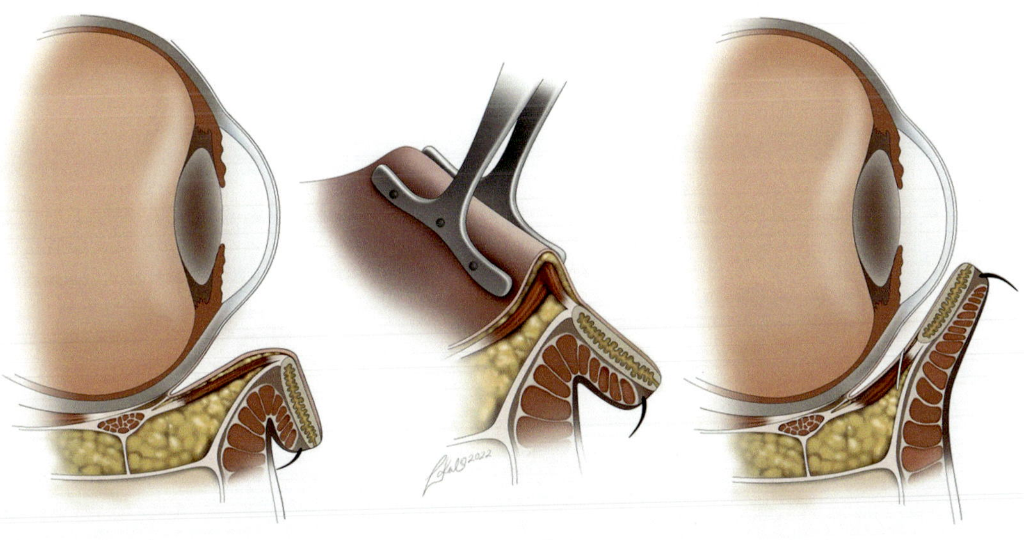

Fig. 1 Repair of tarsal ectropion with the Putterman clamp technique. *(Illustration by Lauren Kalinoski)*

eyelid retractors; however, horizontal laxity also plays a role. As the multifactorial etiology has become better characterized, surgical techniques have been developed that address both horizontal and vertical components. Most involve extensive dissection of the lower eyelid. Repair of tarsal ectropion using the Putterman ptosis clamp in combination with a lateral tarsal strip is a safe and effective approach that addresses disinsertion of the lower eyelid retractors without the need for tedious dissection. This technique is efficient and minimally invasive.

References

1. Fox S. Marginal (Tarsal) Ectropion. Archives of Ophthalmol. 1960;63:660–662.
2. Garza R, Lee G, Press B. Tarsal ectropion repair and lower blepharoplasty: a case report and review of literature. J Plast Reconstr Aesthet Surg. 2012;65:249–51.
3. Tse D. Surgical correction of lower-eyelid tarsal ectropion by reinsertion of the retractors. Arch Ophthalmol. 1991;109:427.
4. White J. Method of Correction of Tarsal Ectropion. Am J Ophthalmol. 1971;72:615–7.
5. Korn B. 2020–2021 Basic and Clinical Science Source (BCSC), Section 7. American Academy of Ophthalmology; 2020.
6. Kakizaki H, Malhotra R, Madge S, Selva D. Lower Eyelid Anatomy. Ann Plast Surg. 2009;63:344–51.
7. Jacono A, Malone M. Transcutaneous Lower Blepharoplasty. Master Techniques in Facial Rejuvenation. 2018;142–151: e1.
8. Hawes M, Dortzbach R. The microscopic anatomy of the lower eyelid retractors. Arch Ophthalmol. 1982;100:1313–8.
9. Kakizaki H, Zhao J, Nakano T, Asamoto K, Zako M, Iwaki M, Miyaishi O. The lower eyelid retractor consists of definite double layers. Ophthalmology. 2006;113:2346–50.
10. Goldberg R, Lufkin R, Farahani K, Jesmanowicz A, Hyde J, James C. Physiology of the lower eyelid retractors: Tight linkage of the anterior capsulopalpebral fascia demonstrated using dynamic ultrafine surface coil MRI. Ophthalmic Plast Reconstr Surg. 1994;10:87–91.
11. Putterman A. Ectropion of the lower eyelid secondary to Müller's muscle-capsulopalpebral fascia detachment. Am J Ophthalmol. 1978;85:814–7.
12. Wesley R. Tarsal ectropion from detachment of the lower eyelid retractors. Am J Ophthalmol. 1982;93:491–5.
13. Singa R, Aakalu V, Putterman A, Epstein G. Lower-eyelid tarsal ectropion repair with the Putterman ptosis clamp for lower-eyelid conjunctival Mueller's muscle resection and lateral tendon tuck. Ophthalmic Plast Reconstr Surg. 2012;28:224–7.
14. Jones S, Aakalu V, Lin A, Perez C, Epstein G, Putterman A, Setabutr P. Surgical microanatomy of lower eyelid tarsal ectropion repair with a Putterman ptosis clamp. Ophthalmic Plast Reconstr Surg. 2017;33:261–3.

Management of Trichiasis

Mahmoud M. Abouelatta, Catherine Y. Liu, Bobby S. Korn and Don O. Kikkawa

Abstract

Trichiasis, the abnormal inward rotation of the eyelashes, is a pathologic condition that commonly causes eye irritation. The treatment includes epilation, electrosurgical or thermal follicle destruction, and surgical resection, depending on the extent of the disease. This chapter highlights the evaluation and management of trichiasis.

Keywords

Trichiasis · Distichiasis · Epilation · Misdirected eyelash · Epilation

M. M. Abouelatta
Division of Oculofacial Plastic and Reconstructive Surgery, Department of Ophthalmology, Faculty of Medicine, Tanta University, Tanta, Egypt

M. M. Abouelatta · C. Y. Liu · B. S. Korn · D. O. Kikkawa (✉)
Division of Oculofacial Plastic and Reconstructive Surgery, Department of Ophthalmology, Shiley Eye Institute, University of California, San Diego, La Jolla, 9415 Campus Point Dr, La Jolla, CA 92093, USA
e-mail: dkikkawa@health.ucsd.edu

1 Introduction

Trichiasis is an abnormal inward rotation of the eyelashes. It can be isolated with aberrant rubbing lashes, but must be differentiated from entropion, distichiasis, and other causes of abnormal lashes. Trichiasis has several causes, with fibrosis and inflammation as common inciting factors. A thorough examination of the eyelid margin and the ocular surface is required to diagnose trichiasis and to differentiate it from other entities.

2 Definitions

Trichiasis is an inward rotation of eyelashes. It may affect an isolated lash or multiple lashes. These misdirected lashes may or may not touch the cornea. While it can be associated with scarring of the tarsus and tarsal conjunctiva, it can exist in the absence of any conjunctival pathology. If touching the ocular surface, especially the cornea, symptoms of foreign body sensation and ocular signs may occur. When left untreated and abrading the cornea, it may lead to epithelial defects, corneal ulceration and scarring, and possible visual loss [1–3].

Distichiasis occurs when there is an abnormal second row of eye lashes originating at or near the meibomian gland orifices. It can occur sporadically or less commonly as an inherited

J. P. Tao (ed.), *Plastic Surgery of the Lower Eyelids*,
https://doi.org/10.1007/978-3-031-36175-3_11

autosomal dominant disorder, known as lymphedema-distichiasis syndrome [4, 5].

Metaplastic lashes arise as a second row of posteriorly rotated lashes originating at or near the meibomian gland orifices. This usually occurs secondary to ocular surface inflammation at or near the orifices of these glands, for example, ocular cicatricial pemphigoid or chemical burns [4, 5].

Entropion is an abnormally rotated eyelid margin that can cause inward turning of lashes. Normally the meibomian gland orifices are visible without eversion of the eyelid. When early entropion occurs, these orifices disappear due to inward posterior rotation (Fig. 1). Cicatricial entropion can be confused with trichiasis. Cicatricial entropion can be caused by ocular surface neoplasia, eyelid malignancy, chemical injury, mucous membrane pemphigoid, Stevens-Johnson syndrome, and infection (trachoma is most common). These entities must be considered if the cause of entropion is unknown [2–5].

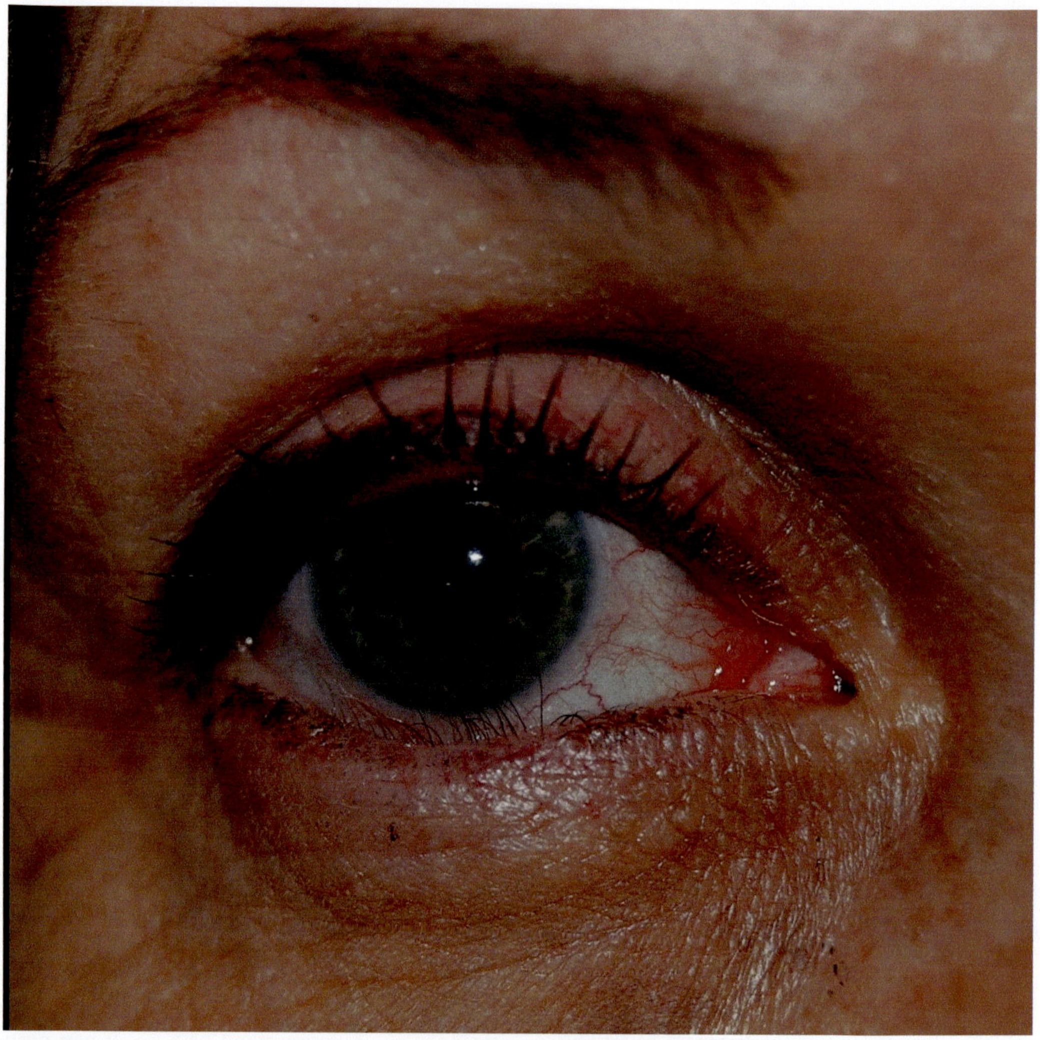

Fig. 1 Patient with right lower eyelid cicatricial entropion with multiple lashes rubbing against the corneal surface protected by a contact lens

3 Other Causes of Trichiasis

There are several other causes of trichiasis. While idiopathic trichiasis is common, other considerations are herpes zoster, chronic blepharoconjunctivitis, erythema multiforme, trauma, post-surgical, and drug induced (sulfonamides, epidermal growth factor receptor (EGFR) tyrosine kinase inhibitors, and prostaglandins analogues have been implicated). Also, trichiasis may be a masquerade of an underlying neoplastic lesion involving the eyelid margin e.g., sebaceous cell carcinoma (Fig. 2) [6, 7].

4 Pathogenesis

The position of the normal eye lashes is dictated by the structure of the lash follicle, the tarsus, and the pretarsal orbicularis oculi. If any of these elements are affected by inciting factors that disturb normative features, trichiasis may occur with or without entropion. Inflammation typically preceding fibrosis is the most significant factor that incites these changes, and it can occur due to several causes. Fibrosis incites shortening or internal disorganization of the posterior lamella and by varying degrees the patient develop trichiasis and/or entropion [8].

5 Classification

Trichiasis can be classified in various ways, which influence choice of treatment [9–14].

Classification may be according to:

1. Etiology: congenital or acquired
2. Association with entropion: segmental or diffuse.
3. Anatomic location: nasal, central, or temporal.
4. Severity: mild (1–4 eyelashes touching globe) (Fig. 3); moderate (5–9 eyelashes touching globe) and severe (>10 lashes touching the globe) (Fig. 4).

6 Diagnosis

A thorough history should be obtained. Specifically, any prior eyelid surgery, trauma, infection, or red eye should be elicited. Symptoms such as foreign body sensation with

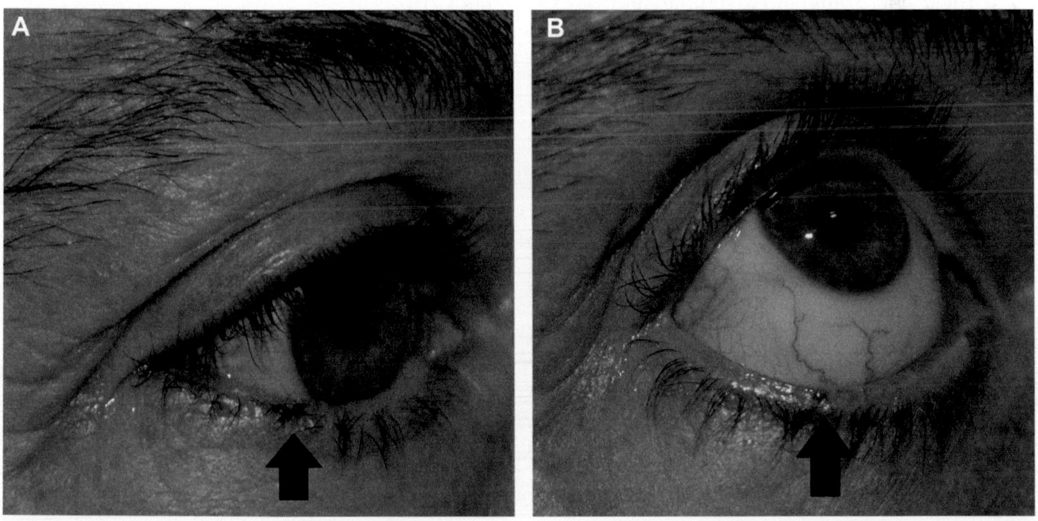

Fig. 2 (A) Trichiasis masquerading a neoplastic lesion of the right lowereyelid. (B) Neoplastic lowereyelid margin lesion (arrow) shown on right lowereyelid eversion

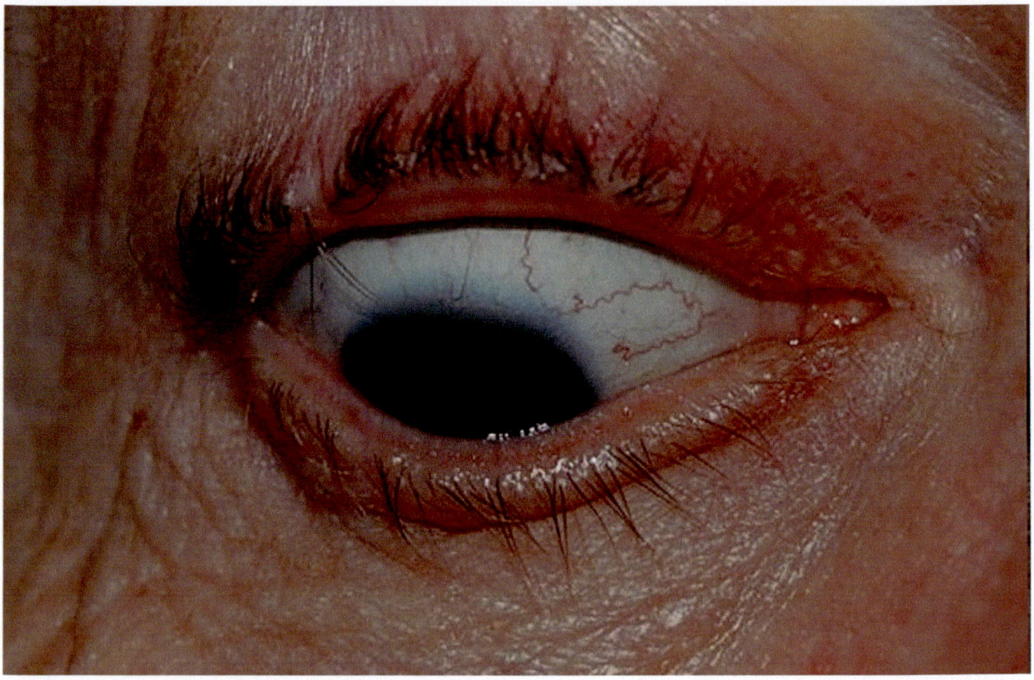

Fig. 3 Mild right upper eyelid trichiasis

lacrimation which becomes aggravated with closure of the eye should be recorded [3].

A slit lamp examination is essential to examine the eyelid margin, the meibomian gland orifices, the lash follicles and their direction, the cornea, and conjunctiva (bulbar and palpebral) [3]. Location and number of misdirected lashes should be noted, and photo documented. Eversion of the eyelids are essential to rule out associated conditions, such as trachoma, malignancy, and ocular surface disorders. Associated entropion must be evaluated as this may alter the treatment plan. Corneal staining and opacity should also be examined and may indicate trachoma [6]. In areas of endemic trachoma, public health programs with community screening are required for early diagnosis and treatment with less invasive modalities [1].

In the absence of a slit lamp, a penlight can be used for external exam, but it is no replacement for a magnified view. Complete absence of lashes in certain area denotes previous prior recent epilation while presence of short lash stubs or broken lashes may indicate incomplete previous epilation or trichotillomania. Combined trichiasis and madarosis with loss of normal eyelid architecture suggest underlying malignancy [6].

7 Treatment

The treatment aim is to remove aberrant lashes to eliminate abrasion of the ocular surface to forestall subsequent ocular sequelae. Several factors may affect treatment outcomes. First, the number of trichiatic lashes correlates with the likelihood of recurrence [15]. Second, associated condition such as cicatricial entropion or trachoma can affect outcomes. Finally, manual epilation should be avoided for several weeks prior to any procedure to ensure follicles are not missed [16]. The treatment plan should follow a stepwise approach according to these factors (Fig. 5).

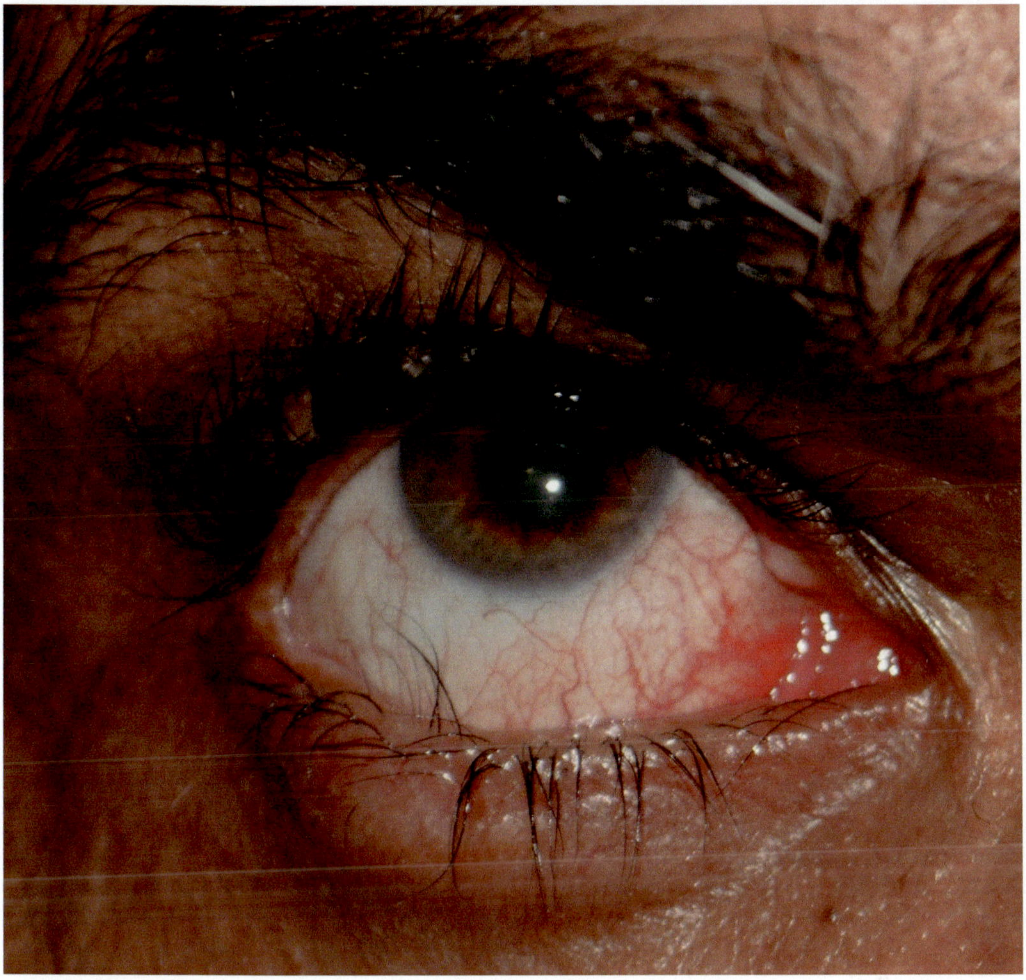

Fig. 4 Severe right lower eyelid trichiasis

7.1 Mechanical Epilation

Mechanical epilation is a simple procedure performed with forceps. It can be performed for trichiasis of any severity and cause but has a high recurrence rate, so it is often used as a temporary procedure. It can also be used to avoid more invasive procedures in high-risk medical patients or in patients that refuse surgery. Use of protective contact lenses with ocular lubricants can also be used as adjuncts until a more definitive procedure can be performed [17, 18].

Until recently, epilation was thought to be in consequential. However, repeated epilation may alter the hair follicle matrix and the keratinocyte apoptosis process that may lead to recurrence of more abnormal lashes. Also, repeated epilation may cause edema and inflammatory changes leading to fibrosis. The net result could be a higher incidence of recurrent post-operative trichiasis and a lower success rate of surgery, in the recurrent epilation group [19].

Another option, in conjunction with epilation, is the Prosthetic Replacement of the Ocular Surface Ecosystem (PROSE), a custom-fit scleral lens used to protect the ocular surface and possibly help with rotation of offending lashes away from the ocular surface [20].

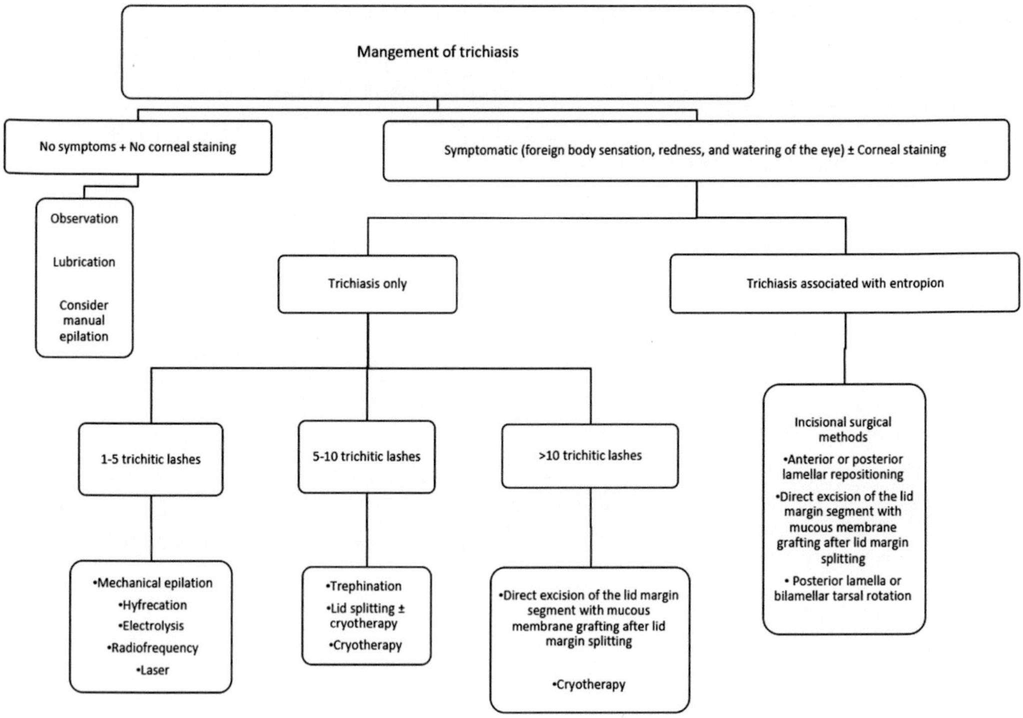

Fig. 5 Flowchart of stepwise approach of trichiasis treatment plan

7.2 Electrolysis and Radiofrequency

Electrolysis and radiofrequency accomplish individual lash follicle destruction with low dose energy utilized via direct intrafollicular application. It is useful for a relatively small number of trichiasis lashes without entropion. Typically, under local anesthesia, a fine needle is placed within the shaft of aberrant lash reaching a depth of approximately 2.5 mm within the hair follicle (Fig. 6). The existing trichiatic lash is used as a visual guide for needle placement and it should be placed either under a loupe magnification or at the slit lamp. A low-power alternating current delivered to produce a thermal reaction, which destroys the follicle one lash root at a time. It is best to use the lowest power setting and titrate upward to effect if needed. Resistance free removal of the lash by a forceps is the goal. If resistance is felt, additional application of energy may be necessary. With higher energy, collateral damage may occur. Recurrence rates of up to 50% have been described [21, 22]. Similar follicle destruction of trichiatic lashes may be accomplished with a 4-MHz dual radiofrequency probe (Cynosure, Westford, MA) [3, 23]. Radiofrequency has a similar success rate. Possible adverse effects include erythema, notching, and granuloma formation [3].

Some have used adjunct mitomycin C (MMC), an anti-metabolite that inhibits cell proliferation throughout the whole cell cycle in attempt to prevent recurrence of the aberrant lashes. To achieve this affect, 0.1 ml of MMC 0.02% is injected using a 27-gauge needle at the site of the lash follicle treated by radiofrequency. Recurrence rates were reduced with no side effects attributable to the MMC [24].

7.3 Laser Thermal Ablation

Laser treatment of trichiasis was first described in 1979. Success rates vary between 39 to 88%

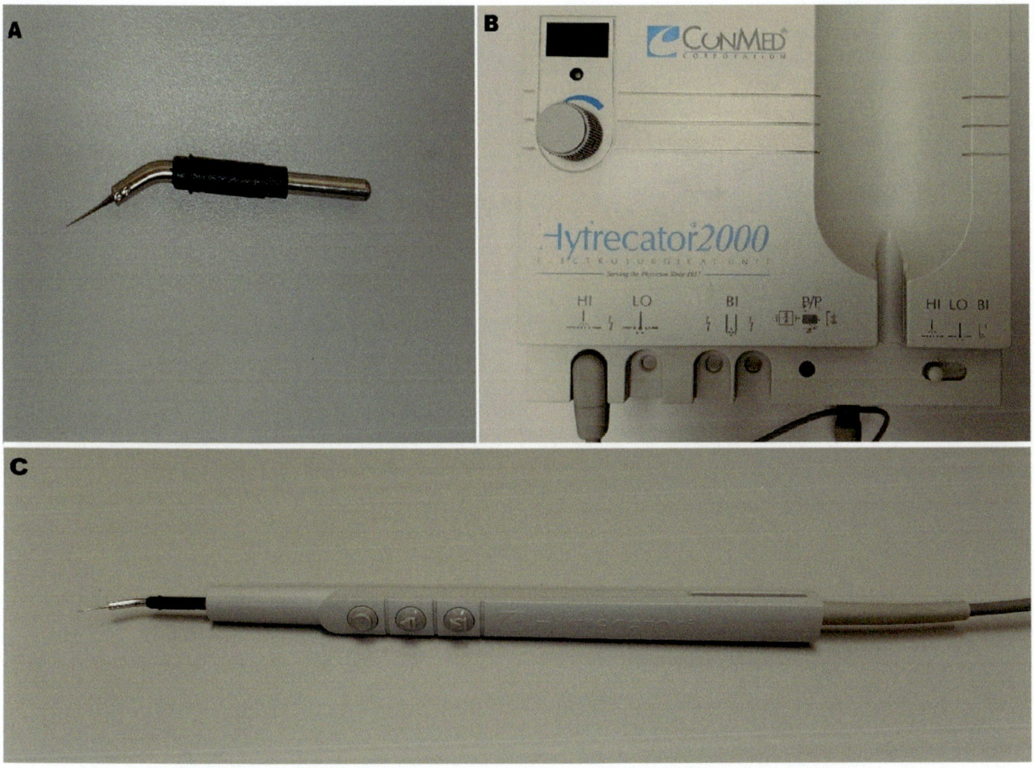

Fig. 6 (A) Electrolysis needle to be placed within the follicle. (B) Electrolysis device. (C) Handle of the device with electrolysis needle attached to it

with a described complication rate of 15%. Laser ablation is performed either under topical anesthesia or local infiltration according to the patient tolerability [3, 25].

The lashes are treated by the argon green 930 nm wavelength. Treatment parameters vary by provider preference: continuous mode or interrupted mode; 50–100 um diameter spot size; 500–760 mW power; 0.2 to 0.3 s duration. Energy is delivered under slit lamp magnification until a white-colored burn is observed [3, 25]. An additional step has been described to increase the absorption of the argon laser energy by using skin marking around the follicle consisting of brilliant green 1%, gentian violet 1%, isopropyl alcohol 48% and 100-ml distilled water [26]. Other wavelengths have been used. The diode green laser has been described for thermal ablation of the aberrant lashes with similar effective results as argon green [27, 28].

Laser ablation is noninvasive and appears to be effective but may be complicated by eyelid notching and hypopigmentation. It also requires the costly laser device and steep learning curve with necessary eye protection to prevent inadvertent intraocular damage [3, 29].

7.4 Eyelash Trephination

Eyelash trephination is a quick, effective, and safe method with a high success rate and minimal scarring. It can be used in ocular cicatrizing conditions without concern for inducing conjunctival scarring or additional fibrosis. No energy is applied, and the lash follicle is directly excised [30].

Under magnification with loupes or the operating microscope, a 21 gauge 0.81-mm diameter micro trephine (BD, Franklin Lakes, NJ) is

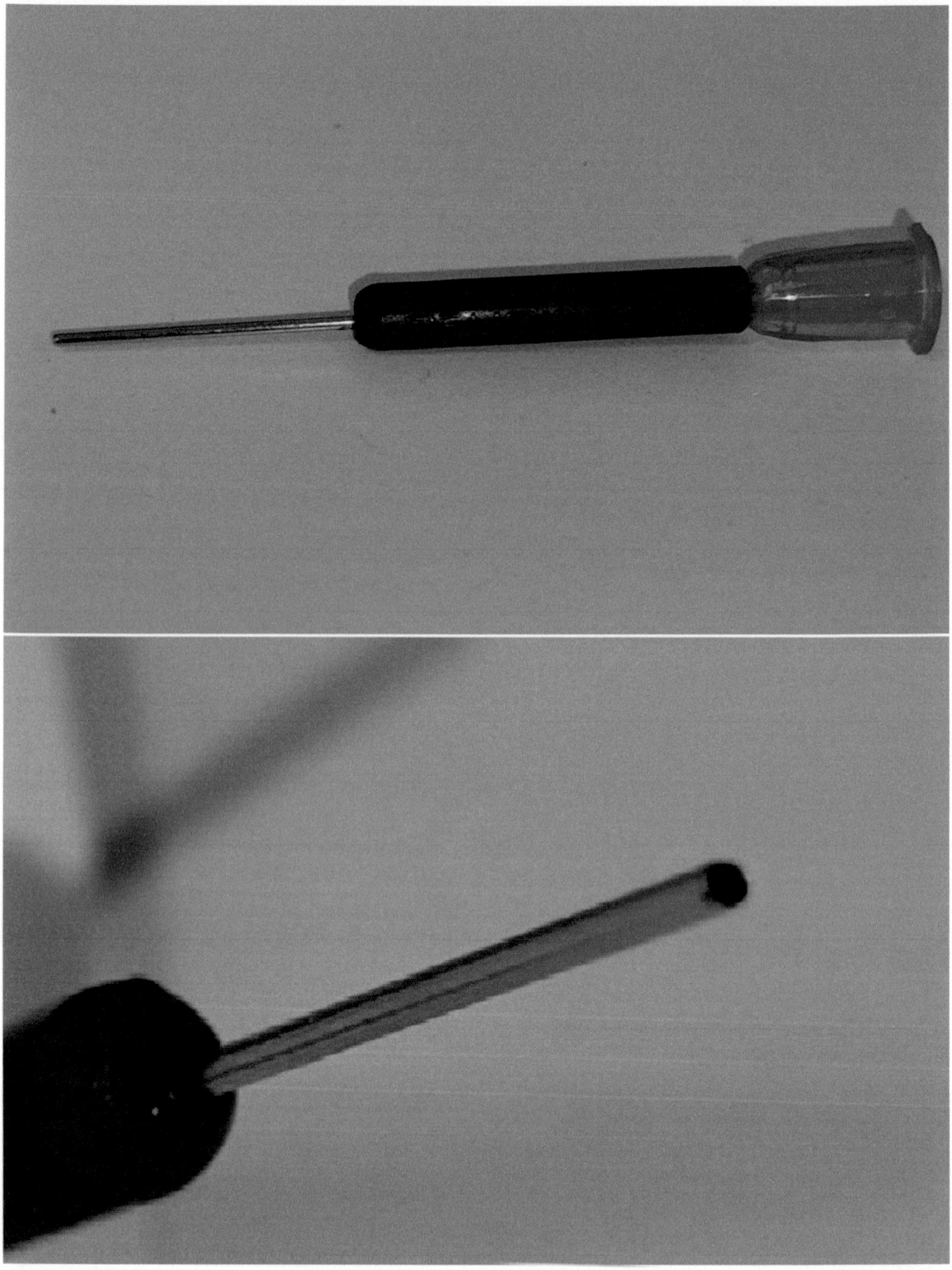

Fig. 7 A 21-gauge 0.8 × 38 mm microtrephine

used to surround the visible portion of the lash and advanced in a circular fashion to depth of about 2 mm to ensure removal of the abnormal follicle with minimal damage to the surrounding tissues (Fig. 7). The procedure can be performed under local anesthesia or general anesthesia in children. It can be used in cases of trichiasis or distichiasis [30].

A modification was described by combining trephination and electrocautery. Following trephination, electrocautery was applied in the trephination site to increase chances of follicle destruction. Success rates up to 89% were achieved with no additional complications [31].

7.5 Cryotherapy

Cryotherapy was first considered as treatment of trichiasis in 1974, after observing that lashes are destroyed permanently when liquid nitrogen was used to treat skin malignancy. Its success rate is variable and reported to be between 34 and to 90% [21].

The procedure is performed under infiltration of local anesthesia. Lidocaine 1% with epinephrine 1:100.000 is used. A rapid freeze and slow thaw cycles are needed to produce follicle destruction. A double freeze–thaw cycle is used with rapid freezing (20–30 s) producing destructive intracellular ice crystallization, followed by slow thawing (several minutes) that produces toxic electrolyte imbalance and osmotic pressure changes. A 5 mm diameter metal cryoprobe (Fig. 8) connected to a cryomachine (Fig. 9) is typically used to produce cooling of the lashes to −20 °C to −30 °C temperature, preferably monitored via a thermocouple attached to the eyelid [21].

Cryotherapy is has several potential side effects. These include eyelid margin necrosis, notching, symblepharon formation, cellulitis,

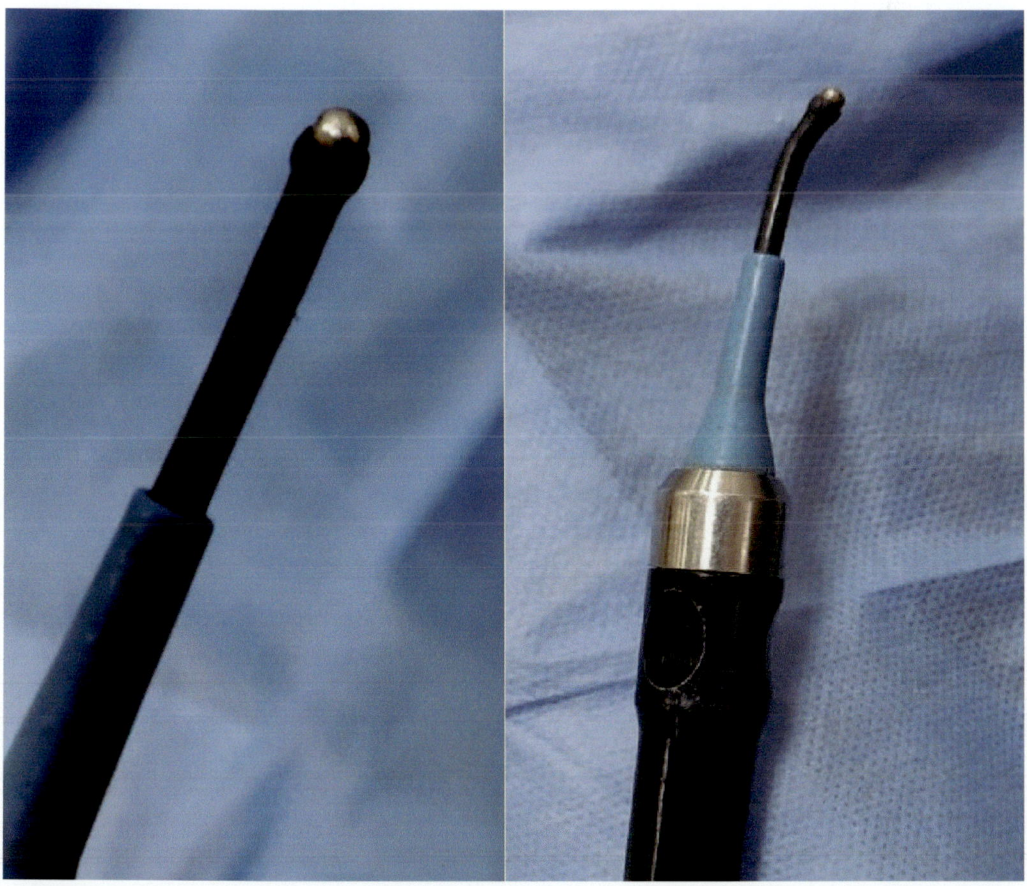

Fig. 8 A 5 mm diameter cryoprobe used for trichiasis treatment

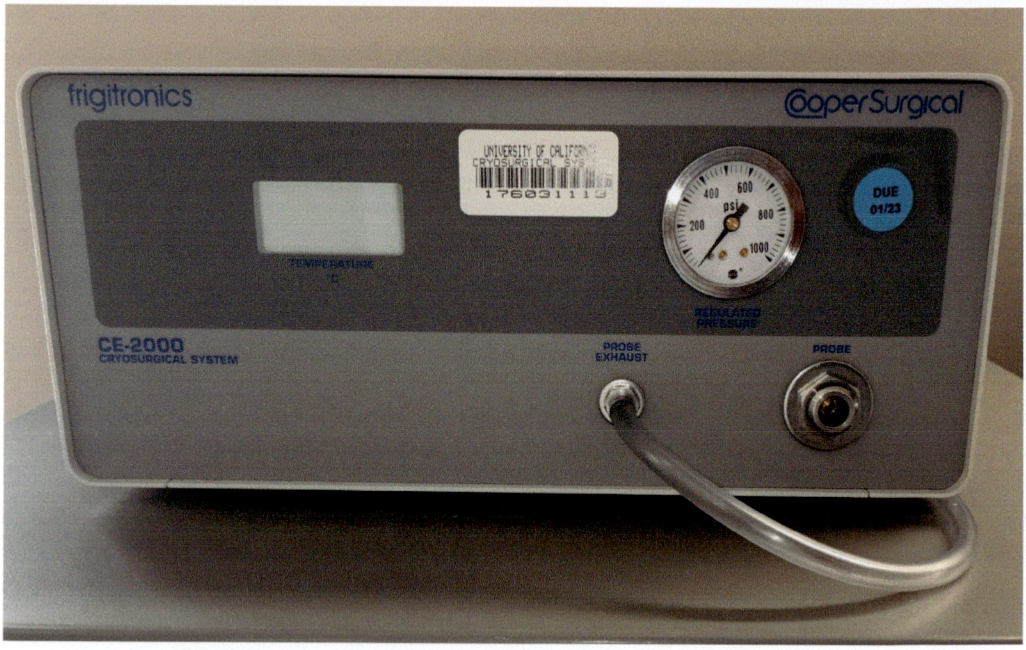

Fig. 9 Cryomachine with temperature gauge

skin depigmentation (worse in the darkly pigmented individuals) and severe soft tissue inflammation. Cicatrizing conditions such as the ocular cicatricial pemphigoid may worsen with cryotherapy, as well as reactivation of herpes zoster. In addition, after cryotherapy, marginal entropion with keratinized skin abrading the ocular surface may occur, which may be just as symptomatic as the trichiasis it was initially intended to treat (Fig. 10). For these reasons, the authors rarely perform cryotherapy and consider it only in severe recalcitrant cases after other methods have been unsuccessful [21, 30].

7.6 Incisional Surgical Methods

Individual follicle treatment with energy devices or direct excision are the preferred initial treatment for trichiasis. A pentagonal wedge excisional technique (described in another chapter) may be useful. If trichiasis persists and other causes of entropion have been ruled out, more invasive surgical procedures may be considered. Most of the surgical methods are variations of cicatricial entropion repair, described in another chapter. They involve anterior and posterior lamellar repositioning or direct excision of the eyelid margin segment with mucous membrane grafting and will be mentioned briefly.

Most of the procedures require eyelid splitting at the gray line with the area of trichiasis being recessed or directly excised [32]. If a large area (over 50% of the eyelid margin) is excised a mucous membrane graft may be harvested intraorally and placed between the anterior and posterior lamellae to provide a smooth surface at the eyelid-ocular surface interface [33].

If there is an element of cicatricial entropion also present, a posterior tarsotomy with placement of everting sutures are used to rotate the posterior lamellar leaving the anterior lamella intact. This rotates the lashes away from the ocular surface but maintains the lash follicles rather than destroying them [34]. For more severe cases, a bilamellar marginal rotation with full thickness blepharotomy (Weis procedure)

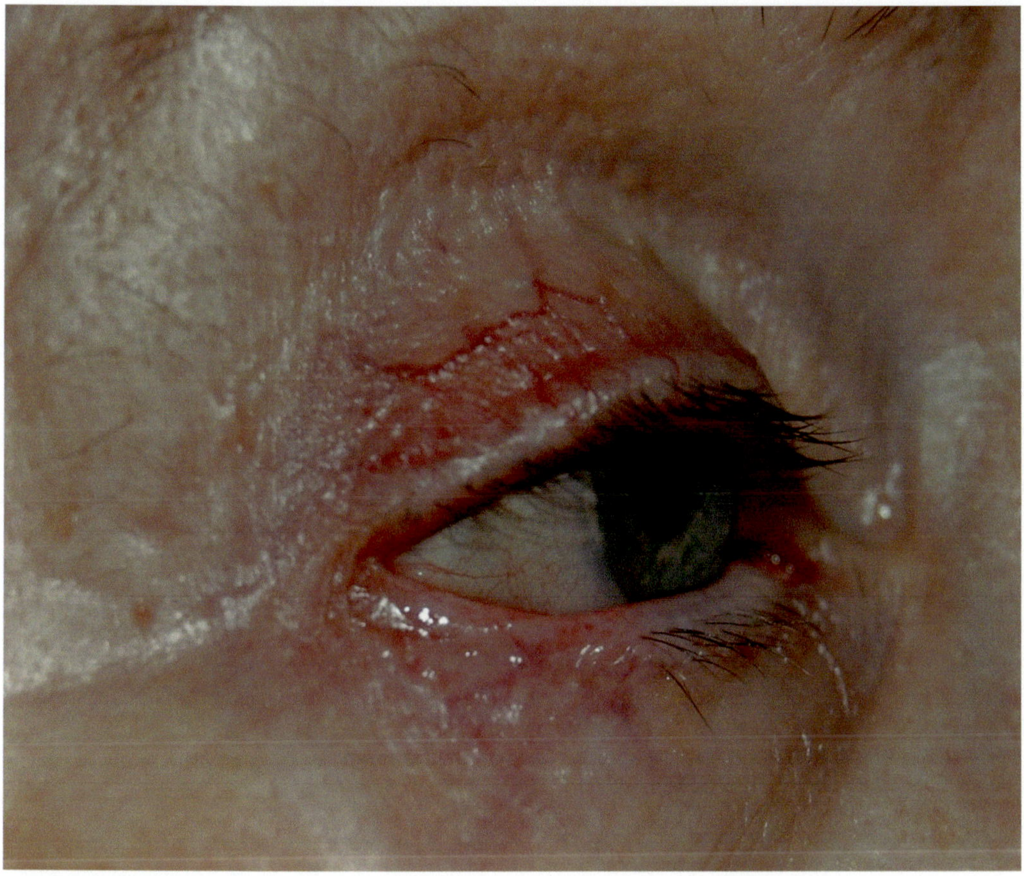

Fig. 10 Keratinized temporal portion of the right lower eyelid margin following cryotherapy

can be used [32, 33]. A modified technique of a beveled incision and eversion of the tarsal segment has produced favorable results in cases of severe trichiasis and entropion. The incised edge of the posterior lamella is advanced to the eyelid margin segment and is secured with horizontal mattress sutures [35].

One technique of re-directing aberrant lashes has been described. Using a supratarsal eyelid crease incision, a dissection between pretarsal orbicularis muscle and tarsus is performed until the roots of the lash follicles are visualized. Each inwardly turned hair follicle root is freed from surrounding tissues by meticulous dissection allowing free rotation. After closure of the eyelid crease incision, the lashes are rotated superiorly with suture fixated to the upper anterior tarsus [36].

7.7 Adjunct Medical Therapy

Adjuvant topical fluorometholone 0.1% drops twice daily for four weeks has been advocated as post-operative medical treatment after surgical procedures for correction of trachomatous trichiasis to reduce inflammation. Monitoring of the intraocular pressure is required to check for IOP spikes [37].

8 Future Directions

Advances in trichiasis management is occurring on various fronts. First, three-dimensional (3D) imaging of trichiasis is now possible to monitor and document abnormal lashes. A digital SLR camera with Loreo 3D macro lens creates 3D images of the eyelid margins in different fields of gaze [38].

At the molecular level, matrix metalloproteinases (MMPs), are a family of zinc-dependent enzymes responsible for degradation of the structural proteins of the extracellular matrix, expressed in the eyelid and conjunctival tissues. They cause collagen matrix remodeling which is implicated in contracture and occurrence of trichiasis. Pharmacologic therapy to inhibit mRNA expression of MMPs with promising agents under study [39].

Pro-inflammatory signaling molecules (IL-1β and S100A7) and pro-fibrotic connective tissue growth factor (CTGF) are mediators and cytokines found in higher levels in the tissues of patients with trichiasis compared to normal individuals, even in the absence of clinically evident inflammation. Future work focusing on detection and new immune modulating drugs to suppress these mediators may be another future pharmacologic option to treat trichiasis [40].

Finally, studies are identifying single nucleotide polymorphisms (SNPs) of the genes that express pro- inflammatory and fibrotic mediators, bringing forth the possibility of gene therapy to modulate the harmful impact of fibrosis in cases of trichiasis and cicatricial entropion [41].

9 Summary

Trichiasis is the most common variant of aberrant lashes. It has a variety of causes and must be differentiated from entropion. A multitude of treatment options exist, including mechanical epilation, cryotherapy, electrolysis, radiofrequency, laser thermal ablation, trephination, and incisional methods. Treatment should be tailored and selected according to the severity and number of aberrant lashes, their location, and status of the patient. Choice of procedure is critical to achieve the best result and decrease the incidence of recurrence and complications. New modalities for treatment are focusing on preventing the cascade of trichiasis development at the genetic and cell biology level.

Disclosures Don O Kikkawa and Bobby S. Korn are former consultants for Horizon Therapeutics and receive book royalties from Elsevier Publishing. Catherine Y. Liu is a site principal investigator for a Horizon Therapeutics-sponsored clinical trial and receives royalties from Wolter Kluwers Health.FundingNo financial interest.

References

1. Mousa A, Courtright P, Kazanjian A, Bassett K. A community-based eye care intervention in southern Egypt: impact on trachomatous trichiasis surgical coverage. Middle East Afr J Ophthalmol. 2015;22(4):478–483.
2. Basar E, Ozdemir H, Ozkan S, et al. Treatment of trichiasis with argon laser. Eur J Opthalmol. 2000;10:273–5.
3. Salour H, Rafati N, Falahi MR, Aletaha M. A comparison of argon laser and radiofrequency in trichiasis treatment. Ophthal Plast Reconstr Surg. 2011;27(5):313–6.
4. Kapantais D, Garrott H, Ford R. Electrolysis outcomes for eyelid trichiasis: Consultants versus trainees. J Fr Ophtalmol. 2022;45(3):298–305.
5. Chi MJ, Park MS, Nam DH, Moon HS, Baek SH. Eyelid splitting with follicular extirpation using a monopolar cautery for the treatment of trichiasis and distichiasis. Graefes Arch Clin Exp Ophthalmol. 2007;245(5):637–40.
6. West ES, Munoz B, Imeru A, Alemayehu W, Melese M, West SK. The association between epilation and corneal opacity among eyes with trachomatous trichiasis. Br J Ophthalmol. 2006;90:171–4.
7. Varajini J, Ophth FRC, Norris FEBO, Ophth JHFRC. (Oxon) Periocular manifestations of afatinib therapy. Ophthalmic Plastic and Reconstruct Surgery 2019;35(1):e12–e13.
8. Lewallen, Courtright P. Anatomical factors influencing development of trichiasis and entropion in trachoma. British J Ophthalmol 1991;75:713–714.
9. Ferreira IS, Bernardes TF, Bonfioli AA. Trichiasis. Semin Ophthalmol. 2010;25(3):66–71.
10. Ferraz LC, Meneghim RL, Galindo-Ferreiro A, Wanzeler AC, Saruwatari MM, Satto LH, et al. Outcomes of two surgical techniques for major trichiasis treatment. Orbit. 2018;37(1):36–40.
11. Kanski JJ, Bowling B. Clinical ophthalmology: a systematic approach. 7th ed. Elsevier; 2012.
12. Kormann RB, Moreira H. Treatment of trichiasis with high-frequency radio wave electrosurgery. Arq Bras Oftalmol. 2007;70(2):276–80.
13. Hirai FE, Shiguematsu AI, Schellini SA, Padovani CR. [Surgical treatment of major trichiasis] Rev Bras Oftalmol. 1998;74(4):357–61.
14. Gower EW, West SK, Harding JC, et al. Trachomatous trichiasis clamp versus standard

bilamellar tarsal rotation instrumentation for trichiasis surgery: results of a randomized clinical trial. JAMA Ophthalmol. 2013;131:294–301.
15. Habtamu E, Wondie T, Aweke S, et al. Predictors of trachomatous trichiasis surgery outcome. Ophthalmology. 2017;124(8):1143–55.
16. Gower EW, West SK, Cassard SD, Munoz BE, Harding JC, et al. Definitions and standardization of a new grading scheme for eyelid contour abnormalities after trichiasis surgery. PLoS Negl Trop Dis. 2012;6(6): e1713.
17. Kirkwood BJ, Kirkwood RA. Trichiasis: characteristics and management options. Insight. 2011;36(2):5–9.
18. Habtamu E, Rajak SN, Tadesse Z, Wondie T, Zerihun M, Guadie B, et al. Epilation for minor trachomatous trichiasis: four-year results of a randomised controlled trial. PLoS Negl Trop Dis. 2015;9(3): e0003558.
19. Talero SL, Munoz B, West SK. Potential effect of epilation on the outcome of surgery for trachomatous trichiasis. Trans Vis Sci Tech. 2019;8(4):30.
20. Scofield-Kaplan SM, Dunbar KE, Campbell AA, Kazim M. Utility of PROSE device in the management of complex oculoplastic pathology. Ophthalmic Plastic and Reconstruct Surgery. 2018;34(3):242–245.
21. Majekodunmi S. Cryosurgery in treatment of trichiasis. Br J Ophthalmol. 1982;66:337–9.
22. Khafagy A, Mostafa MM, Fooshan F. Management of trichiasis with lid margin split and cryotherapy. Clin Ophthalmol. 2012;6:1815–7.
23. Hartzler J, Neldner KH, Forstot SL. X-ray epilation for the treatment of trichiasis. Arch Dermatol. 1984;120(5):620–4.
24. Kim GN, Yoo WS, Kim SJ, Han YS, Chung IY, Park JM, Yoo JM, Seo SW. The effect of 0.02% mitomycin C injection into the hair follicle with radiofrequency ablation in trichiasis patients. Korean J Ophthalmol. 2014;28(1):12–8.
25. Al-Bdour MD, Al-Till MI. Argon laser: a modality of treatment for trichiasis. Int J Biomed Sci. 2007;3(1):56–9.
26. Huneke, JW. Argon laser treatment for trichiasis. Ophthalmic Plastic Reconstruct Surgery 1992;8(1):50–55.
27. Bezerra RG, de Sousa Meneghim RLF, Padovani CR, Schellini SA. Diode green laser in the lid trichiasis treatment. J Ophthalmic Vis Res. 2021;16:320–4.
28. Pham RT, Biesman BS, Silkiss RZ. Treatment of trichiasis using an 810-nm diode laser: an efficacy study. Ophthalmic Plast Reconstr Surg. 2006;22(6):445–7.
29. Yung, Chi-Wah, MD, Massicotte, SJ, Kuwabara Toichiro, MD. Argon laser treatment of trichiasis. Ophthalmic Plastic Reconstruct Surgery 1994;10(2):130–136.
30. McCracken MS, Kikkawa DO, Vasani SN. Treatment of trichiasis and distichiasis by eyelash trephination. Ophthal Plast Reconstr Surg. 2006;22:349–51.
31. Han J-H, Doh S-H. Treatment for trichiasis through a combination of eyelash trephination and electrocautery. Acta Ophthalmol. 2012;90:e211–3.
32. Merbs SL, Harding JC, Cassard SD, Munoz BE, West SK, et al. Relationship between immediate post-operative appearance and 6-week operative outcome in trichiasis surgery. PLoS Negl Trop Dis 2012;6(7): e1718.
33. Zhang H, Kandel RP, Atakari HK, Dean D. Impact of oral azithromycin on recurrence of trachomatous trichiasis in Nepal over 1 year. Br J Ophthalmol. 2006;90:943–8.
34. Abdelaziz et al. Anterior lamellar recession versus posterior lamellar tarsal rotation for lower lid trachomatous trichiasis: a randomized controlled trial. Clinical Ophthalmol 2020;14:2043–2050.
35. Merbs, et al. A new surgical technique for post-operative trachomatous trichiasis. Ophthalmic Plast Reconstr Surg. 2021;37(6):595–8.
36. Karademir S, Agaoglu G. Treatment of trichiasis by releasing follicle roots of eyelashes: a new technique. Plast Reconstr Surg Glob Open. 2021;9(3): e3480.
37. Kempen JH, Tekle-Haimanot R, Hunduma L, Alemayehu M, Pistilli M, Abashawl A, Lawrence SD, Alemayehu W. Fluorometholone 0.1% as ancillary therapy for trachomatous trichiasis surgery: Randomized clinical trial. Am J Ophthalmol. 2019;197:145–155.
38. Hoffman JJ, Habtamu E, Rono H, Tadesse Z, Wondie T, Minas T, et al. 3D images as a field grader training tool for trachomatous trichiasis: a diagnostic accuracy study in Ethiopia. PLoS Negl Trop Dis. 2019;13(1): e0007104.
39. Li H, Ezra DG, Burton MJ, Bailly M. Doxycycline prevents matrix remodeling and contraction by trichiasis-derived conjunctival fibroblasts. Invest Ophthalmol Vis Sci. 2013;54(7):4675–82.
40. Derrick T, Luthert PJ, Jama H, Hu VH, Massae P, Essex D, et al. Increased epithelial expression of CTGF and S100A7 with elevated subepithelial expression of IL-1β in trachomatous trichiasis. PLoS Negl Trop Dis. 2016;10(6): e0004752.
41. Atik B, Skwor TA, Kandel, RP, Sharma B, Adhikari HK, et al. Identification of novel single nucleotide polymorphisms in inflammatory genes as risk factors associated with trachomatous trichiasis. PLoS ONE. 2008;3(10):e3600.
42. Van Millingen E. The tarsocheiloplastic operation for the cure of trichiasis. Ophthal Rev. 1887;6:309–14.
43. Binotti WW, et al. A novel interlamellar oral mucosa graft surgery technique using fibrin glue for the treatment of trichiasis. Arq Bras Oftalmol. 2022—Ahead of Print.

Ectropion Repair and Lateral Canthal Anchoring

Katherine J. Williams and Michael T. Yen

Abstract

Lower eyelid malposition with the eyelid distracted outwards away from the globe is characterized as ectropion. This may lead to ocular surface exposure and symptoms of dry eye. It may also lead to an abnormal facial appearance. Ectropion may be due to horizontal laxity or involutional, mechanical, paralytic, or cicatricial vectors. Treatment for many etiologies of ectropion typically involves horizontal eyelid tightening and lateral canthal anchoring that are described in this chapter.

Keywords

Ectropion · Involutional ectropion · Cicatricial ectropion · Paralytic ectropion · Horizontal eyelid laxity · Lateral tarsal strip · Lateral canthal anchoring · Lateral canthoplasty

Supplementary Information The online version contains supplementary material available at https://doi.org/10.1007/978-3-031-36175-3_12.

K. J. Williams · M. T. Yen (✉)
Cullen Eye Institute, Baylor College of Medicine, 1977 Butler Blvd, Houston 77030, Texas, US
e-mail: myen@bcm.edu

1 Introduction

Ectropion is defined as an eyelid malposition with the eyelid rotated away from the globe. Ectropion most commonly involves the lower eyelid, but can also involve the upper eyelid in cicatricial cases or severe laxity such as floppy eyelid syndrome. Different pathologic vectors may be present and include involutional, cicatricial, paralytic, and mechanical. Ectropion typically presents with ocular irritation, epiphora, photophobia, foreign body sensation, and erythema of the lower eyelid. Over time, ectropion of the lower eyelid may result in exposure keratopathy with associated corneal scarring and vision loss. In many instances, the outturned eyelid contributes to facial disfigurement. Correction of ectropion often requires surgical intervention.

2 Causes of Ectropion

Ectropion of the eyelid can usually be classified as either involutional, cicatricial, paralytic, or mechanical. The proper surgical repair addresses the specific underlying etiology. Therefore, thorough evaluation to ascertain the etiology of the eyelid malposition is crucial to determining the appropriate corrective measures.

Involutional ectropion is most commonly due to horizontal eyelid laxity from aging. The

J. P. Tao (ed.), *Plastic Surgery of the Lower Eyelids*,
https://doi.org/10.1007/978-3-031-36175-3_12

degree of eyelid laxity can be assessed with the degree of distractibility of the lower eyelid, and the rapidity of eyelid snapback. Medial tendon laxity can be assessed with the displacement of the inferior punctum with lateral traction on the lower eyelid. In patients with horizontal lower eyelid laxity without additional anterior lamellar shortening, weakness of the orbicularis, or mechanical causes, ectropion may be classified as involutional (Fig. 1).

Cicatricial ectropion results in vertical anterior lamellar (usually skin) shortening. Cicatricial ectropion may be due to trauma, infection, chronic dermatitis, thermal or chemical injury, or prior surgery (Fig. 2a and b). Midface descent may contribute to the cicatricial ectropion with inferior traction on the eyelid. Eyelid snapback may be appropriate, but the eyelid cannot be positioned against the globe and cannot be elevated to the level of the pupil.

Paralytic ectropion occurs due to decreased orbicularis oculi muscle tone from facial nerve weakness. Etiologies include central nervous system or peripheral neoplasia, infectious, inflammatory, traumatic, congenital, or iatrogenic etiologies of cranial nerve VII palsy (Fig. 3).

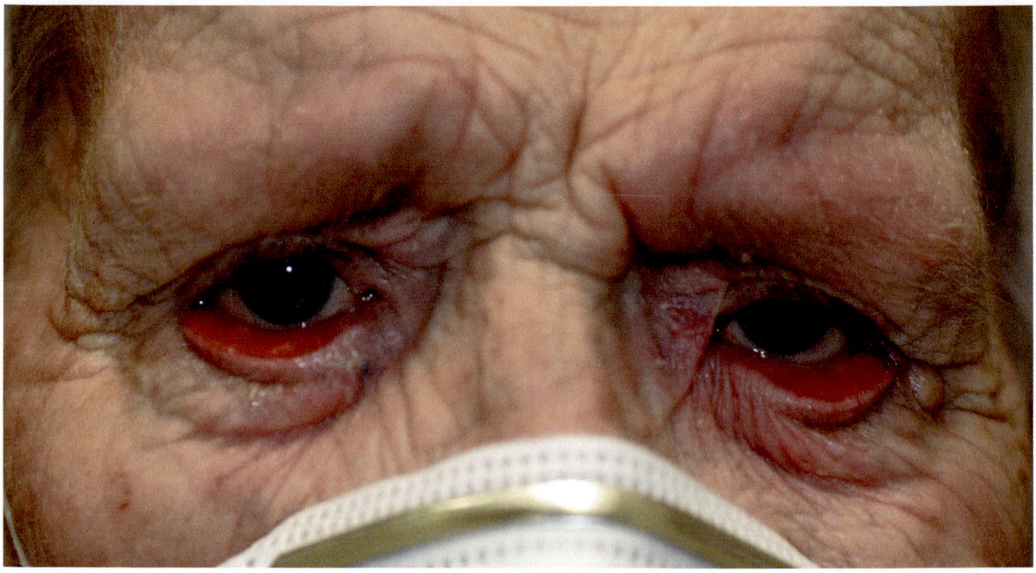

Fig. 1 Involutional ectropion of both lower eyelids resulting in poor eyelid apposition with the globe, exposure of the ocular surface and palpebral conjunctiva, and epiphora with poor lacrimal pump

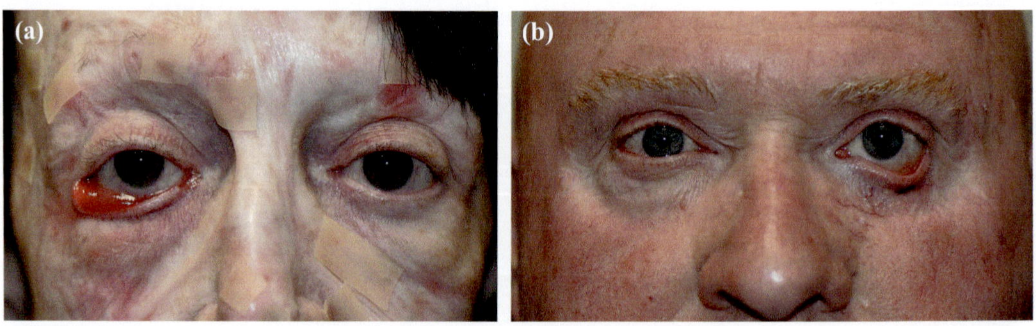

Fig. 2 (**a**) Cicatricial ectropion of the right lower eyelid after treatment for eyelid carcinoma. (**b**) Cicatricial ectropion of the left lower eyelid after surgical repair of an orbital rim fracture with titanium plates

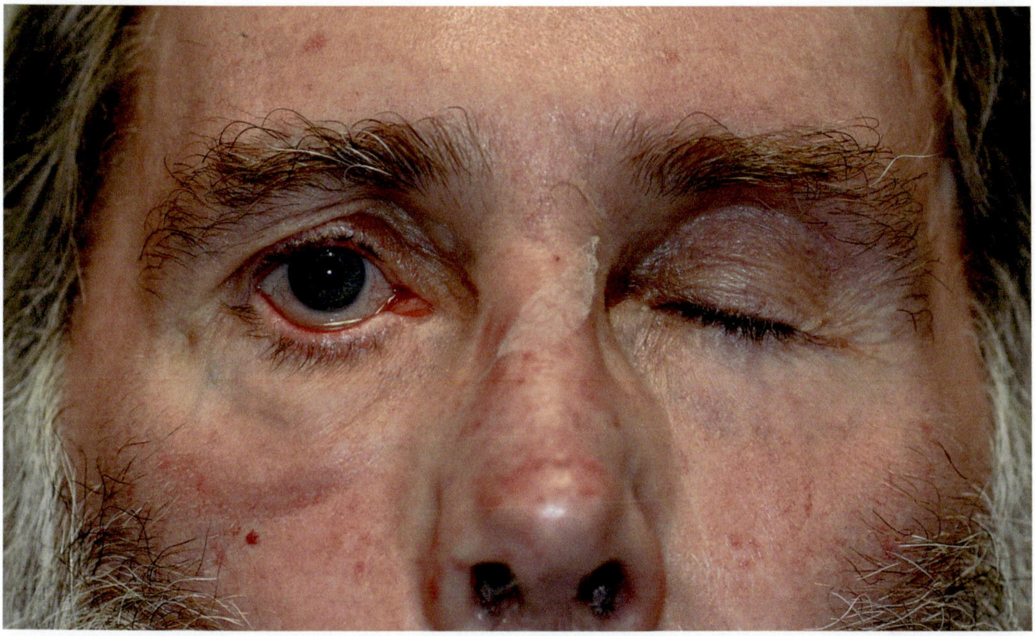

Fig. 3 Paralytic ectropion of the right lower eyelid after acoustic neuroma excision and facial nerve palsy. The patient has significant orbicularis weakness with severe lagophthalmos in addition to the lower eyelid ectropion

Mechanical ectropion is present when there exist forces that pull or push the eyelid into malposition away from the globe. Etiologies include lower eyelid tumors or inflammatory lesions (e.g., chalazion) resulting in downward and/or outward force on the lower eyelid (Fig. 4). Iatrogenic causes of mechanical ectropion can result from orbital implants such as glaucoma drainage devices, scleral buckle elements, and prominent orbital rim and cheek implants.

3 Surgical Techniques for Ectropion Repair

Lateral Tarsal Strip

The lateral tarsal strip is a workhorse for treating horizontal eyelid laxity. The lateral canthal tendon is easily accessible through the lateral canthus where it is fixated to the lateral orbital rim periosteum. In contrast, medial canthal tendon tightening is more difficult owing to the lacrimal drainage system. Therefore, most cases of horizontal eyelid laxity are approached at the lateral canthus.

After administration of local anesthetic, a lateral canthotomy and cantholysis is performed, taking care to fully release the inferior crus of the lateral canthal tendon. With the lower eyelid fully disinserted laterally, the tarsal strip is developed with split between the orbicularis and tarsus between anterior and posterior lamella. The posterior mucocutaneous junction is removed with Westcott scissors. When removing the posterior mucocutaneous junction, small snips with Westcott scissors will allow for smooth removal of the mucocutaneous junction in a single continuous pass. The palpebral conjunctival surface is scraped with a #15 blade to remove epithelial cells. A 4–0 polyglactin or braided polyester suture on a P2 half circle needle is passed to secure the tarsal strip, to the lateral orbital rim periosteum (Fig. 5a). Redundant lower eyelid tissue can be excised if needed. The suture is then tightened to the appropriate tension to fixate the lower eyelid to the lateral orbital rim. The knot of the suture is tied over the loop to prevent slippage off of the tarsal strip (Fig. 5b). The canthal angle is then reformed with 6–0 plain gut suture.

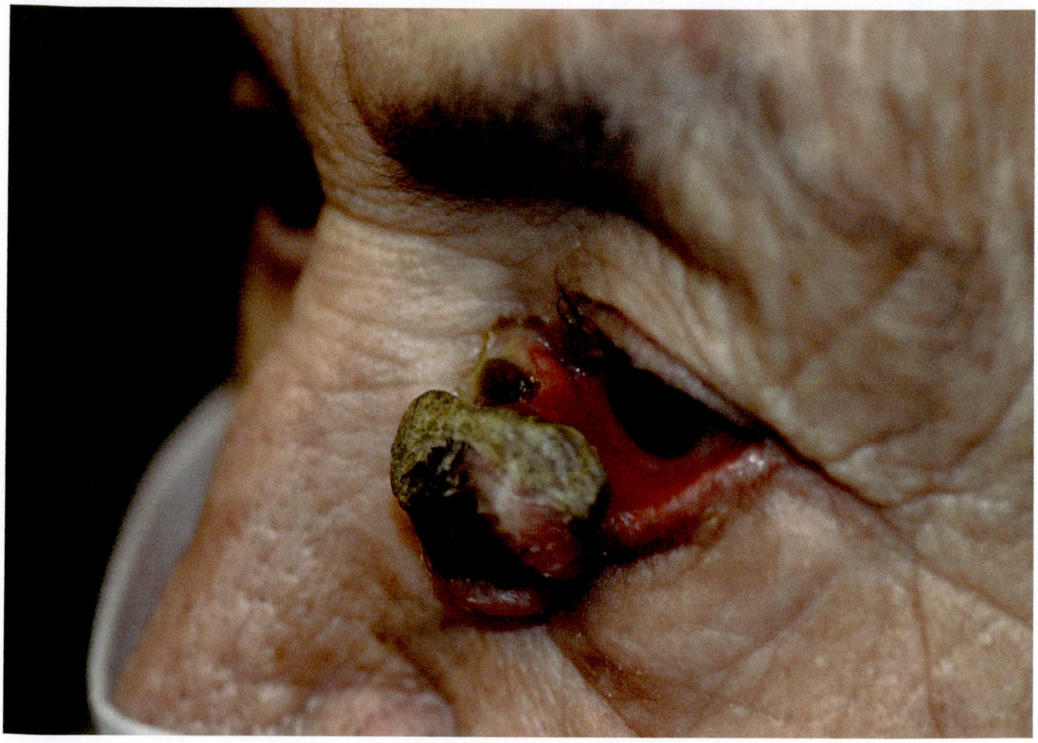

Fig. 4 Mechanical ectropion secondary to a large squamous cell carcinoma of the left lower eyelid

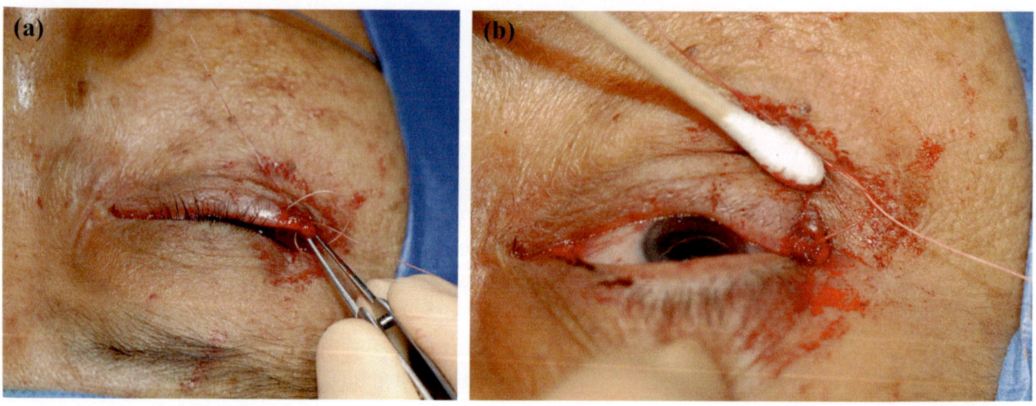

Fig. 5 (**a**) Loop fixation of the lateral tarsal strip. The tarsal strip is pulled through the loop of the suture fixating it to the periosteum of the lateral orbital rim, which allows broad distribution of the fixation across the tarsus instead of point fixation. (**b**) The knot of the suture is tied over the loop which prevents the loop from sliding off of the tarsal strip

For patients with a prominent globe or shallow orbit, a lateral tarsal strip may exacerbate eyelid retraction and inferior scleral show as the horizontal tightening may cause the eyelid margin to slip toward the equator. In these patients, fixation to the superior crus of the lateral canthal tendon or the external orbital rim periosteum may be helpful.

Lateral Canthoplasty (Bick) (Video 12–1)
An alternative to a LTS is a lateral full thickness resection and reattachment. Instead of dissecting out a tarsal strip the free exposed lateral tarsus is simple secured to the lateral rim periosteum using a 4–0 polyglactin or braided polyester suture.

The skin and eyelid margin may be realigned with 6–0 plain suture.

Medial Canthal Tendon Plication (See also Chap. "Medial Canthal Surgery")
In some cases of ectropion, such as paralytic etiologies, lateral canthal tendon tightening may be inadequate, or may cause significant lateral displacement of the punctum. These cases may be better addressed with medial canthal tendon plication or a combination of medial canthal tendon and lateral canthal tendon tightening.

For medial canthal tendon plication, a conjunctival incision just medial to the tarsus and inferior to the punctum can be used expose the medial canthal tendon. Using a double arm suture, the medial canthal tendon is isolated starting at the nasal border of the tarsus. The suture is then passed through the incision and secured to the periosteum of the anterior lacrimal crest. The conjunctival incision is usually well approximated and does not require direct suture closure.

Spindle Procedure (See also Chap. "Medial Canthal Surgery")
An eyelid spindle procedure can also be used to correct ectropion without horizontal laxity, or as an adjunct to horizontal eyelid tightening to further rotate the eyelid margin towards the globe. Using a blade or Westcott scissors or both, an excision from the posterior lamellae is fashioned in a diamond shape horizontally and vertically. Double armed 6–0 chromic gut suture is then used to pass through the inferior border of the tarsus and enter through the center of the posterior lamellar excised diamond, exiting deep in the fornix approximately 15 mm below the lower eyelid margin. The second arm of the 6–0 chromic suture is then used to engage the lower eyelid retractors, and then turned to enter through the center of the posterior lamellar incision and exit next to the previous arm of the gut suture, at the same point deep in the fornix. Both suture arms should be tightened accordingly, and the eyelid position assessed as the suture arms are tied.

Full Thickness Skin Grafting (See also Chap. "Cicatricial Ectropion Repair with Skin Graft")
Full thickness skin grafting serves as a useful adjunct in patients with cicatricial ectropion with significant anterior lamellar deficiency. It is frequently used in conjunction with lateral tarsal strip procedures and temporary tarsorrhaphy such as Frost suture. In a retrospective study, the success rate of the procedure was found to be 76%. In patients who have undergone prior radiation therapy, such as those patients with squamous cell carcinoma with perineural invasion, skin grafts have previously shown to be viable and allow for improvement of lower eyelid ectropion. Donor skin from the ipsilateral or contralateral upper eyelid is preferred for the best match with the lower eyelid skin, if there is sufficient upper eyelid dermatochalasis present to allow for donor tissue. Additional options include skin grafts from post-auricular, preauricular, or supraclavicular donor sites.

Adjunctive Midface Lifting (See also Chap. "Midface Lift")
A midface lift can be used as an adjunctive in cases of severe cicatricial, involutional, or paralytic ectropion. The midface lift can help to reduce downward vertical tension, and can be performed through a transconjunctival or transcutaneous incision, in a supraperiosteal or preperiosteal fashion. With midface lifting, anchoring points can be used to target and support regions of the most severe ectropion. The authors' preference is a dissection performed in the preperiosteal plane, taking care to release all ligaments and maintain dissection posterior to the temporal branch of the facial nerve, extending down to the level of the nasolabial fold (Fig. 6a). A 4–0 polyglactin suture can be used to suspend the midface with anchoring bites to the periosteum at the inferior and lateral orbital rim (Fig. 6b).

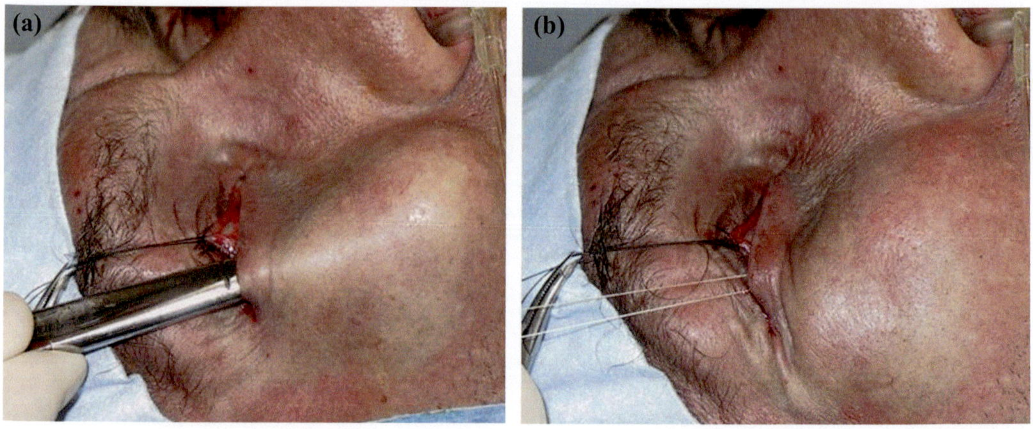

Fig. 6 (**a**) A broad elevator, such as a Sayre elevator used in this Fig. 12., is used to perform the dissection through a transconjunctival incision down to the level of the nasolabial fold. (**b**) The midface is elevated superiorly and fixated to the periosteum of the inferior and lateral orbital rim with polyglactin sutures

4 Summary

Ectropion is a common malposition of the lower eyelid that may result from involutional, cicatricial, paralytic, or mechanical vectors. The majority of cases of ectropion involve horizontal eyelid laxity, hence a lateral canthal anchoring procedure such as the lateral tarsal strip is commonly used. Additional procedures such as medial canthal tendon plication, eyelid spindle procedure, full thickness skin grafting, and midface lifting can also augment lateral canthal tendon anchoring in select cases.

References

1. Marx DP, Yen MT. Management of ectropion and floppy eyelids. In: Yen MT, editor. Surgery of the eyelids, lacrimal system and orbit. 2nd ed. New York: Oxford University Press; 2012. p. 91–101.
2. Choi CJ, Bauza A, Yoon MK, Sobel RK, Freitag SK. Full thickness skin graft as an independent or adjunctive technique for repair of cicatricial lower eyelid ectropion secondary to actinic skin changes. Ophthalmic Plast Reconstr Surg. 2015;31:474–7.
3. Chung JE, Yen MT. Midface lifting as an adjunct procedure in ectropion repair. Ann of Plast Surg. 2007;59:635–40.
4. Jacono AA, Stong BC. Combined transconjunctival release and midface-lift procedure for post blepharoplasty ectropion repair. Arch Facial Plast Surg. 2010;12:206–8.
5. Jordan DR, Anderson RL. The lateral tarsal strip revisited: the enhanced tarsal strip. Arch Ophthalmol. 1989;107:604–6.
6. Kam KYR, Cole CJ, Bunce C, et al. The lateral tarsal strip in ectropion surgery: is it effective when performed in isolation? Eye. 2012;26:827–32.
7. Kim HJ, Hayek B, Nasser Q, Esmaeli B. Viability of full thickness skin grafts used for correction of cicatricial ectropion of lower eyelid in previously irradiated field in the periocular region. Head Neck. 2013;35:103–8.
8. Kopecky A, Rokohl AC, Wawer Matos PA, Němčanský J, Heindl LM. Cheek-midface lifting with lateral canthoplasty for repair of complex iatrogenic lower eyelid ectropion. Eur J Ophthalmol. 2022;32:2085–92.
9. Lee H, Park M, Chang M, et al. Clinical characteristics and effectiveness of the lateral tarsal strip and medial spindle procedure. Ann Plast Surg. 2015;75:365–9.
10. Lee S, Marx D, Yen MT. Transeyelid supraperiosteal (preperiosteal) midface lifting. In: Holck DEE, editor. Hartstein ME. New York: Midfacial Rejuvenation Springer; 2012. p. 83–8.
11. Rubin P, Mykula R, Griffiths RW. Ectropion following excision of lower eyelid tumours and full thickness skin graft repair. Br J Plast Surg. 2005;58:353–60.

Medial Canthal Surgery

Emily Sarah Charlson, Christopher Dermarkarian and Maria A. Belen Camacho

Abstract

The medial canthus is key for proper positioning of the lower eyelid to the globe as well as for facial appearance. The medial canthus includes important tendinous structures as well as the proximal lacrimal drainage apparatus. Externally, the medial canthus abuts the medial orbit and nose in a concavity that is highly prone to web formation. Medial canthal surgery is challenging, owing to the complexities in anatomy including the delicate lacrimal outflow structures as well as the highly visible nature. Surgery may be indicated for reconstructive indications—namely eyelid malpositions stemming from age-related, paralytic or cicatricial post traumatic causes. Cosmetic surgery may be desired for epicanthal folds, often in conjunction with blepharoplasty. This chapter details various medial canthus surgeries.

Keywords

Epicanthoplasty · Medial Canthus · Medial Canthal Tendon · Epicanthus · Telecanthus · Medial Canthal Web · Medial Ectropion

1 Introduction

Surgery of the medial canthus may be indicated for aesthetic or functional indications. This chapter details relevant anatomy and functional and aesthetic surgeries. (Reconstruction of medial canthal defects are covered in Chapter "Repair of Full Thickness Lower Eyelid Defects").

2 Anatomy

The medial canthal tendon is a band of fibrous connective tissue arising from the medial orbicularis oculi muscle and inserting into the medial orbital wall. The medial preseptal and pretarsal components of the orbicularis oculi muscle fibers from both the upper and lower

Illustrations by Michael Han

Supplementary Information The online version contains supplementary material available at https://doi.org/10.1007/978-3-031-36175-3_13.

E. S. Charlson (✉)
Oculofacial, Orbital, and Aesthetic Plastic Surgery, California Pacific Medical Center, Van Ness Pacific Eye Associates, 2100 Webster Street Suite 214, San Francisco, CA 94115, USA
e-mail: emily.charlson@pacificeye.com; emily.charlson@gmail.com

C. Dermarkarian · M. A. Belen Camacho
Gavin Herbert Eye Institute, University of California, Irvine, USA

J. P. Tao (ed.), *Plastic Surgery of the Lower Eyelids*,
https://doi.org/10.1007/978-3-031-36175-3_13

eyelids meet to form the common medial canthal tendon. The common tendon then splits into anterior and posteriors limbs prior to insertion onto the medial orbital wall [1].

Both the anterior and posterior limb have an intimate relationship with the nasolacrimal sac. The anterior limb courses in front of the nasolacrimal sac and inserts into the frontal process of the maxillary bone, as well as the anterior lacrimal crest of the lacrimal bone (Fig. 1). The posterior limb courses behind the nasolacrimal sac and inserts into the posterior lacrimal crest of the lacrimal bone [1].

Traditionally, the posterior limb is most important to the proper apposition of the medial eyelid to the globe. The posterior limb has also been described as the smaller/weaker of the two limbs [2]. Many techniques to reconstruct the medial canthal tendon after traumatic avulsion, aim to secure the remaining portion of the medial canthal tendon to the periosteum of the posterior lacrimal crest, or surgical plate placed in the same location, to ensure proper eyelid position relative to the globe. The anterior limb is known as the larger/stronger limb and is important for ensuring the puncta of the nasolacrimal system are in place [2].

Cadaveric dissections have proposed alternative configurations of the medial canthal tendon. In two studies, the posterior limb of the medial canthal tendon was unable to be identified [2, 3]. The posterior limb, as traditionally described as the a tendon arising from the pretarsal and preseptal orbicularis oculi muscle, may actually be a fibrous condensation of Horner's muscle inserting into the posterior lacrimal crest [2–4].

Others have described an additional superior limb of the medial canthal tendon [2, 5]. Also based on cadaveric dissections, a proposed superior limb of the medial canthal tendon may insert onto the frontal bone. This superior limb, along with the anterior limb, may be responsible for the majority of the structural support that the medial canthal tendon provides the medial eyelid [2, 5].

3 Medial Canthal Tendon Plication for Mild-Moderate Laxity

Repair of a lax medial canthal tendon may be indicated to improve the position of the medial eyelid. The anatomical position of the lower eyelid punctum is just sightly lateral to the superior punctum. Mild medial canthal tendon laxity has been defined as lateral displacement of the lower eyelid punctum by 4 mm or less with lateral traction of the nasal eyelid. Others have defined laxity as mild if distraction of the lower eyelid punctum does not permit encroachment on the medial corneal limbus [6].

Severe medial canthal laxity is encountered when the lateral distraction moves the puncta beyond to the medial corneal limbus. In these more severe cases, lateral distraction of the medial eyelid necessary to correct the laxity may result in extreme lateral displacement of the lower eyelid puncta negatively affecting cosmesis, functionality, or both [6].

If mild medial canthal tendon laxity is noted, shortening or tightening the lateral canthal tendon alone may be sufficient [7]. The lateral canthal tendon is thought to be weaker than the anterior limb of the medial canthal tendon. Cases of mild medial canthal laxity may be due to the weakening of the lateral canthal tendon. Tightening of the lateral canthal tendon is commonly performed in conjunction with a medial spindle procedure [6].

When moderate medial canthal tendon laxity is noted, surgery to the medial canthal tendon is undertaken, most commonly via medial canthal tendon plication. Surgery to the anterior limb of the tendon is often limited because tightening of the anterior limb alone can result in undesired distraction/tenting of the eyelid away from the globe [6]. Procedures to tighten the anterior limb are done under specific circumstances of trauma or congenital telecanthus, such as blepharophimosis [6, 8].

Anterior limb plication can be undertaken via a transcutaneous approach (Fig. 2). A curved

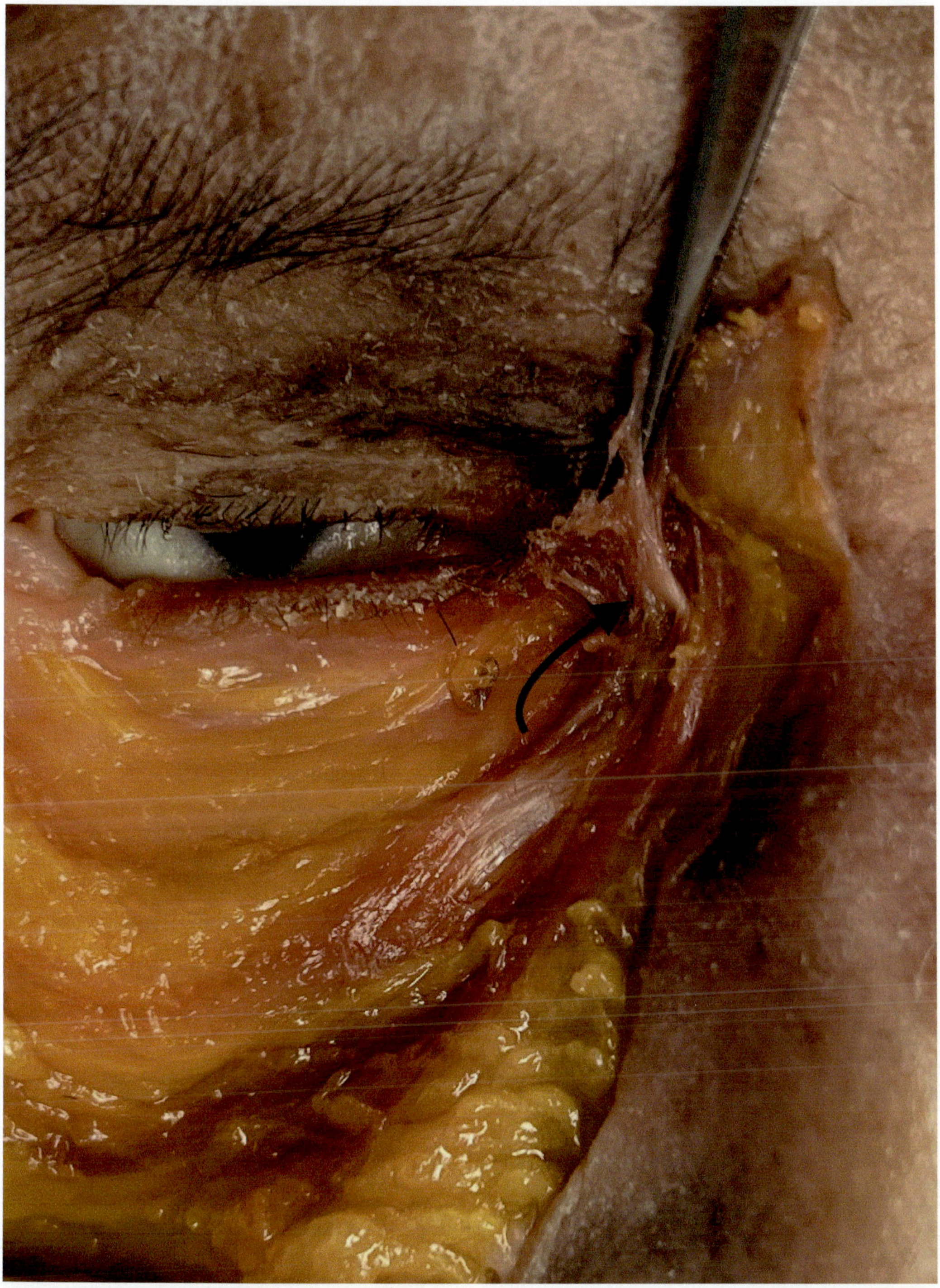

Fig. 1 Anterior limb of medial canthal tendon exposed on a cadaver dissection

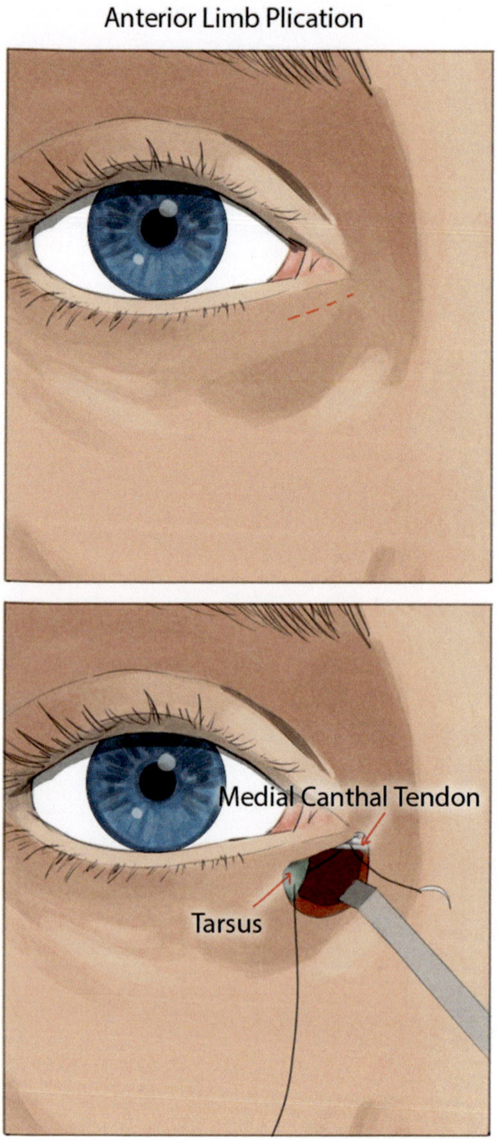

Fig. 2 Anterior approach to medial canthal tendon plication

vertical incision through skin is made with a 15-blade starting just over the superior boarder of the medial canthal tendon and ending at a position 2–3 mm inferior to the medial eyelid margin at the level of the puncta [9]. A Bowman probe can be introduced through the punctum to protect the canaliculus. The most medial aspect of the inferior tarsus and the medial canthal tendon are exposed by blunt dissection through the orbicularis oculi muscle with a periosteal elevator. The authors recommend a double armed non-absorbable suture with half circle needles. In this example, each arm of a double armed 4-0 braided polyester suture on a S-2 half circle needle is passed full thickness through the either the superior or inferior border of the medial aspect of the lower eyelid tarsus then passed beneath the orbicularis muscle. The needle should stay anterior to the Bowman probe to prevent canalicular injury and exit at the superior margin of the medial canthal tendon insertion. The suture is tied, taking care to avoid bunching up the inferior canaliculus and displacing the punctum away from the globe [9].

Plication of the posterior limb of the medial canthal tendon is the preferred option for repair of medial canthal laxity as risk of inadvertent canalicular injury or displacement is less. Plication can occur via a transconjunctival/transcaruncular method (Fig. 3). A conjunctival incision is made at the inferior tarsal margin of the most medial aspect of the inferior tarsus with a 15-blade [10]. A vertical conjunctival incision is made posterior to the caruncle with a 15-blade and blunt dissection with a Freer periosteal elevator is undertaken to expose the medial orbital wall periosteum including the posterior lacrimal crest. Each arm of a double armed non-absorbable suture with half circle needles is passed full thickness through the either the superior or inferior border of the medial aspect of the lower eyelid tarsus. The needs are then buried subconjunctival to the medial incision overlying the medial orbital wall. Each arm is then passed through the periosteum posterior to the posterior lacrimal crest and tied. The desired tension is carefully considered to ensure proper placement of the lower eyelid punctum relative to the superior punctum and good approximation of the eyelid to the globe. The conjunctival and caruncular incisions are then closed with fast absorbing suture and the knots buried [10].

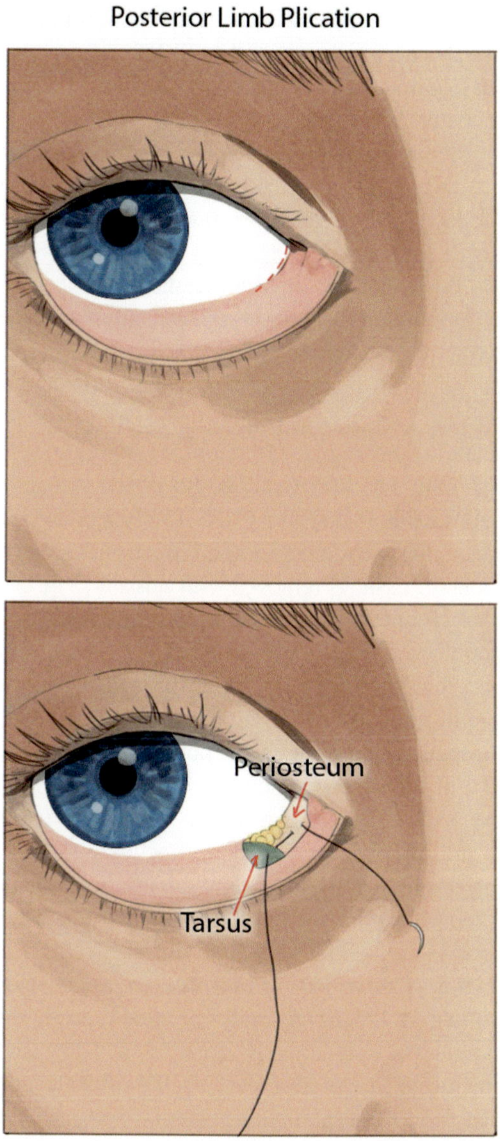

Fig. 3 Plication of the posterior limb of thre medial canthal tendon through a transconjunctival incision

4 Medial Canthoplasty/ Full Thickess Resection for Moderate to Severe Laxity

In cases of severe medial canthal tendon laxity often to due severe involutional or paralytic changes, a medial canthoplasty via full thickness eyelid resection may be indicated. This approach is combined with lower eyelid punctum rotation and lateral canthal shortening/tightening procedures. With full thickness medial canthal resection the inferior canaliculus is resected and it must be repaired, usually with lacrimal intubation (see Chapter “Canalicular and Tearing Considerations”) (Fig. 4).

Scissors are used to make a full thickness incision vertically just lateral to the caruncle through the medial canthal tendon and the

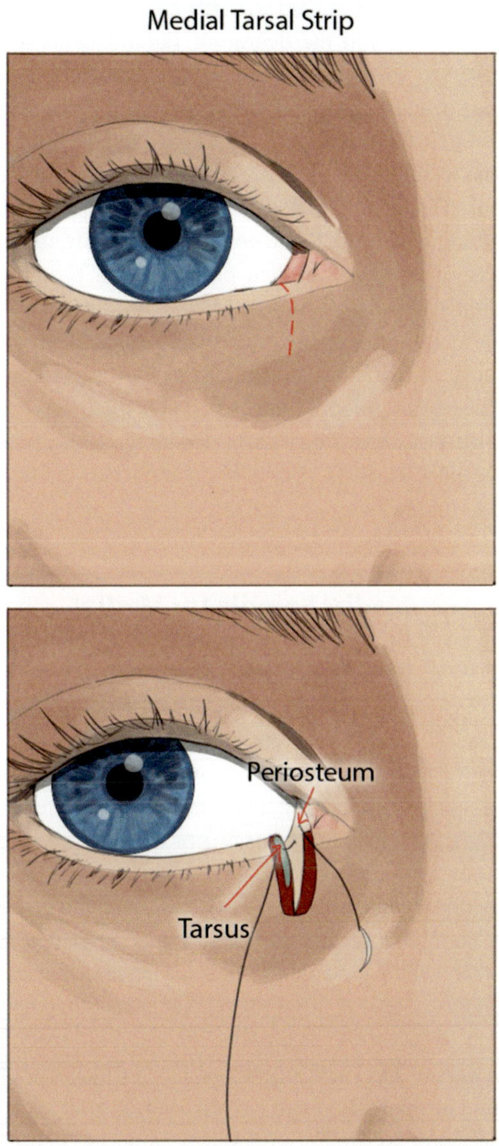

Fig. 4 Medial full thickness resection canthoplasty. In this technique, the canaliculus is included in the full thickness eyelid resection and the canaliculus is repaired, usually with silicone tube intubation

inferior canaliculus [11]. Blunt dissection using a Freer periosteal elevator is then undertaken within the medial canthus to expose the posterior lacrimal crest. Each arm of a double armed non-absorbable suture with half circle needles is passed through the periosteum of the posterior lacrimal crest, 2 mm apart from each other at the level of the posterior limb of the medial canthal tendon. The lateral (temporal) edge of the cut margin is then pulled towards the posterior lacrimal crest and the degree of redundant tissues assessed and then excised. Each arm of the double armed suture is then passed full thickness through the cut edge of the lower eyelid tarsus, one at the superior boarder and one the inferior boarder. Bicanaliculus intubation with silicone tubing retrieved from under the inferior turbinate in the nose is then preformed to preserve proper tear drainage post-operatively. Intubation also helps maintain lower eyelid punctal alignment after medial attachment of the tarsal strip. The eyelid margin and skin are then sutured with fast absorbing suture. Redundant and prolapsed caruncule tissue, if present, can also be resected [11].

5 Medial Spindle for Medial Ectropion of the Lower Eyelid and Punctum

Medial ectropion of the lower eyelid often presents with complaints of tearing. Epiphora and exposure keratopathy may be noted on exam due to malposition (eversion) of the lower eyelid puncta. Medial ectropion is best treated with a medial spindle procedure. Depending on the cause of ectropion, medial spindle can be combined with other eyelid procedures such as lateral canthoplasty via lateral tarsal strip, medial canthal tendon plication for involutional or paralytic medial ectropion, and a skin graft or flap in the case of anterior lamellar cicatrix when clinical exam findings support the use of surgical adjuncts [12]. At times, punctoplasty, or widening of the lower eyelid puncta may be performed simultaneously to allow for improved tear drainage. Occasionally, isolated medial punctal ectropion without any of the aforementioned clinical exam findings may be noted. This is a poorly understood phenomena but may be related to dehiscence of the lower eyelid retractors within the medial eyelid.

Medial spindle involves the shortening of the posterior lamella of the eyelid and tightening of the lower eyelid retractors directly inferior to the lower eyelid puncta. Often, a Bowman probe is placed within the inferior canaliculus to protect it. A diamond fusiform wedge of conjunctiva and retractors is marked below the inferior margin of the tarsal plate centered on the lower eyelid puncta. The vertical height of the wedge should relate to the degree of ectropion, approximately 4–6 mm. The horizontal length of the wedge is approximately 6–8 mm [9]. A 15 blade is used to make incise conjunctiva and retractors. This diamond of tissue is removed with scissors (Fig. 5).

A double armed absorbable suture such as a double armed 5-0 chromic on a P-2 needle may be used. Each arm is passed through the lower eyelid retractors along the inferior incision then through the inferior tarsal border and conjunctiva of the superior incision. When pulled tight, the suture brings the lower eyelid retractors to the inferior tarsal border, effectively shortening the retractor band below the inferior puncta. The needles are then passed deep into the lower eyelid fornix and exits the lower eyelid full thickness about 10–15 mm inferior to the eyelid margin [15]. The sutures are tied tight on the skin surface effectively creating a downward and posterior-anterior pull on the lower eyelid that rotates the punctum posteriorly against the globe. The suture, once absorbed, is thought to create a cicatricial band within the lower eyelid that helps to maintain the proper punctal position [9, 15]. Alternatively, the posterior lamella defect may be closed with absorbable sutures buried in the wound and not exiting externally.

6 Tissue Rearrangement Flaps for Medial Canthal Webbing

Medial canthal webbing can results from trauma, iatrogenic causes, or it may be congenital (Fig. 6). When congenital, webbing is

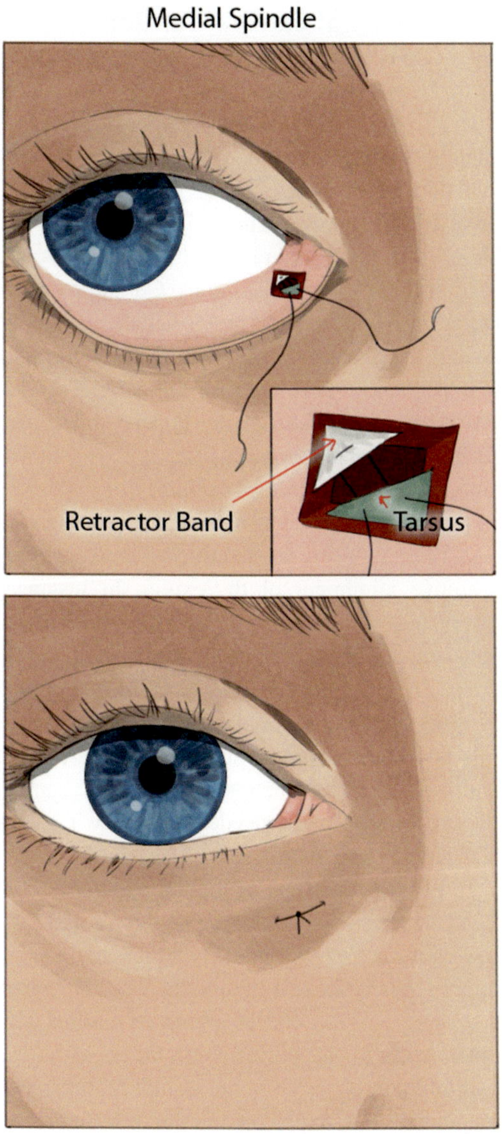

Fig. 5 Medial spindle conjunctivoplasty. A Diamond or ellipse of posterior lamella is resected and the conjunctiva and retractor band are tightened to rotate the medial eyelid margin toward the ocular surface

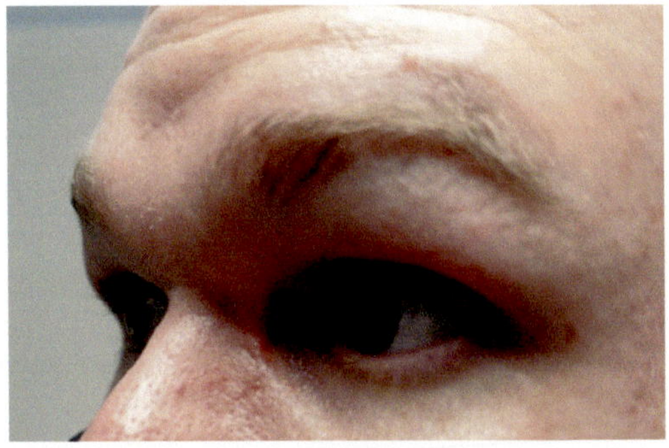

Fig. 6 Medial canthal web after external dacryocystorhinostomy

referred to as an epicanthal fold and is often associated with the Asian eyelid. These webs may be associated with retraction or ectropion of the medial lower eyelid can result causing tearing and ocular exposure.

Cicatricial webs, especially in the early months after trauma or prior surgery, may be treated medically with massage or injection of corticosteroids or injection of 5-fluorouracil. When medical management is inadequate, surgical correction of medial canthal webbing may be indicated. Surgical repair attempts to lengthen the area of vertical shortening. If the vertical vector of inferior pull is confined to just one vector, a Z-plasty is often the procedure of choice (Fig. 7). Alternatively, if the anterior lamellar shortening is not due to a vertical cicatrix but rather is an amorphous tightness with downward pull, a skin graft is the more appropriate option.

A Z-plasty lengthens the area of vertical shortening by transposing the tension to different directions. To start, the area of linear vertical pull (the scar tension line) is marked. Two triangles with are marked on the superior and inferior ends of the scar line at a 60° angle [13]. Incisions are made over the skin markings through the skin. Any subcutantous scar tissue or adhesion is lysed with sharp dissection. The skin flaps are widely undermined and then transposed. Deep sutures may be placed to secure the flaps to the deep medial canthal tissue. The skin is then closed.

Apposing Z-plasties in a jumping man configuration may be of particular benefit for broader medial canthus webs with telecanthus (Fig. 8). In this configuration, there exists a lateral to medial Y to V plasty that pulls the canthus toward the midline.

Multiple V-Y advancements and multiple and/or modified Z-plasties may be employed for extensive webs extending on to the midface

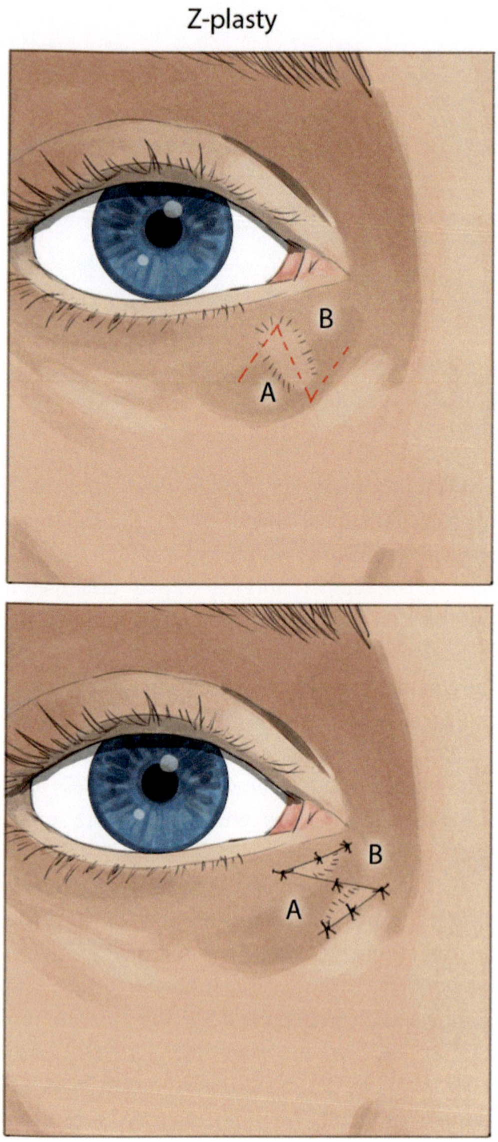

Fig. 7 Z-plasty tissue rearrangement on the medial lower eyelid

or forehead (18). Massry described additional Z-plasties hinged om the arms of the Y that well transpose triangular skin segments from their relative horizontal excess to the vertical plane to further flatten large webs.

7 Medial Canthal Tendon Avulsion Repair

Injury to the medial canthus can result in medial canthal tendon avulsion. Medial canthal tendon avulsion occurs when all or part of the eyelid involving the medial canthus has been disrupted. On clinical exam, there may be telecanthus and rounding of the medial canthus. Common causes including blunt trauma (motor vehicle accidents, assault, etc.), animal bites, surgical resection due to malignant tumors with medial canthal tendon involvement, or iatrogenic damage sustained during oculoplastic (external dacryocystorhinostomy) or ortolaryngology surgery.

It should be noted that medial canthal tendon repair is not always needed to obtain proper postoperative alignment of the eyelid. In instances where the naso-lacrimal system has been damaged, intubation with a bi-canalicular stent is indicated. The posterior and medial traction provided by a bi-canalicular nasolacrimal stent can provide good tissue alignment; separate or extensive suturing and reconstruction of the medial canthal tendon is not always needed [14] (see Chapter "Canalicular and Tearing Considerations").

In general, the type of medial canthal tendon repair depends on the degree of the medial canthal injury and the availability of residual tissue/bone in the canthus. If the medial canthal tendon is severed and the distant stump of tendon with attachments to the periosteum can be identified a simple non-absorbable horizontal mattress can be placed to reapproximate the proximal and distal ends. In situations with the distal stump cannot be identified, the posterior lacrimal crest is exposed with blunt dissection and two sutures passed between the stump of medial canthal tendon and the periosteum of the posterior lacrimal crest, one each at the anatomic sites of tendon attachment [14] (Video 1).

If the periosteum is not present for reconstruction (as is often the case with tumor

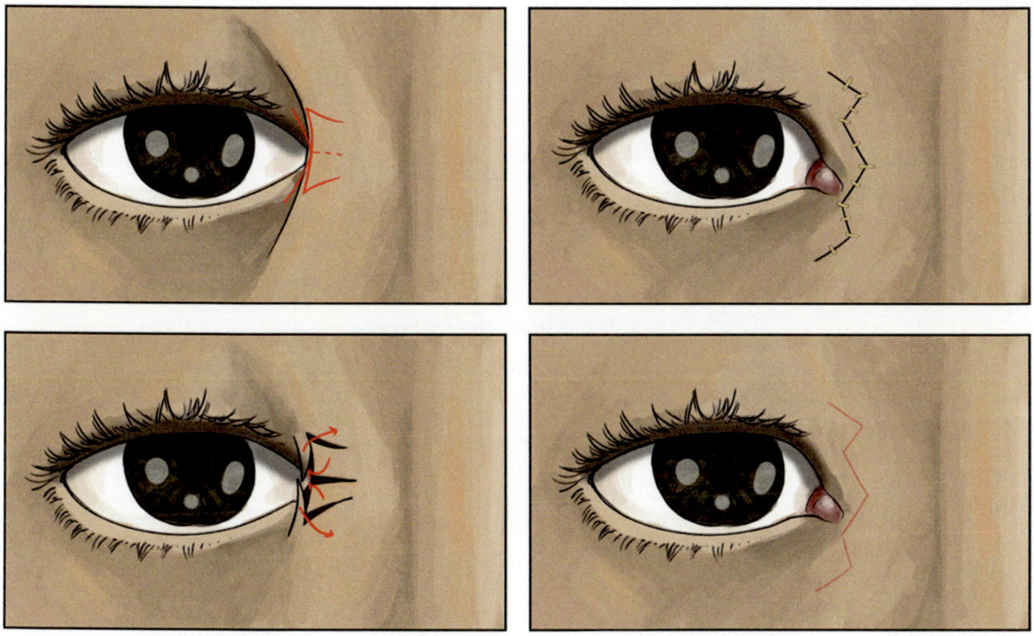

Fig. 8 Jumping man opposing Z-plasty rearrangement for broad medial web

resections, trauma etc.) and the bone comprising the posterior lacrimal crest is missing (naso-orbito-ethmoid fractures) then microplates, direct drill hole fixation, or transnasal wiring can be used for fixation of the medial canthal tendon [14–17]. Proper alignment of the medial lower eyelid to the globe requires a very posterior fixation point. Modern microplating devices have largely obviated the need for transnasal wiring, an older technique used to create a posterior suture fixation point to re-attach the medial canthal tendon.

8 Epicanthoplasty

The epicanthal fold is a skin flap over the lacrimal lake in the medial corner of the eye. It is an extension of the upper eyelid skin and is generally seen among East Asians [19]. There are multiple types and varying degrees of severity of epicanthal folds. In more severe cases, the lacrimal lake and caruncle are covered almost completely by the skin fold. For moderate severity epicanthal folds, the authors recommend a Z-epicanthoplasty as described by Park et al. [19] (Video 2). This technique consists of a blepharoplasty incision for a "double eyelid" crease formation operation in combination with a Z-epicanthoplasty (Fig. 9). In particular, the technique involves a triangle-shaped pretarsal skin resection medially with transposition of the epicanthal fold into this defect in a Z-plasty tissue rearrangement. This lengthens skin along the epicanthal fold. The excision and rearrangement also pull skin superiorly and medially to expose the underlying canthus and caruncle. Many other flap designs have been described for epicanthal folds including the jumping man opposing Z plasties described above [18]. However, these and others are less preferred in aesthetic epicanthoplasty owing to increased number of resultant scars.

9 Conclusion

Medial canthal surgery is one of the most intricate on the face owing to the complex anatomy including the lacrimal drainage apparatus and

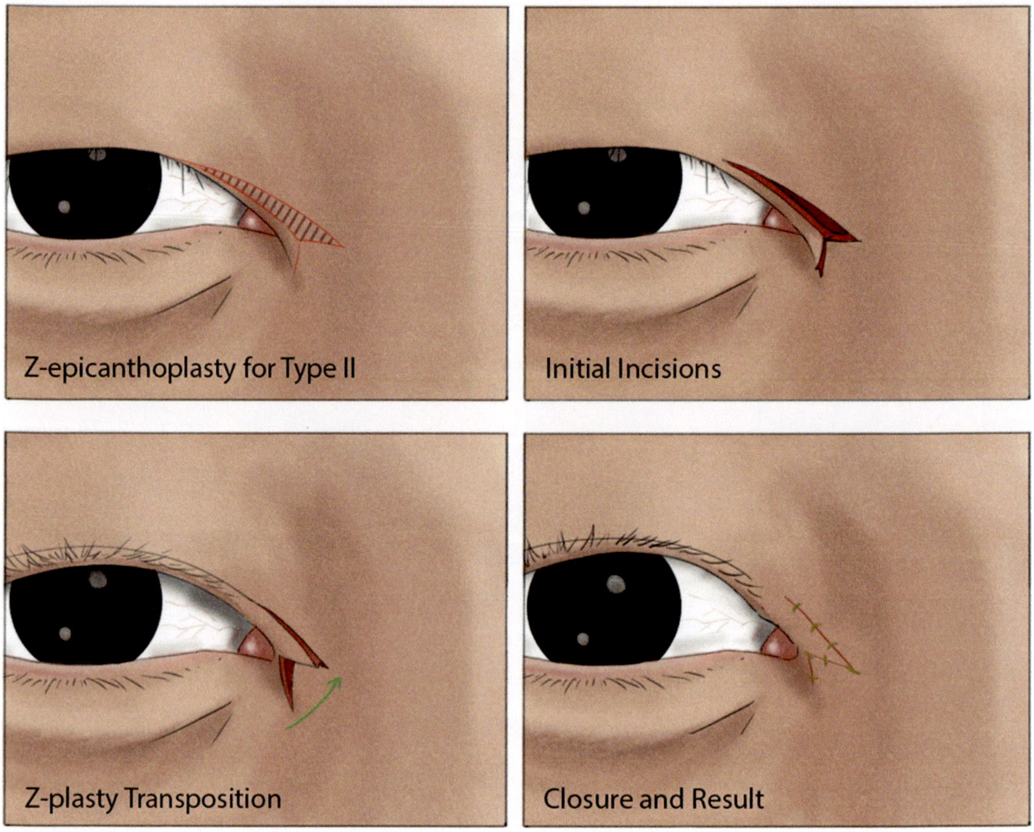

Fig. 9 Z-epicanthoplasty for mild-moderate epicanthal fold

since it is highly conspicuous. The general principles of posterior medial tendon fixation so that the eyelid hugs the globe and maintaining patency of the lacrimal drainage apparatus are key. Tissue rearrangements that flatten webs or epicanthal folds while leaving minimal scars are ideal.

References

1. Robinson TJ, Stranc MF. The anatomy of the medial canthal ligament. Br J Plast Surg. 1970;23(1):1–7.
2. Anderson RL. Medial canthal tendon branches out. Arch Ophthalmol. 1977;95(11):2051–2.
3. Poh E, Kakizaki H, Selva D, Leibovitch I. Anatomy of medial canthal tendon in Caucasians. Clin Exp Ophthalmol. 2012;40(2):170–3.
4. Ahl NC, Hill JC. Horner's muscle and the lacrimal system. Arch Ophthalmol. 1982;100(3):488–93.
5. Jones LT, Reeh MJ, Wirtschafter JD. Ophthalmic anatomy. Rochester, NY: American Academy of Ophthalmology and Otolaryngology; 1970. p. 39–48.
6. O'Donnell BA, Anderson RL, Collin JR, Fante RG, Jordan DR, Ritleng P. Repair of the lax medial canthal tendon. Br J Ophthalmol. 2003;87(2):220–4.
7. Anderson RL, Gordy DD. The tarsal strip procedure. Arch Ophthalmol. 1979;97:2192–6.
8. Amer AA, Abdellah MM, Hassan NHF, et al. Surgical outcome of epicanthus and telecanthus correction by C-U medial canthoplasty with lateral canthoplasty in treatment of Blepharophimosis syndrome.
9. David TT. Color atlas of oculoplastic surgery. Lippincott Williams & Wilkins; 2012.
10. Elner VM, Demirci H, Morton AD, Elner SG, Hassan AS. Transcaruncular medial canthal ligament plication for repair of lower eyelid malposition. Arch Ophthalmol. 2007;125(3):374–9.

11. Sullivan TJ, Collin JR. Medical canthal resection: an effective long-term cure for medial ectropion. Br J Ophthalmol. 1991;75(5):288–91.
12. Nowinski TS, Anderson RL. The medial spindle procedure for involutional medial ectropion. Arch Ophthalmol. 1985;103(11):1750–3.
13. Codner MA, McCord CD Jr, editors. Eyelid and periorbital surgery. CRC Press; 2016.
14. Tint NL, Alexander P, Cook AE, Letherbarrow B. Eyelid avulsion repair with bi-canalicular silicone stenting without medial canthal tendon reconstruction. Br J ophthalmol. 2011;95:1389–92.
15. Medra AM, Ashour EM, Shehata EA. Medial canthopexy using mini-screws &/or micro plates for the surgical treatment of post traumatic telecanthus associated with naso-orbito-ethmoidal fractures. Adv Oral Maxillofac Surg. 2021;2:100051.
16. Lauer G, Pinzer T. Transcaruncular-transnasal suture: a modification of medial canthopexy. J Oral Maxillofac Surg. 2008;66(10):2178–84.
17. Mustarde JC. Repair and reconstruction in the orbital region: a practical guide. London, United Kingdom: Churchill Livingstone, Publishing; 1966. p. 292–8.
18. Massry GG. Cicatricial canthal webs. Ophthal Plast Reconstr Surg. 2011;27:426–430.
19. Park JI, Park MS. Park Z-Epicanthoplasty. Facial Plastic Surgery Facial N Am. 2007;15:343–52.

Cicatricial Ectropion Repair with Skin Graft

Mary Alex Parks and Jeremy Clark

Abstract

Cicatricial ectropion occurs when the eyelid is abnormally rotated outward due to shortening of the eyelid or midface skin. This eyelid malposition causes exposure of the ocular surface that can result in irritation, corneal dryness, conjunctival injection, and other visual complaints. Treatment typically involves replacement or recruitment of skin combined with lateral canthal anchoring procedures.

Keywords

Skin graft · Cicatricial ectropion · Eyelid scarring

1 Introduction

Cicatricial ectropion is the abnormal rotation of the eyelid away from the ocular surface. It may be both disfiguring and medically significant. In addition to dry eye and ocular irritation, corneal damage and loss of vision are possible due to this eyelid maloposition.

There are many causes of anterior lamellar disease that lead to cicatricial ectropion. Actinic damage from chronic sun exposure, dermatologic conditions such as rosacea, and even iatrogenic anterior lamellar shortening post blepharoplasty or Mohs reconstruction are all common causes of cicatricial ectropion.

1.1 Systemic Diseases

Bilateral cicatricial ectropion can be a result of a variety of systemic diseases such as ichthyosis and psoriatic arthritis. Ichthyosis is an inherited group of dermatoses characterized by dry and scaly skin due to impaired keratinization which can, over time, cause contracture of the lower eyelid leading to ectropion. Psoriatic arthritis is a common chronic inflammatory condition affecting the skin and joints of those with an underlying genetic predisposition. It is characterized by concomitant symptoms of erythematous, scaly, pruritic plaques most commonly on the extensor surfaces of the knees and elbows along with arthritis of the fingers and lower spine. Ocular manifestations of psoriatic arthritis vary, but the eyelids can be affected by chronic blepharitis and loss of eyelid tissue leading to ectropion. Because of long-term nature and systemic manifestations of these conditions,

Supplementary Information The online version contains supplementary material available at https://doi.org/10.1007/978-3-031-36175-3_14.

M. A. Parks (✉) · J. Clark (✉)
University of Louisville, Louisville, KY, USA

J. Clark
e-mail: jdclar13@louisville.edu

J. P. Tao (ed.), *Plastic Surgery of the Lower Eyelids*,
https://doi.org/10.1007/978-3-031-36175-3_14

symptom recurrence and a potential need for repeated surgery may be necessary.

1.2 Dermatologic Conditions

Dermatologic conditions such as ocular rosacea and discoid lupus erythematosus should be considered for anyone presenting with cicatricial ectropion. Discoid lupus erythematosus accounts for the large majority of chronic cutaneous lupus erythematosus. It is rarely associated with systemic disease, and it typically presents with erythematous, inflammatory scaly plaques affecting areas with exposure to UV light that heal but cause significant scarring and atrophy which can ultimately result in cicatricial ectropion.

1.3 Post Blepahroplasty

Post blepharoplasty lower eyelid ectropion is common owing to the pervasiveness of cosmetic lower eyelid or midfacial surgery. Overaggressive resection or poor technique or both can cause the lower eyelid to pull away from the globe.

1.4 Infectious Diseases

Periocular infections and associated inflammation may induce cicatricial changes to the skin that can cause ectropion. Surgical repair of ectropion should be delayed until the active infection is resolved and the tissues are quiescent. However, a tension suture tarsorrhaphy (i.e., Frost) may be useful to counteract vectors actively pulling they eyelid away from the globe.

1.5 Medications

Antineoplastics, bisphosphonates, and topical anti-glaucoma agents have been associated with the development of cicatricial ectropion. Cetuximab, a monoclonal antibody that inhibits cell-signaling pathways used primarily in colorectal cancer treatment, is associated with madarosis and cicatricial ectropion. Cases of cicatricial ectropion with cetuximab have been described as soon as one week after beginning treatment with resolution six week after discontinuation of therapy. Similar ocular reactions have been described with the use of erlotinib, an antineoplastic agent used to treat non-small-cell lung cancer, and 5-flurouracil, a fluorinated pyrimidine used to treat cancers of the breast, colon, and skin. Notably, both topical and systemic 5-fluorouracil have been implicated in the occurrence of cicatricial ectropion. Another medication class commonly prescribed to treat osteoporosis, bone metastasis, multiple myeloma and Paget's disease that has been associated with cicatricial ectropion is bisphosphonates. These drugs have the potential to cause maxillary osteonecrosis ultimately leading to cicatricial ectropion. Lastly, anti-glaucoma agents dorzolamide and brimonidine have rarely been associated with ectropion. Of note, compared to other causes of cicatricial ectropion which typically require surgical correction, most causes of medication-induced cicatricial ectropion resolve with discontinuation of the offending medication.

1.6 Trauma

Cicatricial ectropion can occur as a consequence of direct eyelid injury or facial burns. Cicatricial ectropion is a common iatrogenic problem from orbitofacial fracture repair with poor orbitotomy technique.

1.7 Other

Radiation to the head and neck poses a significant risk for cicatricial ectropion through skin contraction and distortion along with muscle atrophy. Treatment should be delayed until radiation therapy has been completed and after adequate revascularization and maturation of cicatricial changes.

2 Clinical Evaluation

Patients may experience epiphora, foreign body sensation, redness, and irritation. Eversion of the lower eyelid can cause lacrimal outflow failure and if chronic, these patients can show complete or partial punctal stenosis. Because the palpebral conjunctiva can be chronically everted, keratinization may ensue. Prolonged ocular exposure can ultimately cause corneal decompensation and in severe cases corneal ulceration or infection. Furthermore, there may be co-existing neurotrophic disease or follicular keratitis that warrant separate treatments.

The exam should include assessing for skin shortening. For instance, vertically oriented anterior lamellar striae are a sign of skin tightening. Other signs include limited movement of the lower eyelid with upward gaze and decreased skin recoil upon manual downward lower eyelid distraction. Orbicularis oculi tone can be assessed by having the patient squeeze their eyes closed forcefully. Then, the examiner will manually try to open the eyelids of the patient. The force required to open the eyelids can be graded.

3 Surgical Management with Full Thickness Skin Graft (FTSG)

Full-thickness skin grafts lengthen the anterior lamella and aid in returning the lower eyelid to a more normal anatomic position. Common donor sites for the skin graft include the upper eyelid, post-auricular, supraclavicular, and upper inner arm areas. It is important to consider the color and thickness of the donor graft and the upper eyelid is generally the best match. In addition to donor site considerations, patient selection is key because a skin graft can leave a conspicuous scar or be associated with color and other mismatch with the surrounding recipient site.

For most anterior lamellar skin grafting procedures, skin grafting is combined with a lateral canthal anchoring procedure such as a lateral tarsal strip. Initially, local anesthesia is injected into the anterior lamella along with the area of the skin graft (Fig. 1). A subciliary incision is made to release the area of anterior lamellar deficiency. Further dissection is performed to release the lower eyelid completely so that it can be freely mobilized superiorly along with releasing any residual deep cicatricial bands (Figs. 2 and 3). Complete dissection through middle and deep posterior lamella structures to the level of conjunctiva is often useful to ensure complete release of cicatricial vectors (Figs. 3 and 4). This more adequately mobilizes the eyelid and forestalls ectropion recurrence.

Horizontal tightening is usually performed to treat any laxity as well as anchor the eyelid. A lateral canthotomy is performed with inferior cantholysis and further dissection between the anterior and posterior lamella for approximately 5–10 mm. The released lateral canthal tendon is anchored in the appropriate position along the internal lateral orbital rim at the level of the lateral orbital tubercle (Fig. 5). Once all cicatricial bands are released, the eyelid should be easily elevated and rotated to a normal anatomical position flush with eyeball. A Frost suture tarsorrhaphy is placed on upward tension to counter inferior contractile forces from healing as well as gravity. An appropriately sized graft is then measured and harvested from the donor site (Fig. 6). The graft is removed of all subcutaneous fat so that only dermis and epidermis remain (Fig. 7). The skin graft is placed into position and trimmed to best fit the area of

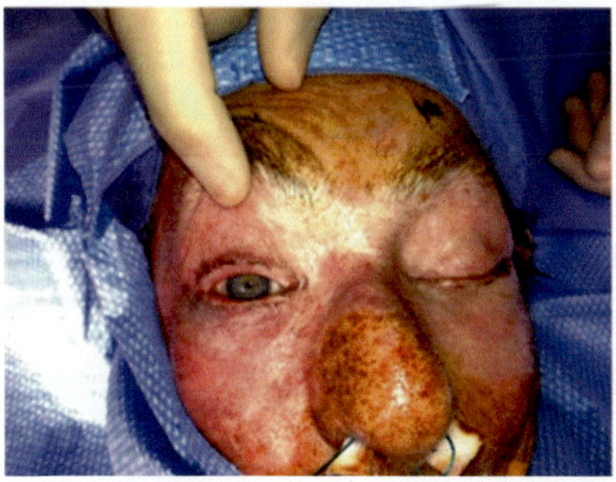

Fig. 1 Right lower eyelid cicatricial ectropion with eversion. Local anesthetic is administered into the anterior lamella along with the area of the graft harvest site

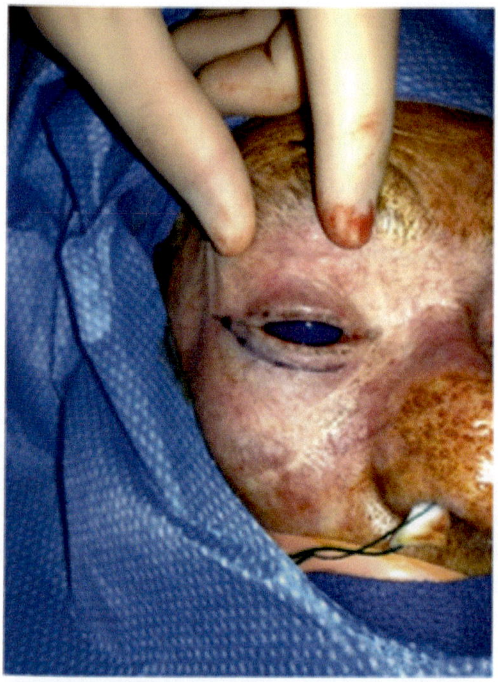

Fig. 2 A subciliary incision is planned across the horizontal extent of the lower eyelid. The subciliary incision should extend 5-10 mm past the lateral canthus

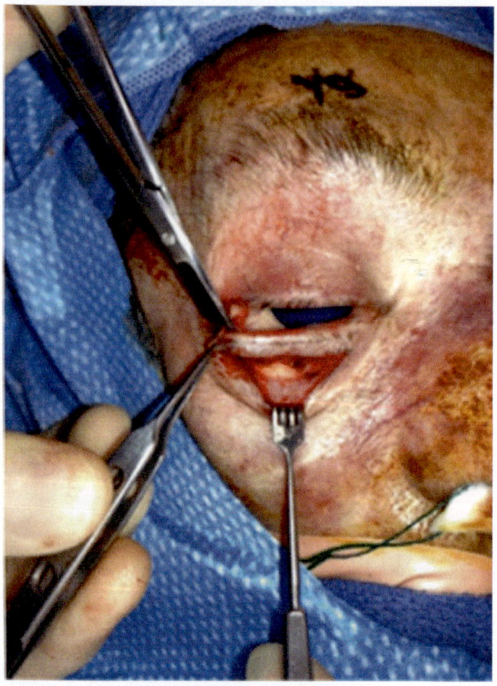

Fig. 3 A subciliary incision is created and extended past the canthus. Through this wound cicatricial bands are released. The inferior crus of the lateral canthal tendon is released

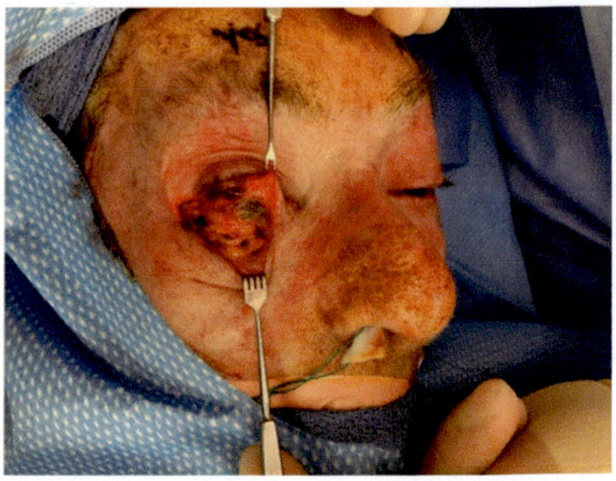

Fig. 4 Further dissection is performed through cicatricial bands (often through all eyelid layers except conjunctiva) to freely mobilize the lower eyelid

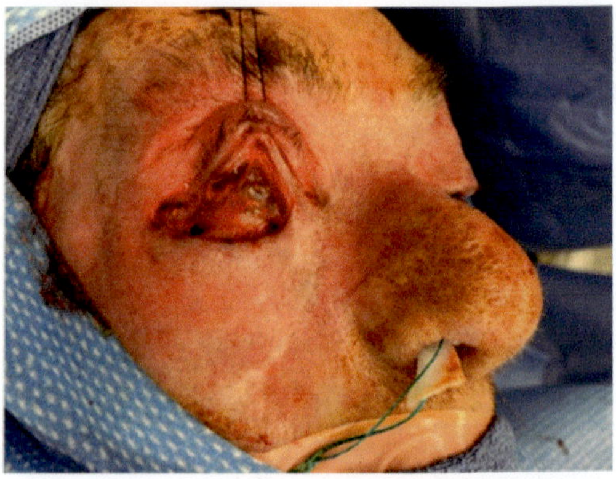

Fig. 5 A Frost suture tarsorrhaphy is placed to keep the lower eyelid on upward tension and then an appropriately sized graft is measured

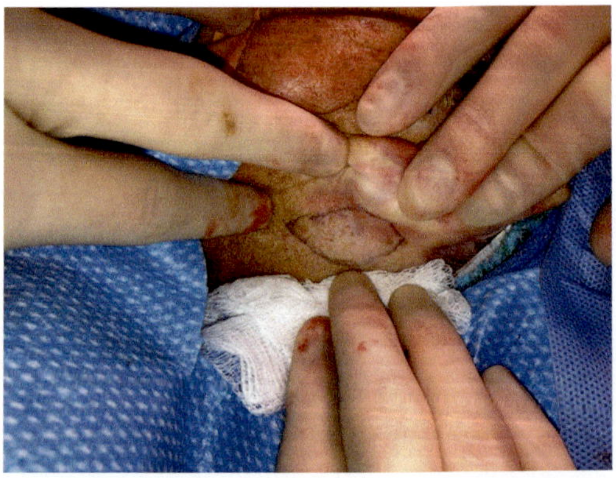

Fig. 6 The anterior lamellar defect is measured and an appropriately-sized graft is harvested from the donor site (postauricular shown here)

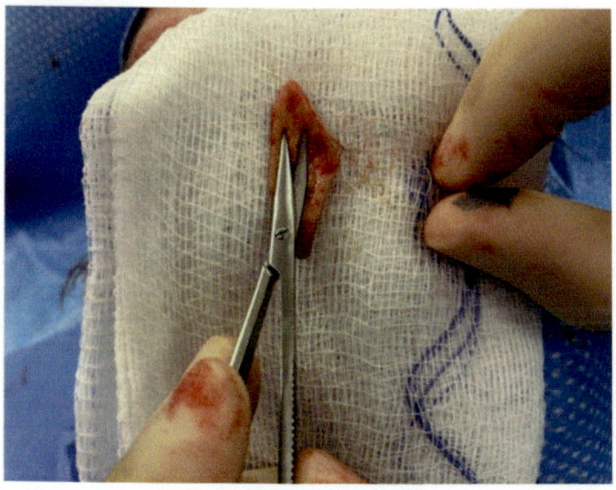

Fig. 7 The graft is thinned

the defect. It is secured with 5-0 or 6-0 plain gut suture (Fig. 8). A pressure patch is placed over a nonadherent dressing to prevent collection of fluid or dislocation (Video 1).

With good technique and proper patient selection, good results can be achieved (Figs. 9, 10, 11 and 12). However, patients should be prepared for the potential need for scar modulation or revision described below.

3.1 Other Therapies

Surgical management remains the gold standard for treatment of cicatricial ectropion; however, other nonsurgical treatments have been described and, as aforementioned, include the use of hyaluronic acid, corticosteroid, or 5-fluorouracil injections.

A midface lift (also known as a suborbicularis oculi fat lift (SOOF) lift can obviate a skin graft in some instances. This approach is often pursued in the post cosmetic blepharoplasty setting in which a patient is still seeking an excellent aesthetic outcome. These are performed with or without posterior lamella spaces. Additional canthoplasty or tarsoconjunctival suspension flaps are other adjuncts. These are described in other chapters.

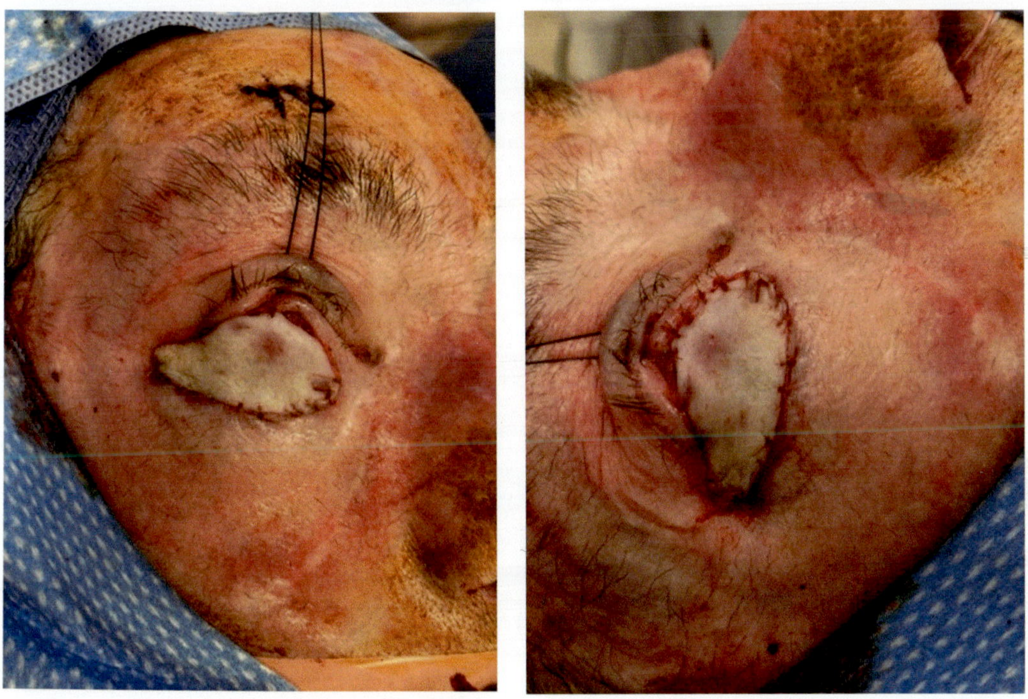

Fig. 8 The skin graft is placed into position and secured along the perimeter of the defect with a 6-0 plain or 6-0 chromic suture. A 4-0 silk Frost suture is placed to achieve upward tension for approximately 1 week. After topical antibiotic is applied to the surgical site, a moderate pressure dressing is applied (not shown; the authors place a nonadherent Telfa® dressing under two-folded eyepads, secured with paper tape)

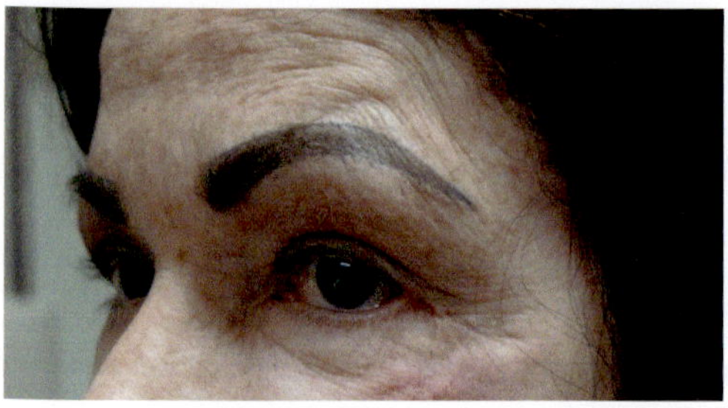

Fig. 9 Cicatricial retraction and ectropion after cosmetic blepharoplasty

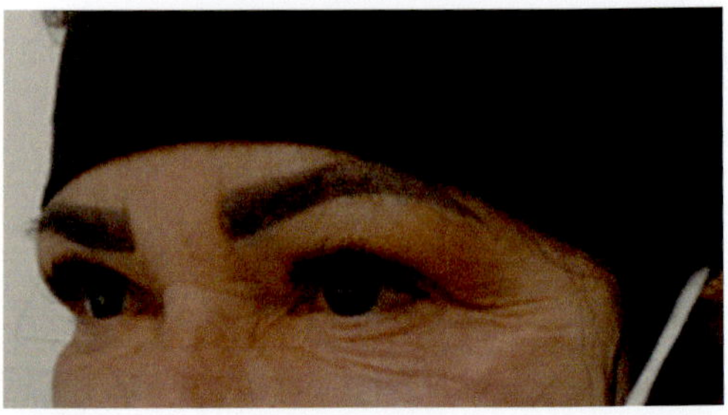

Fig. 10 3 years post lower eyelid ectropion repair with skin graft from upper eyelid. Fair complexion and fine rhytids contribute to good aesthetic result and minimally conspicuous scarring

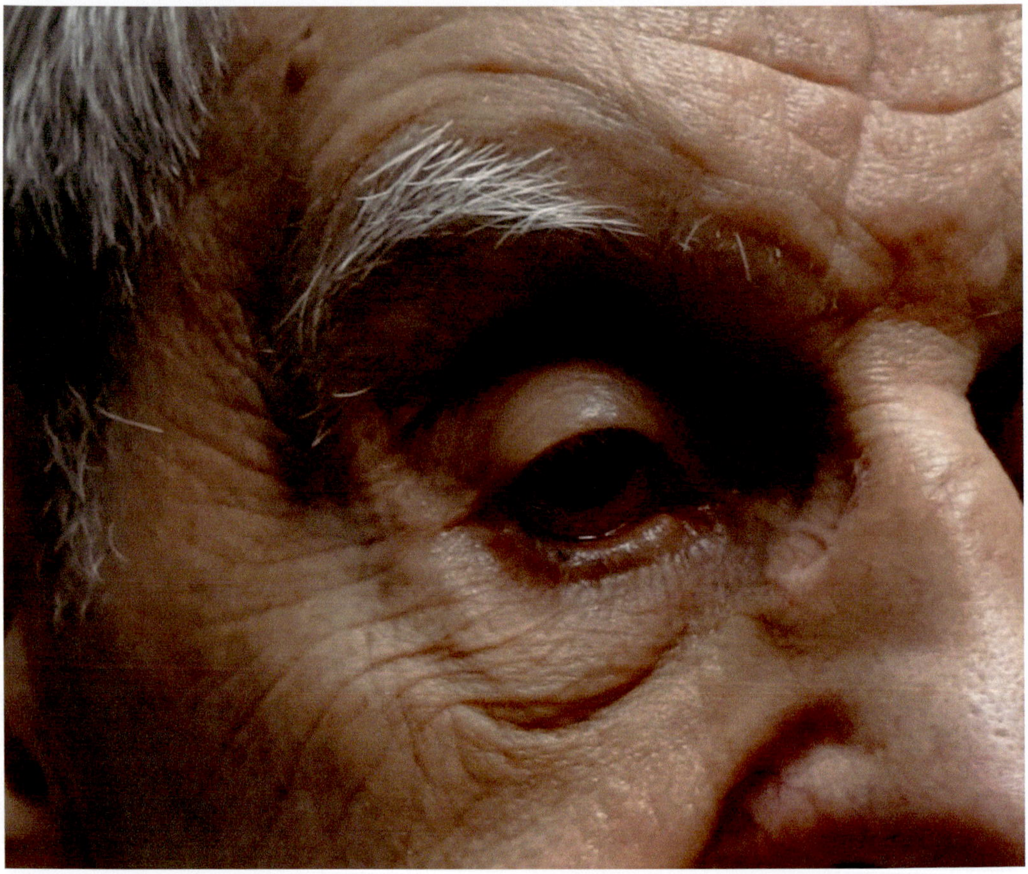

Fig. 11 Combined involutional and cicatricial retraction and ectropion

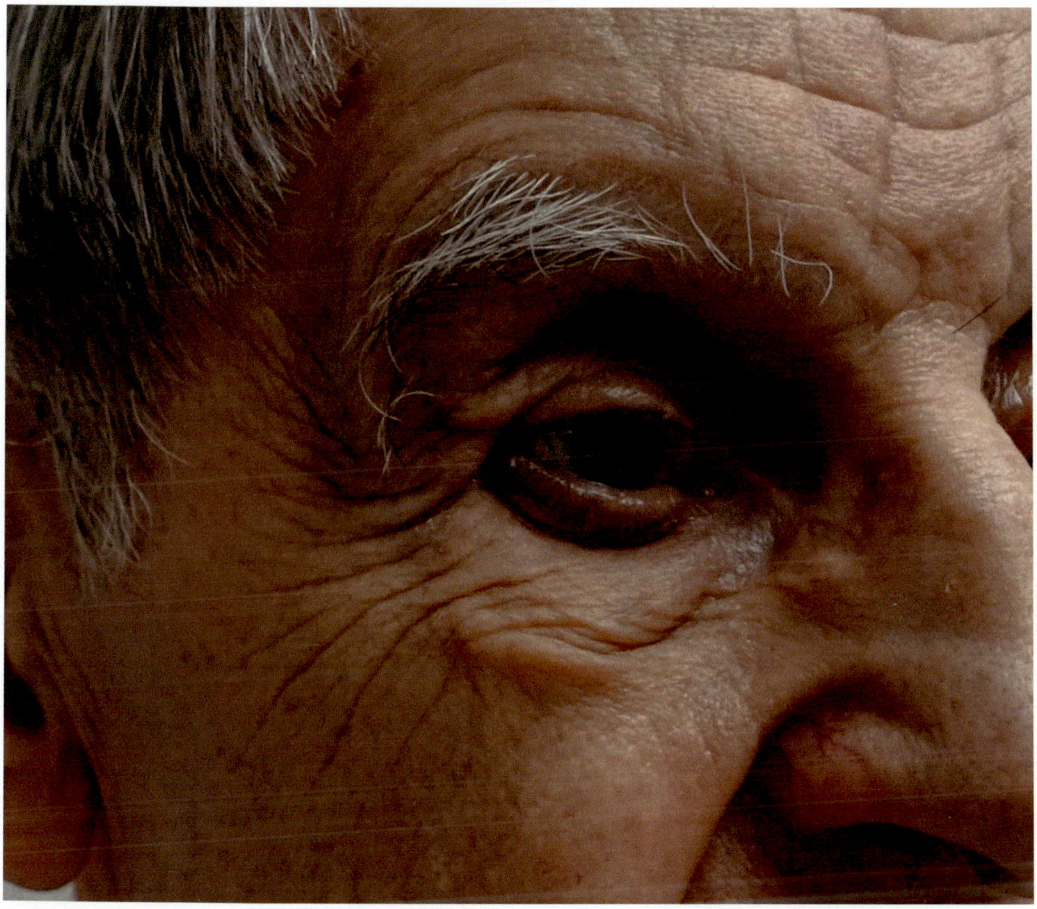

Fig. 12 Patient in Fig. 11 4 months post lower eyelid ectropion repair with skin graft from upper eyelid. Fair complexion and thin skin with inferior edge of graft place near the palpebromalar groove contribute to good aesthetic result and minimally conspicuous scarring

4 Complications

Cicatricial ectropion repair with full thickness skin graft typically has a high success rate with minimal graft failure or necrosis. However, it is important to consider some of the complications that can occur with skin grafting.

4.1 Graft Failure or Necrosis

A hematoma or seroma can separate the graft from the wound bed. This prevents the graft from receiving vital nutrition from the donor site and increases the risk of graft failure. Appropriate pressure dressing or anchoring sutures can help decrease this risk. Some surgeons also advocate for providing slit incisions to allow egress of fluid and promote adherence and graft-donor opposition. Graft infection can also occur and may lead to graft failure.

If graft failure is evident it may require debridement or repeat surgery. However, the authors advocate expectant management and leaving the graft as a biological dressing to cover the wound until the time of revision surgery. In some instances, portions of the graft may take and other areas healed through second intention may result in a stable, adequately positioned eyelid.

5 Primary Contracture/ Secondary Contracture

The full-thickness-skin graft (FTSG) is more likely to have primary contracture after harvest due to the passive recoil of elastin fibers in the dermis. This will reduce the amount of added anterior lamellar support and makes recurrence more likely or cicatricial retraction a possibility. To avoid this, it is important to harvest a graft that is 1–2 mm larger than the lamellar defect. Split thickness skin grafts (STSG) may not have as much primary contracture because they have a smaller proportion of the dermis.

Unlike STSG, full thickness grafts are less likely to shrink with time because there is usually a less robust myofibroblast deposition. However, it is possible to see FTSG shrink with time, especially in cases of facial burns or cutaneous chemical injuries.

5.1 Scarring

Skin grafts may lead to conspicuous scarring at the graft interface or may result in skin tone or texture mismatch. The use of upper eyelid skin may minimize these risks owing to the more similar and thinner skin. Nevertheless, hypertrophic scarring can be managed medically or surgically. In general, within 6 months, corticosteroid or 5 fluorouracil injections may be useful. Surgical revision may have a role in mature scars.

5.2 Donor Site Morbidity

Ipsilateral or contralateral upper eyelid skin is an ideal tissue match for the lateral eyelid defect; however, large grafts may cause anterior lamellar shortage to the upper eyelid. Hence upper eyelid skin harvest should obey resection parameters and principles of blepharoplasty. Additionally, harvesting skin laterally may be more resistant to upper eyelid malposition or lagophthalmos.

The retroauricular site is also a common harvest site. It is usually thin, non-hair-bearing and camouflages a surgical incision well. If a patient wears spectacles, the harvest site should be inferior and away from the resting position of the spectacle temple piece.

5.3 Overcorrection

Although rare, it is possible to overcorrect the lower eyelid. Entropion or reverse ptosis can be seen and usually requires raising and debulking the graft to shorten the subciliary anterior lamellae.

6 Conclusion

Cicatricial ectropion is common. Surgical release of all cicatricial vectors followed with full-thickness skin grafting and horizontal eyelid tightening remains one of the most effective treatments but can leave a conspicuous scar. Patient selection, skin graft harvest site choice and good technique are important variables. In special scenarios, other procedures including midface lift, spacer graft placement, canthoplasty, or eyelid suspension flaps, may be indicated.

Surgical Management of Cicatricial Entropion

Jacob Lifton, Elana Meer and M. Reza Vagefi

Abstract

Cicatricial entropion arises from contracture of the posterior lamella of the eyelid. It may occur in response to chemical insult, infection, inflammatory disease, surgery, or trauma. Inward misdirection of eyelashes towards the globe may lead to ocular surface decompensation. This chapter describes evaluation and surgical management of cicatricial entropion.

Keywords

Cicatricial entropion · Conjunctival scarring · Trichiasis · Trachoma

Illustrations by Maureen Lifton

Supplementary Information The online version contains supplementary material available at https://doi.org/10.1007/978-3-031-36175-3_15.

J. Lifton · E. Meer
Department of Ophthalmology, University of California San Francisco, San Francisco, CA, USA

M. R. Vagefi (✉)
Department of Ophthalmology, Division of Oculofacial Plastic and Orbital Surgery, Tufts University School of Medicine, Boston, MA, USA
e-mail: reza.vagefi@tuftsmedicine.org

1 Introduction

Cicatricial entropion arises from vertical shortening of the posterior lamella of the eyelid, resulting in non-reducible, posterior rotation of the eyelid margin. Tarso-conjunctival scarring and contracture may occur in response to chemical insult, infection, inflammatory disease, surgery, or trauma. Inward malposition of the eyelid margin will misdirect eyelashes posteriorly towards the globe, predisposing the ocular surface to breakdown and, ultimately, decompensation if not promptly recognized and addressed.

The goal of surgical treatment is to alleviate patient discomfort, protect the ocular surface, and minimize the risk of future reversion. Definitive treatment of cicatricial entropion may be difficult since the underlying etiologies can be chronic and progressive. Recurrence rates after surgical correction are high, and many patients require multiple procedures over their lifetime. This chapter will aim to provide an overview of the various etiologies of cicatricial entropion as well curate surgical approaches that may be used to correct it.

2 Clinical Presentation

Cicatricial entropion usually presents with signs and symptoms of tearing, foreign body sensation, conjunctival injection, and mucoid discharge in the presence of persistent internal

J. P. Tao (ed.), *Plastic Surgery of the Lower Eyelids*,
https://doi.org/10.1007/978-3-031-36175-3_15

rotation of the upper and/or lower eyelid. Generally, the internal rotation of the eyelid cannot be manually reduced. This is a key feature that distinguishes cicatricial and involutional etiologies. There can also be varying degrees of eyelid retraction, as the tarsus may become thickened and shortened; and the vectors of scar contracture will generally act to pull the eyelid margin towards the fornix, away from the limbus.

Examination at the slit lamp may reveal distichiasis, trichiasis, posterior displacement of the meibomian gland orifices, conjunctivalization of the eyelid margin, palpebral subconjunctival fibrosis, symblephara, shortening of the fornix, and/or keratopathy. It should be noted that there may be cases of combined cicatricial and involutional entropion in which a component of horizontal eyelid laxity is also present. In such patients, both etiologies of entropion should be addressed with a combined surgical procedure.

3 Etiologies

Cicatricial entropion may be divided into two distinct categories: those which are stable and unlikely to progress; and those which are chronically active and prone to progression. It is crucial to differentiate between these two subsets prior to intervening, as stable disease lends itself well to surgical correction alone, whereas progressive disease may require more complex procedures in conjunction with local and/or systemic immunotherapy to control the underlying cicatricial process.

4 Non-progressive Cicatricial Entropion

Non-progressive cicatricial entropion is typically due to an isolated external insult, such as chemical injury, trauma, surgery, infection, or radiation (Fig. 1). Management of such cases involves correction of the underlying anatomical derangement with the choice of procedure depending on the location and severity of the entropion.

4.1 Medical Management of Non-progressive Cicatricial Entropion

Topical Therapy

Medical therapy in non-progressive cicatricial entropion typically consists of supportive ocular lubrication with artificial tears, emollients, and/or ointments with the goal of maintaining the ocular surface integrity until surgical correction can be performed.

Local Antifibrotic Therapy

Local injection of antifibrotic agents such as 5-fluorouracil (5-FU) and mitomycin C (MMC) have long been used in ophthalmology to prevent unfavorable conjunctival scarring in glaucoma filtering procedures [1, 2] 5-FU may also be employed to remodel cutaneous hypertrophic healing, contractures, and keloids in an off-label dermatologic application [3–5]. Local antifibrotic therapy has not been described as a surgery-sparing treatment for non-progressive cicatricial entropion. However, given its successful use as an adjunct in chronic progressive cicatricial disease, it may be reasonable to consider its application within the acute healing phase after an initial insult or as a post-operative measure when significant or repeat conjunctival manipulation may result in robust wound healing.

5 Chronic Progressive Cicatricial Entropion

The leading cause of progressive cicatricial entropion in the world is infection secondary to *Chlamydia trachomatis*. Nonetheless, a variety of mucosal inflammatory disorders are known to elicit progressive tarso-conjunctival scarring leading to similar consequences. These

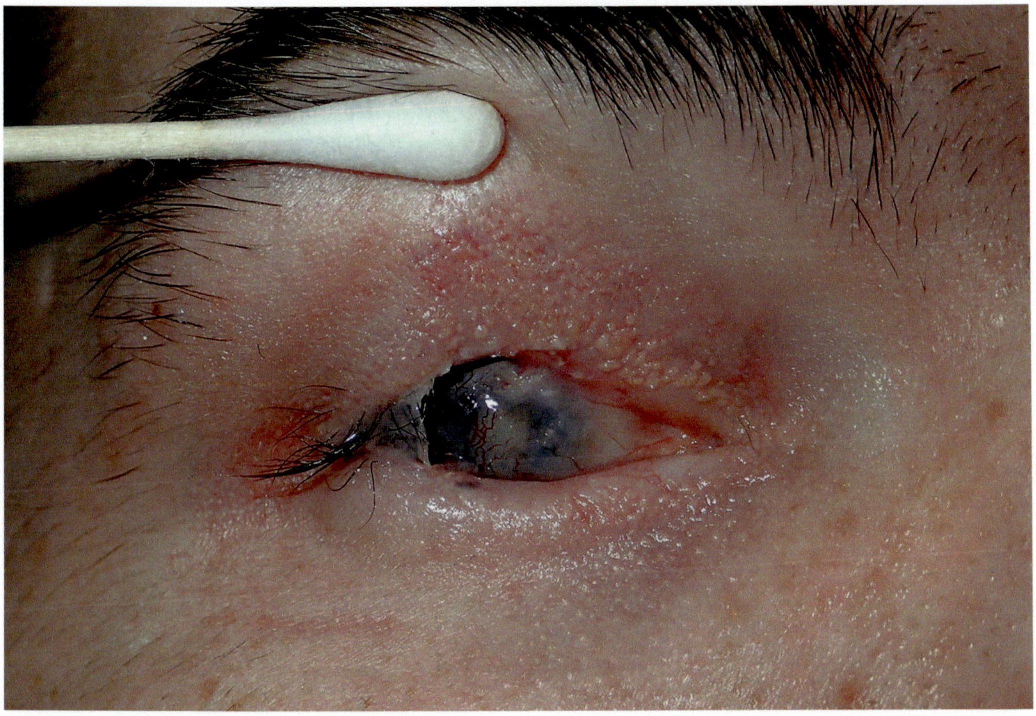

Fig. 1 Nonprogressive cicatricial entropion in the setting of an alkali injury: 29-year-old man with alkali injury of the right eye resulting in a cicatricial entropion of the lower eyelid, upper eyelid adhesion to cornea, and corneal opacification with neovascularization (*Photo courtesy* Steven Couch)

inflammatory conditions tend to be chronic and may require long-term immunomodulatory therapy, as uncontrolled disease activity can lead to further contracture of the palpebral conjunctiva and worsening of the entropion. Because their causes are usually systemic in nature, they may require a multidisciplinary approach involving ophthalmology, dermatology, and/or rheumatology.

5.1 Ocular Cicatricial Pemphigoid (See also Chapter "Inflammatory Symblepharon")

Ocular cicatricial pemphigoid (OCP) is a subtype of a mucous membrane pemphigoid (MMP), and is one of the more common causes of progressive cicatricial entropion [6]. As with other variants of pemphigoid, OCP is thought to be governed by a type II hypersensitivity reaction of auto-antibodies directed against integrins and laminins located in the hemidesmosomes of the conjunctiva and squamous epithelium [7, 8]. The resulting local inflammatory response leads to the formation of epithelial bullae, migration of inflammatory cells into the substantia propria, followed by fibroblast activation and subepithelial fibrosis.

OCP presents primarily as a relapsing–remitting conjunctivitis that can scar the conjunctiva and tarsus, resulting in shortened fornices, symblephara, cicatricial entropion, meibomian or lacrimal gland dysfunction, limbal stem cell deficiency, and keratinization of the ocular surface (Fig. 2) [9, 10]. Disease staging has been described using the degree of conjunctival scarring and associated findings or forniceal depth (Tables 1 and 2) [11, 12]. If the disease involves the eyelid margin and lash follicles, trichiasis may result [9]. Despite carrying the moniker "ocular", it commonly involves the skin (~25% of

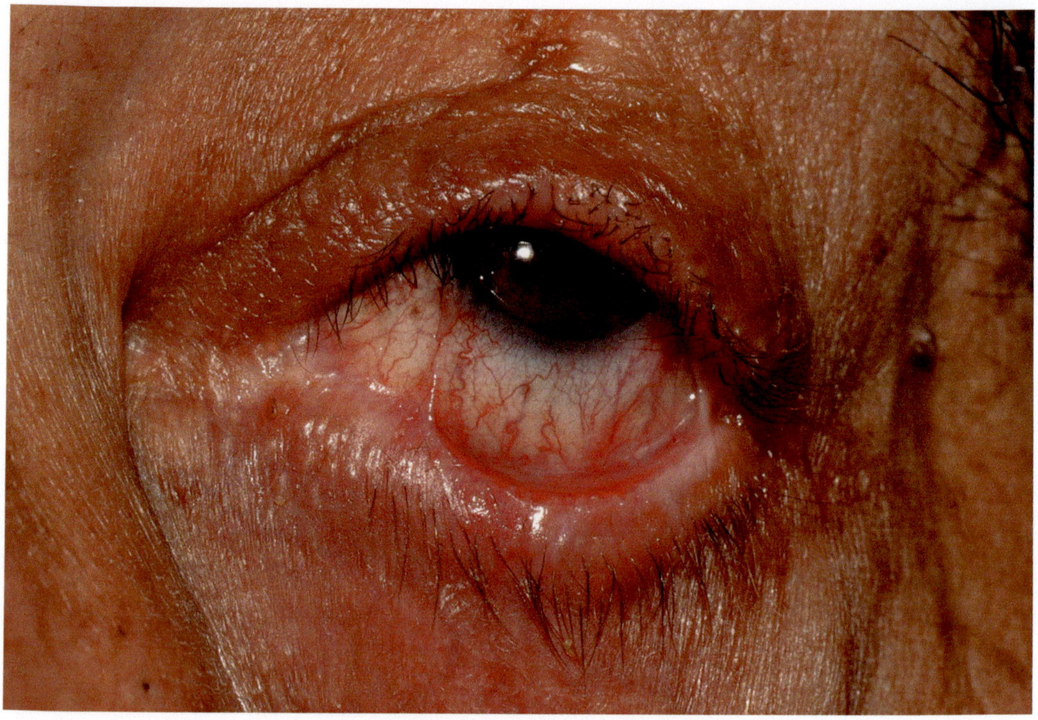

Fig. 2 Progressive cicatricial entropion in setting of ocular cicatricial pemphigoid (OCP): 65-year-old man with OCP resulting in symblephara and contraction of inferior fornix, keratinization of the lower eyelid margin, and upper eyelid entropion on the left side

Table 1 Foster classification of ocular cicatricial pemphigoid [11]

	Clinical findings
Stage I	Chronic mild conjunctivitis, tear dysfunction, subconjunctival fibrosis
Stage II	Cicatrization with conjunctival shrinkage, distorted anatomy, forniceal shortening
Stage III	Symblepharon formation, subepithelial scarring, cicatricial entropion
Stage IV	Keratoconjunctivis sicca, ankyloblepharon, restricted motility from symblephara, conjunctival and corneal keratinization

Table 2 Mondino and Brown classification system for ocular cicatricial pemphigoid [12]

	Clinical findings
Stage I	Loss of forniceal depth ≤25%
Stage II	Loss of forniceal depth 25–50%
Stage III	Loss of forniceal depth 50–75%
Stage IV	Loss of forniceal depth >75%

cases) and other mucous membranes, including the oral mucosa (85–100% of patients), esophagus, pharynx/larynx, and genitourinary tracts [6].

A diagnosis of OCP can be confirmed by a conjunctival biopsy with direct immunofluorescence (DIF), revealing linear accumulation of immunoglobulins along the epithelial basement membrane. However, due to skip lesions and the variability of local disease activity, a negative biopsy result does not exclude a diagnosis of OCP [13, 14]. Therefore, accurate diagnosis requires high clinical suspicion, and repeat biopsy may be indicated.

5.2 Stevens-Johnson Syndrome/ Toxic Epidermal Necrolysis (See also Chapter "Inflammatory Symblepharon")

Stevens-Johnson Syndrome/Toxic Epidermal Necrolysis (SJS/TEN) is a spectrum of severe type IV hypersensitivity reaction that can lead to mucocutaneous blistering, sloughing, and progressive mucosal scarring. It is typically triggered by an offending drug (i.e., antibiotics, anti-epileptics), and in its acute phase requires inpatient admission for systemic immunosuppression and wound care [15, 16].

Ocular involvement is seen in 40–84% of patients in the acute phase of the disease, manifesting as hyperemia and ulceration of the conjunctiva and eyelid margin [16–18]. Long-term sequelae primarily result from destruction of the conjunctival goblet cells, limbal stem cells, accessory lacrimal tissue, and meibomian glands, leading to dry eyes and refractory ocular surface disease. However, SJS/TEN also has the propensity to cause cicatricial changes to the eyelid and conjunctiva including symblephara, cicatricial entropion, forniceal shortening, keratinization, trichiasis, and/or distichiasis (Fig. 3).

While these findings may remain stable after resolution of the acute phase, many patients develop chronic recurrent cicatrizing conjunctivitis despite removal of the offending trigger [19]. In severe cases, the cicatrizing conjunctivitis of SJS can be clinically indistinguishable from that of OCP with reports of DIF demonstrating linear immunoglobulin deposition along the basement membrane in SJS patients similar to OCP [19]. The pathophysiology of such chronic conjunctival inflammation in SJS is unclear, but is thought to be due to a combination of persistent endogenous inflammation

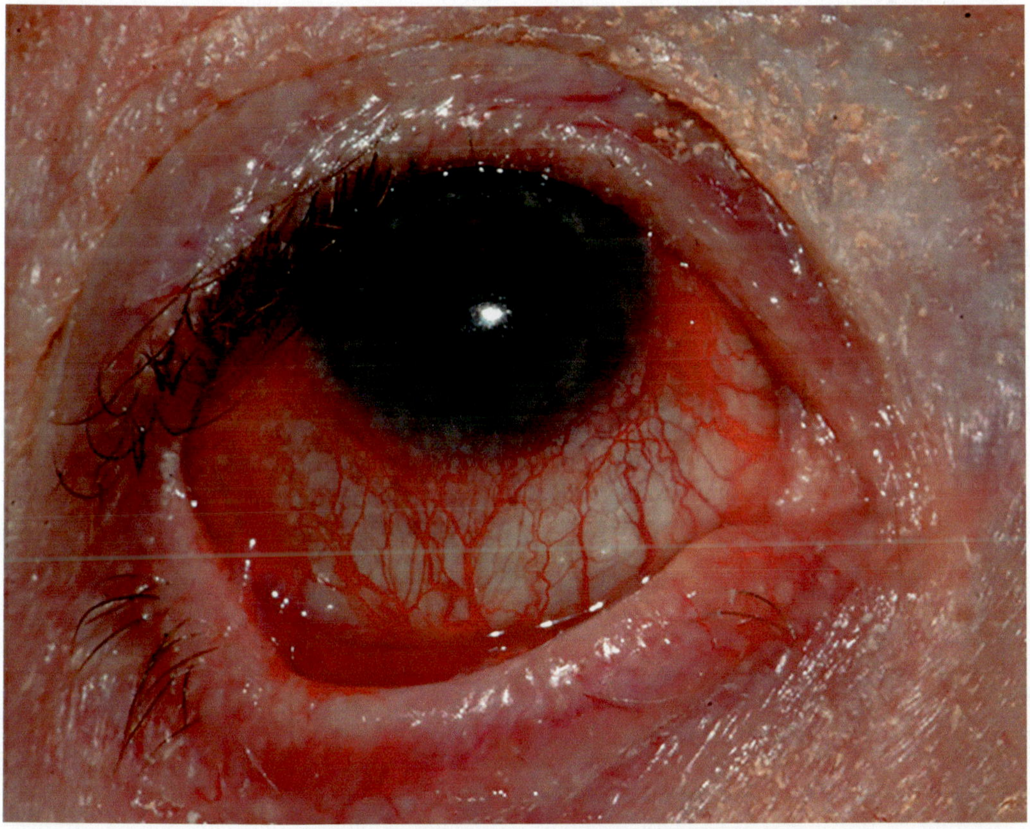

Fig. 3 Progressive cicatricial entropion in setting of Stevens-Johnson Syndrome (SJS): 55-year-old woman with history of SJS resulting in a cicatricial entropion of right upper eyelid, symblepharon of right lower eyelid, keratoconjunctivitis sicca and limbal stem cell deficiency (*Photo courtesy* Gerami Seitzman)

triggered by the inciting agent as well as chronic mechanical irritation (i.e., from keratoconjunctivitis sicca, trichiasis, distichiasis or eyelid margin keratinization). As such, the aim of treatment should be to neutralize these external irritative factors and suppress the endogenous immune response.

5.3 Trachoma

Trachoma is an infectious disease caused by the gram-negative bacterium *Chlamydia trachomatis* (serovars A-C) which through repeated bouts of severe keratoconjunctivitis can cause conjunctival scarring, trichiasis, cicatricial entropion and ultimately corneal opacification. An estimated 1.9 million people across developing countries suffer from some degree of visual impairment from trachoma, most of whom are concentrated in the poorest rural areas of Africa, Asia, Australia, and the Middle East [20, 21]. As such, trachoma is the leading infectious cause of preventable blindness in the world.

C. trachomatis is spread via direct inoculation of the conjunctiva with live bacteria, be it through contact with contaminated secretions, fomites (e.g., towels, bedding), or species of eye-seeking flies such as *Musca sorbens*, which feed on human mucus and discharge. Active infection presents as a follicular conjunctivitis with preferential involvement of the palpebral conjunctiva of the upper eyelids. Large conjunctival follicles of the upper eyelid may leave depressions in the superior cornea known as Herbert pits which are pathognomonic for trachoma. Active, untreated infection can last between three to eight weeks, but there can be persistent smoldering conjunctival inflammation for many weeks after clearing the bacterium [22, 23]. Re-infections are extremely common in endemic areas, and with each episode, the likelihood of developing conjunctival scarring and its associated sequelae increases. It is estimated that over 150 bouts of trachoma are needed to precipitate trichiasis or cicatricial entropion [22, 23]. Once trachomatous trichiasis has developed, the chronic conjunctival inflammation associated with lash-globe touch predisposes the patient to further re-infection and conjunctival scarring. Examination at this stage may reveal white bands of palpebral conjunctival fibrosis just posterior to the eyelid margin (Arlt line), varying degrees of entropion, and if left untreated, ulcerative keratitis, corneal opacification, and neovascularization. Thus, visual impairment from trachoma is often quite delayed from the time of initial infection, presenting ample opportunity to intervene prior to vision-threatening stages.

The World Health Organization (WHO) has proposed the SAFE strategy as a framework for managing trachoma: 'S' for surgical correction of trichiasis, 'A' for antibiotics (usually with mass azithromycin distribution at a community level), 'F' for facial cleanliness, and 'E' for environmental changes to sanitation [20]. Surgical correction can be undertaken via a bilamellar or posterior lamellar fracture with marginal rotation (both described later in this chapter) with similar levels of efficacy [24].

While it remains unclear whether the chronic conjunctival inflammation in trachoma is due to mechanical irritation, a smoldering auto-inflammatory reaction, and/or some degree of active infection, trachomatous trichiasis is more likely to recur if surgery is performed on inflamed conjunctiva [25–28]. Some studies have suggested that administering perioperative azithromycin may lessen the chance of recurrence; however, this evidence remains limited and heterogeneous [25, 29, 30]. Systematic review of the literature found no clear role for perioperative antibiotics [24].

5.4 Other Etiologies

While OCP, SJS/TEN, and trachoma are the most common causes of chronic progressive cicatricial entropion, clinicians should be aware of other etiologies that can present similarly (Table 3) [31–47].

Table 3 Other etiologies of chronic progressive cicatricial entropion

	Description	Clinical findings	Medical management
Lichen planus [31]	Chronic immune-mediated disease of unknown etiology that affects the skin, nails, hair, and mucous membrane. More commonly seen in women with peak onset between the ages of 30 to 60	Cicatricial conjunctivitis with subepithelial fibrosis, fornix shortening, and symblepharon formation ± involvement of lacrimal drainage system	Long-term immunosuppressive therapy Topical cyclosporine and corticosteroid for ocular involvement
Reactive infectious mucocutaneous eruption (RIME) [32, 33]	Classically seen in adolescent patients with prodromal cough followed by severe mucositis of two or more mucous membranes with or without a cutaneous rash. Most commonly secondary to mycoplasma pneumoniae infection	Conjunctival shrinkage, corneal ulceration, blindness, synechiae, dry eyes, loss of lashes	No standardized treatment. Trials of therapy with topical corticosteroids, cyclosporine, intravenous immunoglobulin, and oral corticosteroids
Atopic keratoconjunctivitis [34–36]	Chronic inflammatory disease affecting the conjunctiva and cornea seen in patients with atopic dermatitis. Peak incidence is between 30 to 50 years of age. Pathophysiology is incompletely understood but felt to represent a combination of genetic predisposition, immune dysregulation of IgE mediated pathways, and type IV delayed hypersensitivity reactions	Eyelids and periorbital skin may show evidence of eczematous dermatitis (erythematous, thickened dry skin with blistered patches), tylosis with crusting and scaling, and meibomian gland disease. Conjunctiva, cornea, and anterior segment findings are also common	Mild disease: hand hygiene, cold compresses, antihistamines, mast cell stabilizers Moderate disease: topical steroids, topical calcineurin inhibitors (cyclosporine, and tacrolimus) Severe/recalcitrant disease: oral steroids, supratarsal triamcinolone, systemic cyclosporine
Allergic conjunctivitis [37]	One of the most common forms of conjunctivitis occurring because of host immune response to environmental allergens through IgG4 mediated hypersensitivity reactions	Hyperemic and edematous conjunctiva with prominent tarsal papillae (papillary conjunctivitis), mucoid discharge, occasional scarring and symblepharon ± Horner-Trantas dots	Mild disease: hand hygiene, cold compresses, antihistamines, mast cell stabilizers Moderate disease: topical steroids, topical calcineurin inhibitors (cyclosporine, and tacrolimus) Severe/recalcitrant disease: oral steroids, supratarsal triamcinolone, systemic cyclosporine
Ocular rosacea [38–41]	A subtype of rosacea which is a chronic inflammatory acneiform skin condition. Ocular involvement seen in up to 60% of patients. Pathophysiology is attributed to an altered immune response with upregulation of specific cytokines and metalloproteinases with associated vascular dysregulation	Erythematous changes involving malar region, nose eyelids, ranging from mild discoloration to severe violaceous changes to skin tone with telangiectasias of the eyelid margin, and meibomian gland dysfunction. Late findings may include rhinophyma, Morbihan syndrome, and corneal damage ranging from mild punctate epithelial keratitis (PEK) to corneal neovascularization, infiltration, ulceration and perforation	Conservative management with lifestyle modification, warm compresses, eyelid scrubs, and digital massage. Medical management includes artificial tears and lubricating agents, systemic tetracyclines or macrolides. Immunosuppressive agents such as cyclosporine may also be used to reduce chronic eyelid and corneal inflammation

(continued)

Table 3 (continued)

	Description	Clinical findings	Medical management
Linear IgA dermatosis [42]	A rare subepidermal vesiculobullous disease that occur in both adults and children caused by circulating IgA anti-basement membrane zone antibodies. In the adult form of the disease, a drug induced etiology should be considered with vancomycin responsible for 50% of cases	Chronic cicatricial conjunctivitis with subconjunctival fibrosis and symblepharon formation. Direct immunofluorescence of conjunctiva positive for IgA and C3 in a linear pattern along the epithelial basement membrane	Discontinue vancomycin if offending agent. Disease is exceptionally responsive to dapsone. Antibiotic therapies (e.g., tetracycline class, dicloxacillin, and trimethoprim-sulfamethoxazole) have also shown to control disease. Nicotinamide may be used as adjunctive treatment
Ocular graft-versus-host disease [43–45]	Graft-versus-host disease (GVHD) occurs because of an overactive systemic inflammatory response after allogenic hematopoietic stem cell transplantation and can lead to destruction of normal host tissue. About 40% to 90% of patients with chronic GVHD develop ocular symptoms	Meibomian gland obstruction, anterior and posterior blepharitis, associated scaring of the lacrimal gland leading to decreased tear production. Conjunctival hyperemia with pseudomembrane and/or membrane formation. Chronic inflammation may lead to conjunctival necrosis, cicatrical scarring, and fibrosis. Severe disease may progress from PEK and filamentary keratitis to corneal erosions, thinning, ulceration, and possible perforation	Localized treatment with topical lubricants with preservative-free artificial tears, and/or autologous serum tears. Topical anti-inflammatories are first line and the mainstay of treatment (e.g., topical corticosteroids, topical tacrolimus, topical cyclosporine A, and serum tears). Punctal plugs or punctal cautery may also be applied. Systemic steroids may show efficacy
Pseudopemphigoid medicamentosa [46, 47]	Similar in presentation to ocular cicatricial pemphigoid, but due to long-term use of a topical ophthalmic medication, most commonly for glaucoma. Conjunctival biopsy may show linear staining of conjunctival basement membrane zone	Chronic conjunctival hyperemia and scarring resulting in shortened fornices, symblephara, and eventual cicatricial entropion	Discontinue offending agent

5.5 Medical Management of Non-infectious, Chronic Progressive Cicatricial Entropion

Topical Therapy

Topical therapy is generally supportive and aims to prevent excessive breakdown of the ocular surface due to eyelid malposition, trichiasis and/or distichiasis, all of which will worsen the local inflammatory milieu and produce greater scarring. As with non-progressive entropion, this involves the use of aggressive lubrication with artificial tears, gels, or ointments, and may include scleral contact lenses. However, topical steroid medications such as prednisolone acetate or fluorometholone are often used as adjuncts as well as topical steroid-sparing immunosuppressants such as tacrolimus or cyclosporine.

Bandage Contact Lens

Contact lenses may be used to forestall further ocular surface irritation or damage. They come in various types including standard soft lenses. Scleral lenses vault the cornea and rest on the surrounding sclera. The reservoir anterior to the cornea may be filled with preservative free normal saline to create a tear lens reservoir. Contact lenses are generally not favored for long term use owing to other side effects but they are often an excellent stop gap before surgery.

Local Antifibrotic Therapy

Systemic therapy alone may not adequately control non-infectious, chronic progressive cicatricial entropion, and as such, it may be difficult to performsurgical repair without inducing significant local inflammation.

Jovanovic et al. described injecting subconjunctival 5-FU in a series of 25 eyes with cicatrizing conjunctivitis due to SJS/TEN or OCP, either in tandem with or instead of systemic therapy [48]. The technique involves injection of 0.50–1.0 mL of 5-fluorouracil at 50 mg/mL directly into and beneath scarred conjunctiva. The injections may be repeated every three to five weeks. Over a median follow-up period of 18 months (range: 6 to 36 months) and while adjusting for age, sex, race, and systemic therapy, the patients who were treated with 1 to 4 injections of 5-FU tended to have a greater improvement in visual acuity, lesser requirement for repeat mucous membrane grafting, fewer instances of symblephara, and less corneal scarring compared to those who did not receive injections. Injection of 5-FU also demonstrated a dose-dependent relationship with less corneal scarring and less symblephara at the time of the final encounter [48].

As a corollary, it may be reasonable to utilize local therapy with subconjunctival 5-FU in chronic progressive cicatricial entropion, particularly when it is to establish quiescence prior to surgery, or postoperatively to counteract fibroblast activation and collagen deposition. 5-FU may also be considered as a conservative, first-line treatment in those unable or hesitant to undergo surgery.

Systemic Immunosuppression

Common systemic therapies for systemic inflammatory diseases causing cicatrizing conjunctivitis include corticosteroids, intravenous high-dose immunoglobulin (IVIG), infliximab, mycophenolate mofetil, cyclophosphamide, cyclosporine, and dapsone, either alone or in combination therapy. Generally, these medications should be prescribed collaboratively with an experienced rheumatologist or dermatologist.

Role of Medical Management in Preparing for Surgery

It is generally recommended to defer surgical repair in patients with chronic progressive cicatricial disease until disease quiescence has been established for at least two months prior to surgery, using any combination of the medical treatment options. With disease inactivity, a surgical procedure can hopefully be undertaken with less risk of reactivation or progression, even for those requiring direct incision of the conjunctiva. That said, if selecting between two otherwise comparable procedures, it may be prudent to select the one that minimizes conjunctival trauma. In addition, while evidence is lacking, an intravenous methylprednisolone pulse may be employed on the day of surgery as well as intraoperative steroid injection into the wound bed to further control the post-operative healing response.

6 Grading Scheme and Treatment Algorithm

A grading scheme for cicatricial entropion has not been prospectively validated. However, Kemp and Collin have proposed a classification system for upper eyelid cicatricial entropion that provides a useful framework for stratifying cases of both upper and lower eyelid, progressive and non-progressive entropion [49, 63]. Their grading scheme has been modified to reflect a more granular approach to the disease and to more precisely guide the choice of procedure (Table 4).

When deciding on an approach, it is critical to first determine whether the cicatricial entropion is due to a chronic progressive disease. Once that has been established, a procedure can be selected based on the presence and extent of trichiasis, eyelid retraction, forniceal or tarsal involvement, mucosal keratinization, and distortion of the eyelid margin.

Surgical procedures for cicatricial entropion generally fall into one of three categories: (1) dissociating the anterior from the posterior lamellae via a gray-line eyelid margin split, (2)

Table 4 Proposed cicatricial entropion grading scheme and treatment algorithm

	Characteristics	Procedural/surgical Management
Degree of entropion	Mild: posterior migration of meibomian gland orifices, lash-globe contact in up- or down-gaze	Tarsotomy Alternatives: • Transverse blepharotomy with marginal rotation/ Bilamellar tarsal rotation (Wies procedure) • Excision of skin and orbicularis muscle with tarsal fixation (modified Hotz procedure)[a] • Lower eyelid retractor plication (Jones procedure)[a]
	Moderate: Conjunctivalization of the lid margin, thickening and fibrosis of tarsal plate, lash-globe contact in primary gaze	Tarsotomy Alternatives: • Transverse blepharotomy with marginal rotation/ Bilamellar tarsal rotation (Wies procedure) • Lower eyelid retractor plication (Jones procedure)[a] • Tarsal wedge resection[a]
	Severe: Lash-globe contact in primary gaze with gross tarsal deformity	Modified tarsotomy Alternatives: Tarsal marginal rotation with posterior lamellar super-advancement Posterior lamellar grafting
Special case		**Adjunct procedure**
Eyelid retraction/ posterior lamellar contraction	Severe: >1.5 mm lid retraction, symblepharon, forniceal shortening >50%	Posterior lamellar excision with grafting
Isolated lash-globe contact	Focal trichiasis	Epilation[a] Electrolysis[a] Argon laser ablation[a]
	Broad trichiasis	Cryotherapy Gray line split with cryotherapy[a] Gray line split with anterior lamellar recession[a]
	Metaplastic	Excision of metaplastic lashes with mucous membrane grafting
Mucosal keratinization	Broad area, contacting globe, leading to ocular surface breakdown	Excision of keratinized mucosa with mucous membrane grafting

[a] Conjunctiva-sparing procedures (i.e., those less likely to reactivate chronic progressive cicatrizing disease)

lengthening of the posterior lamella, or (3) rotation/eversion of the eyelid margin. Techniques may be combined with each other as deemed necessary.

7 Procedural and Surgical Management of Cicatricial Entropion

7.1 Removal of Misdirected Eyelashes (See also Chapter "Management of Trichiasis")

Eyelash removal is the least invasive means of preventing the sequelae of lash-globe contact. It is particularly useful when the trichiasis or distichiasis is focal and limited. These procedures can also be performed as a temporizing measure if the patient is unable to undergo surgery in an appropriate time frame. However, the disadvantage of eyelash removal includes induction of a local inflammatory response with ablative therapies, intermediate success rate with a proclivity for recurrence, and inability to address eyelid margin malposition. For this reason, surgical repair is typically the preferred approach, especially when there is a broad area of misdirected lashes or accompanying eyelid malposition.

Epilation

Misdirected eyelashes may be removed manually at the slit lamp by grasping them at their base with fine, non-toothed forceps and pulling them from their follicle. This technique has the advantage of being easy, relatively safe, and non-inflammatory. It also does not require subcutaneous anesthesia. Epilation is considered a temporizing measure, as eyelashes will grow back within four to ten weeks [50]. For some patients, this is preferable to more invasive procedures, or it may serve to bridge them until the trichiasis can be more definitely addressed.

Cryotherapy

More permanent eyelash follicle destruction can be achieved with application of a cryoprobe to the skin overlying the eyelash follicles. Freezing the affected eyelid area twice to -20 degrees Celsius has been demonstrated to be effective and relatively safe. Special instrumentation (thermocouple) will allow precise achievement of the ablative temperature; however, many clinicians simply wait until the underlying skin whitens before removing the cryoprobe.

While effective, cryotherapy is a blunt instrument that is unable to isolate the eyelash follicles from the surrounding eyelid tissue. As such, cryotherapy is prone to complications including local skin depigmentation, eyelid margin notching, destruction of the Meibomian glands, and tarsal atrophy [51, 52]. Cryotherapy can also be painful for the patient, thus adequate topical and subcutaneous anesthesia should be used.

Cryotherapy has been demonstrated to successfully ablate aberrant eyelashes in 84 to 90% of treated eyelids with non-cicatricial disease [51]. For cicatricial trichiasis, success rates appear to be as low at 49% at six months [51, 53]. Due to the diffuse inflammatory response that it produces, cryotherapy should be avoided in cases of uncontrolled cicatrizing conjunctivitis with progression of symblepharon and posterior lamellar scarring observed in up to 77% of such cases [54]. Reactivation of disease after cryoablation appears to be unlikely when OCP is adequately controlled with immunosuppressive therapy. Success rates are still lower than those in non-cicatrizing disease, reaching 40% at 12 months with repeat treatments frequently needed during that time [55].

Electrolysis

In contrast to cryotherapy, electrolysis is highly controlled and targeted, allowing for isolated ablation of eyelash follicles and producing less local inflammation. This makes it a more favorable choice for cases of cicatrizing conjunctivitis. Still, it must be emphasized that cicatrizing disease must be inactive at the time of treatment.

After administration of subcutaneous anesthesia, the slit lamp is used for visualization. The needle electrolysis probe is inserted along the eyelash shaft to the depth of each hair follicle and then 2.0–3.5 mA of current is applied for several seconds. Once a follicle is sufficiently treated, the eyelash will become loose. This is repeated for each eyelash until the desired number have been ablated.

While the effects of electrolysis are precise, they are often temporary. Recurrence rates after a single treatment may be as high as 70% [56]. Repeat treatments can be undertaken to increase the chance of success, but excessive delivery of energy may result in eyelid scarring or notching [57].

Argon Laser Ablation

Argon laser ablation involves applying a blue-green argon laser beam to the base of each eyelash follicle to destroy the eyelash germinal cells. This is ideally done using an Argon laser that is coupled to a slit lamp. The patient's eyelids can then be rotated outward such that the eyelash follicle is oriented in parallel with the laser beam, while the patient looks in the opposite direction of the treatment area. Typically, a laser spot size of 50–200 μm is used with 0.3 s duration and 0.50 Watts of power. Repeated laser burns are applied, starting at the eyelash root and continuing along the shaft of the hair follicle until reaching an approximate depth of two to three millimeters, yielding a small crater at the previous site of the follicle. This may require between 10 to 40 burns per eyelash.

Success rates after one or two treatment sessions range from 54% to 67.9% with recurrence most often being attributable to insufficient deep treatment or failure to apply the beam coaxially with the eyelash [58–62]. Complications include mild eyelid notching and faint hypopigmentation [57]. Furthermore, argon laser appears to be safe in patients with well-controlled cicatrizing conjunctivitis such as OCP (albeit in small case series), without risk of inducing worsening conjunctival shrinkage or symblepharon [62].

7.2 Conjunctiva-Involving Surgical Procedures

Tarsotomy/Tarsal Fracture

Tarsal fracture, also termed tarsotomy is indicated for mild-to-moderate cases of cicatricial entropion. The procedure consists of incising the posterior lamella horizontally to create a hinge, about which the distal eyelid can be rotated outward into its proper position. This approach is particularly effective in cases where the terminal tarsus is selectively contracted. It also does not require cutaneous incisions or grafting, making it more efficient and potentially more aesthetically favorable.

After infiltration with local anesthetic, the lower eyelid is everted over a Desmarres retractor or cotton-tip applicator such that the palpebral conjunctiva is exposed, and the eyelid is held in place with either skin hooks or a eyelid traction suture. A horizontal incision is then made through the palpebral conjunctiva and tarsus, approximately two milimeters proximal to the eyelid margin, until the plane of the orbicularis is reached (Fig. 4). The incision should be extended medially and laterally several millimeters beyond the horizontal extent of any entropion. Blunt dissection between the orbicularis and tarsus may be performed to release any adhesions, allowing for free movement of the anterior and posterior lamella relative to each other. Each end of a double-armed absorbable suture is then passed anteriorly through the palpebral conjunctiva three to four millimeters apart just inferior to the tarso-conjunctival incision. The needles are then directed superiorly through the orbicularis and skin, exiting near the lash line (Fig. 5). Alternatively, instead of passing the needles anteriorly through the palpebral conjunctiva, one end of the double-armed suture may be passed through the proximal cut edge of tarsus parallel to the tarsal plate before each arm is passed through the orbicularis and eyelid skin. Either method of suture placement may be repeated with additional double-armed sutures

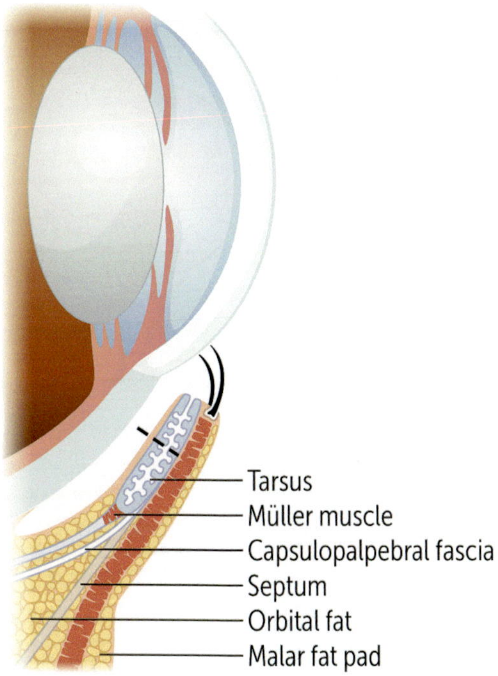

Fig. 4 Tarsotomy: Position of posterior lamellar incision

if the entropion spans the entire eyelid, and their locations adjusted as necessary. The suture is then secured to itself with enough tension to evert the lash line and induce a moderate ectropion, as subsequent contracture during the healing period will tend to cause recurrent inward rotation of the eyelid. The everting sutures may be removed in clinic during the ensuing postoperative weeks if the overcorrection is deemed excessive.

Tarsotomy has been shown to successfully repair mild-to-moderate cicatricial entropion in up to 94% of cases. However, this technique is much less effective for severe cicatricial entropion (defined as gross entropion with tarsal deformity and conjunctival scarring), yielding success rates of 55% [63, 64].

In severe cases of entropion, a simple modification can be made to the standard tarsotomy to increase the likelihood of success. Upon making the horizontal incision through the posterior aspect of the tarsal plate below the eyelid margin, two additional vertical relaxing incisions can be made at both ends of the tarsotomy and carried towards the eyelid margin, yielding a free-floating tarsal island (Fig. 6). This free segment of tarsus should be separated from the orbicularis oculi up to the level of the eyelid margin using meticulous blunt dissection. The everting sutures can then be placed as described above and tied with enough tension to overcorrect the entropion. This approach has been demonstrated to effectively repair severe cicatricial entropion in 81.8% of cases [65].

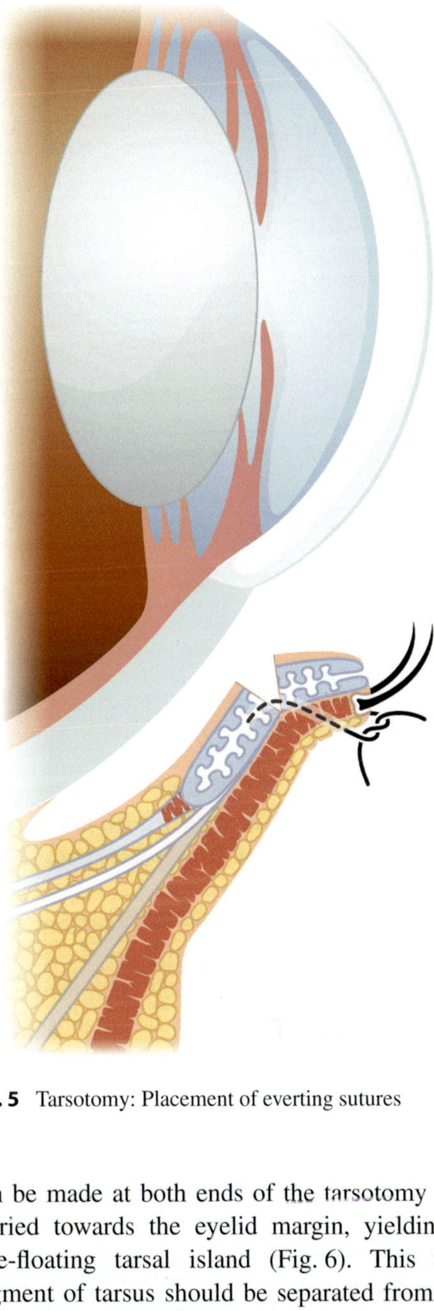

Fig. 5 Tarsotomy: Placement of everting sutures

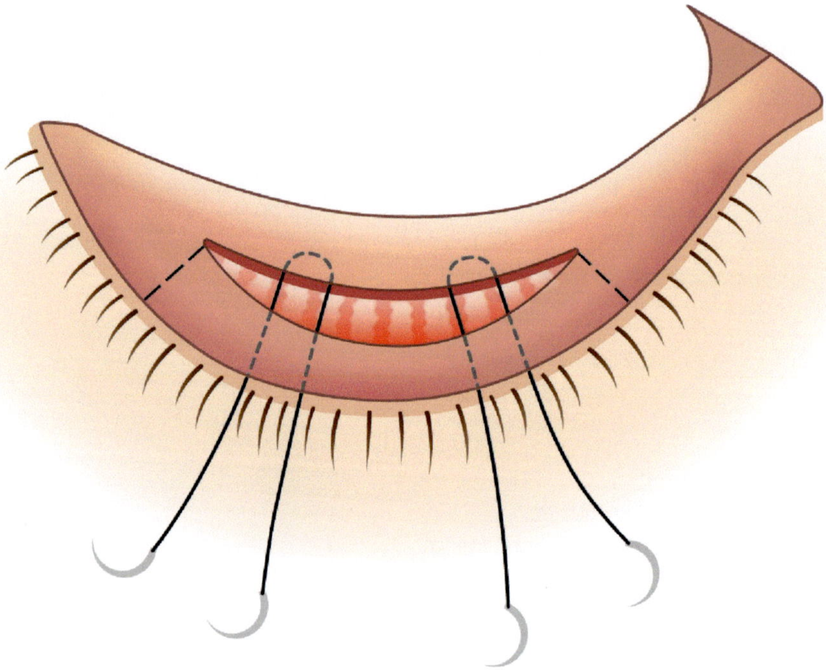

Fig. 6 Modified tarsotomy with incorporation of back-cuts to create a tarsal island

Transverse Blepharotomy with Marginal Rotation/Bilamellar Tarsal Rotation (Wies Procedure)

The basis of the transverse blepharotomy with marginal rotation or bilamellar tarsal rotation is similar to that of the tarsotomy with the goal of creating a hinge through the eyelid about which the distal eyelid margin can be rotated [66, 67]. However, unlike the tarsotomy, this procedure does involve a cutaneous incision and may be less favorable from an aesthetic standpoint. It is known to be effective for mild-to-moderate cicatricial entropion. It is also the endorsed surgery to correct cicatricial entropion secondary to trachoma by the WHO.

The entire length of the eyelid involved by entropion is marked with a surgical pen four millimeters from the eyelid margin. After local anesthetic is injected, a traction suture may be placed in the eyelid. Using a scalpel, a full thickness horizontal eyelid incision is made four millimeters proximal to the eyelid margin. This blepharotomy wound can then be extended temporally and nasally to match the extent of entropion. Double-armed absorbable sutures are passed partial-thickness through the eyelid in a horizontal mattress fashion, starting subconjunctivally through the proximal fragment of tarsus and/or eyelid retractors and then through the orbicularis and eyelid skin of the distal eyelid to exit near the lash line. Of note, sutures exiting closer to the lash line will provide a greater degree of eyelid margin eversion. These suture passes may be repeated to match the horizontal extent of the blepharotomy with each suture placed about two millimeters from its neighbor. The sutures may be passed through silicone bolsters to prevent cheese-wiring through the eyelid skin. The skin edges are closed with an absorbable suture, and the everting sutures are tightened and tied to achieve the desired level of eyelid margin rotation.

Transverse blepharotomy with marginal rotation has been shown to have overall success rates as high as 85%, and with repeat surgeries in cases of recurrent entropion it can reach closer to a 100% success rate [67–69]. A head-to-head randomized clinical trial comparing transverse blepharotomy with marginal rotation to tarsotomy demonstrated equivalent rates of recurrence, but with the former procedure yielding significantly more complications such as eyelid notching or pyogenic granulomas [68, 69].

Tarsal Margin Rotation with Posterior Lamellar Super-Advancement

The tarsal margin rotation with posterior lamellar super-advancement is an upper eyelid surgical procedure [70, 71]. A full-thickness horizontal incision is made in the posterior tarsus approximately three millimeters superior to the eyelid margin along the extent of entropion. The levator aponeurosis is dissected from the anterior face of tarsus distally to prevent lagophthalmos. The freed distal fragment of tarsus is then rotated outwards 180 degrees, hinging on the eyelid margin and thereby displacing the lash line superiorly (Fig. 7). Three sets of double-armed absorbable suture are passed and tied in a horizontal mattress fashion through the anterior lamella—entering above the lash line, engaging Müller muscle just superior to the posterior tarsus while staying in the subconjunctival space. A final set of double-armed horizontal mattress sutures are used to fixate the remaining tarsus to the rotated tarsal fragment such that the posterior lamella is advanced two to three millimeters past the cut end of the fragment. While placing these sutures, care must be taken to prevent tarsal buckling.

A small case series of patients who underwent this procedure suggest it is highly effective at treating cicatricial entropion regardless of etiology with none of the 19 patients developing recurrent entropion or requiring a second surgery [71]. Five eyes exhibited recurrent trichiasis that was successfully addressed with subsequent cryoablation.

Posterior Lamellar Grafting

For severe cases of entropion, the above surgical techniques will prove insufficient in restoring the vertical height of the posterior lamella. Instead, this is typically achieved by way of a posterior lamellar graft. A variety of tissues can be used for this purpose, including donor sclera, hard palate mucosa, nasal or auricular cartilage, orolabial mucosa, or acellular dermis allo- or xenograft. Surgeon familiarity with the donor

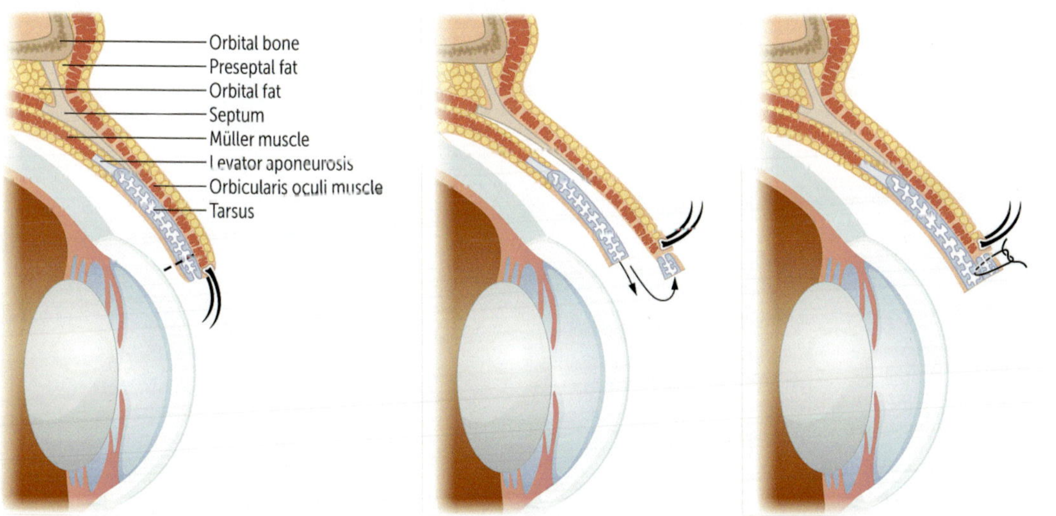

Fig. 7 Tarsal margin rotation with posterior lamellar super-advancement

Table 5 Tissue options for posterior lamellar grafting [72]

Graft tissue	Tissue considerations	Advantages	Disadvantages
Tarsus ± conjunctiva	Graft harvested from ipsi- or contralateral upper lid with preservation of at least 4 mm of remaining tarsus; donor site allowed to heal by second intent	Optimal for exact posterior lamella tissue match with ability to restore eyelid margin	Donor site morbidity, possible graft shrinkage and/or postoperative contraction leading to exacerbation of entropion and ocular surface irritation
Sclera	Tissue banked sclera	Elastic rigidity, biocompatibility, availability, malleable tissue, avoids donor site morbidity	Minor keratopathy, scleral tissue degrades overtime and is quickly replaced by fibroblasts and connective tissue leading to inability to provide long-term elastic support
Auricular cartilage	Cartilage harvested from the scaphoid, root of the helix, or perichondrium of the auricular concha	Minimal donor site morbidity, no size/dimension limitation of donor graft, eventual mucosalization of the perichondrium	Initial lack of mucosal layer leading to ocular surface irritation and discomfort, greater thickness and rigidity compared to tarsus
Nasal cartilage	Cartilage and overlying mucosa harvested from the nasal turbinates or septum	Can include mucosal layer to allow reconstruction of both layers of the posterior lamella, no size/dimension limitation of donor graft, underlying mucosa thicker than buccal mucosa with a lower incidence of contraction	Donor site pain/morbidity, risk of bleeding during harvest, more challenging harvest technique
Hard palate	Mucous membrane graft harvested from the hard palate while avoiding the greater palatine neurovascular bundle originating from the greater palatine foramen	Donor graft tissue matching, donor site not visible, no size/dimension limitation of donor graft, collagen-rich and robust tissue able to recapitulate the structural integrity of the tarsus, low rate of cicatricial contracture	Donor site pain/morbidity, risk of bleeding
Buccal mucosa	Oral mucosa harvested from the lip or cheek	Donor site not visible, soft and flexible, reliable source for reconstructing palpebral mucosa	Painful donor site, lack of structural support necessary to reconstruct tarsal plate, postoperative contraction with increased risk of further exacerbating entropion
Acellular dermis allograft	Acellular dermal matrix of human origin	Spacer for posterior lamella, similar rigidity and plasticity to native tarsus providing structural integrity, biocompatible serving as a matrix for conjunctival tissue growth; no donor site morbidity	Possible keratopathy, tissue degradation by host collagenase, need for further research on long-term outcomes
Acellular dermal collagen xenograft	Acellular bovine or porcine dermal collagen implant	Spacer for posterior lamella with similar rigidity and plasticity to native tarsus; provides a scaffold for fibroblast infiltration and vascularization; no donor site morbidity	Possible keratopathy, host inflammatory response to xeno-tissue, and tissue degradation by host collagenase, need for further research on long-term outcomes

site and tissue preference can help dictate the choice of graft material (see Table 5) [72].

To perform posterior lamellar grafting, the palpebral conjunctiva and tarsus are first split horizontally as in the initial steps of a tarsotomy procedure. A combination of blunt and sharp dissection is used to separate the orbicularis from the posterior lamella, allowing for distraction of the distal tarso-conjunctival fragment away from the proximal fragment and creation of a crescent-shaped recipient bed. The graft of preferred tissue is then prepared such that the horizontal width matches that of the recipient bed, and the vertical height is *oversized* by approximately 50%. This will accommodate postoperative contraction that would otherwise tend to re-invert the eyelid.

Interrupted absorbable sutures are used to secure the borders of the graft to the proximal and distal tarso-conjunctival fragments. Double-armed absorbable sutures are passed through the middle of the graft through the orbicularis and eyelid skin, exiting anteriorly. The arms are then secured over bolsters on the eyelid skin that serve to support the graft, preventing the formation of potential space between the graft and anterior lamella that may lead to graft failure. A symblepharon ring or bolster may be placed in the fornix at the conclusion of the procedure and can be removed at two to four weeks postoperatively.

Evaluation of surgical success rates is limited by sample size. Case series and retrospective cohort studies have demonstrated success rates reaching 85%, with recurrences primarily occurring due to shrinkage of the grafts [72, 73].

7.3 Conjunctiva-Sparing Procedures

Excision of Skin and Orbicularis Muscle with Tarsal Fixation (Modified Hotz Procedure, Hotz-Celsus Procedure), Epiblepharon Repair

An ellipse is marked along the length of the eyelid with the first incision one to two millimeters from the eyelash line and the second incision two to three millimeters away from the primary. After local anesthetic injection, an elliptical incision is made, and the anterior lamellar tissue is excised. Dissection is also performed to expose the anterior tarsal surface. This skin is then closed with an absorbable suture in an interrupted fashion, incorporating passes through the anterior tarsal surface, resulting in rotation of the eyelid margin. Surgery is typically used in the lower eyelid but may be employed in the upper eyelid as well (Fig. 8; Video 1).

Lower Eyelid Retractor Plication (Jones Procedure)

Like the above technique, this procedure incorporates lower eyelid retractor plication and omits resection of the anterior lamella. After

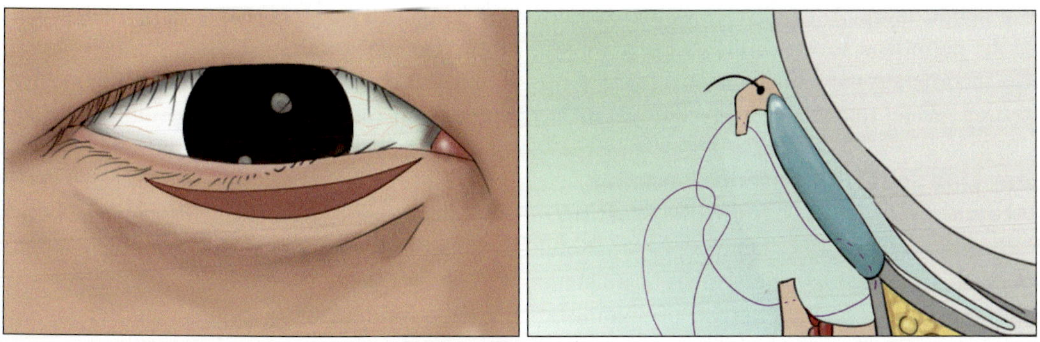

Fig. 8 Epiblepharon repair (illustration by Michael Han)

infiltration with local anesthetic, a horizontal incision is made through skin and orbicularis muscle four to five millimeters inferior to the lower eyelid margin, spanning the width of the eyelid from the lateral canthus to a position lateral to the punctum. The inferior edge of tarsus is exposed along with the orbital septum which is divided to reveal the lower eyelid retractors. Several interrupted absorbable sutures are placed first through the eyelid skin inferior to the wound, then piercing the retractors before being directed anteriorly through the inferior tarsal plate, orbicularis, and skin superior to the incision. The sutures are then secured to themselves resulting in eversion of the eyelid margin.

Tarsal Wedge Resection

Tarsal wedge resection aims to evert the distal tarsus by resecting a wedge of tarsal tissue and placing everting sutures, all without disturbing the palpebral conjunctiva [63, 74]. It may be particularly useful if the tarsus is significantly thickened and contracted.

Local anesthesia is applied subcutaneously along the eyelid. A horizontal skin incision is made along the length of the tarsus in the upper eyelid crease. Scissors may be used to facilitate the sub-orbicularis dissection for exposure of the tarsus. A wedge of tarsal tissue is then removed to create a trough in the central tarsus. Interrupted absorbable sutures may then be passed through the edges of the created tarsal wedge and when secured, result in eversion of the eyelid margin. Skin is then closed with an absorbable suture over the everting tarsal sutures in a single layer. Alternatively, wound closure can be performed in which the everting sutures also incorporate the skin incision in one pass, creating greater rotation of the eyelid margin.

Gray Line Split with Anterior Lamellar Recession ± Mucous Membrane Grafting

Recessing the anterior lamella is a useful approach when there are broad areas of trichiatic eyelashes—either in the absence of significant eyelid inversion that would be better addressed with a tarsotomy or transverse blepharotomy with marginal rotation. Anterior lamellar recession may also be used as an adjunct in cases where eyelid-everting procedures do not sufficiently address the trichiasis. Another benefit of this approach is that it is conjunctiva-sparing, making it a suitable first-line option for cases of chronic progressive cicatricial entropion. Anterior lamellar recession may be done with or without placement of a mucous membrane graft (MMG) to the exposed tarsal plate.

After infiltration with local anesthetic, a scalpel is used to incise the grey line from the lateral canthus to a position lateral to the punctum. Blunt dissection along the submuscular plane is performed using scissors until reaching the proximal edge of tarsus. An assistant may aid with visualization of the dissection planes by exerting mild traction on the posterior lamella.

Once the anterior and posterior lamellae are adequately dissociated, the anterior lamella (namely, the skin, orbicularis muscle, and eyelash follicles) should be recessed vertically along the tarsus 3 to 4 mm inferior to the tarsal margin for the lower eyelid, and 5 mm superior to the tarsal margin for the upper eyelid. The anterior lamella is affixed to the anterior tarsal plate through the lash line with interrupted absorbable sutures. It is useful to evert the lash line inferiorly when securing to the anterior, inferior tarsus. By recessing the anterior lamella, dermatochalasis may worsen. A combined or staged blepharoplasty has been shown to be a reasonable option for such instances [75].

The bared tarsus usually needs a MMG (i.e., oral mucosa) as a spacer to forestall recurrence [76]. An oversized MMG is harvested usually from the inner lower lip (Fig. 9). The graft is thinned accordingly, and a combination of interrupted and running absorbable sutures are then used to fixate it to the tarsal bed and eyelid margin (Fig. 10). The host site may be left bare to heal by second intention. Interrupted, buried 5–0 chromic sutures may help with patient comfort during healing of the this oral donor site. A bolstered temporary suture tarsorrhaphy can then be placed to support the graft in place as it heals for the first postoperative week (Video 2).

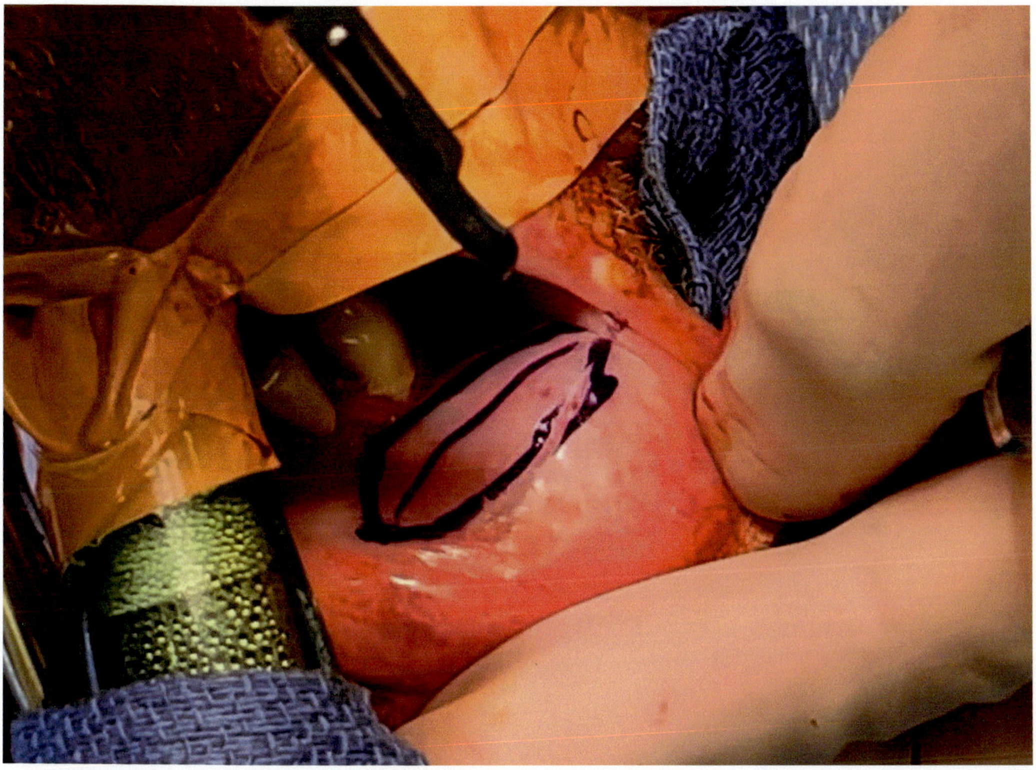

Fig. 9 Mucous membrane graft from the lower lip

Small retrospective case series of anterior lamellar recession have demonstrated recurrence rates between 20 and 40% [75–77].

8 Conclusion

Cicatricial entropion arises from vertical shortening of the posterior lamella of the eyelid, resulting in non-reducible, posterior rotation of the eyelid margin. It can be due to an isolated insult such as trauma or chemical injury, or it can result from a chronic inflammatory process leading to fibrosis, scarring, and shortening of the lamella. Depending on the etiology, cicatricial entropion has the potential to progress or recur, making it one of the more challenging types of eyelid malposition to treat definitively.

Given the wide range of possible presentations and disease severities, surgical approach is best guided by the degree of entropion and tarsal deformity, the amount of posterior lamellar shortening, the presence of isolated lash-globe contact, and whether there is mucosal keratinization. Non-progressive cicatricial entropion may be addressed according to a graduated surgical algorithm. For chronic progressive cases, the surgeon should establish disease quiescence ideally for a minimum of two months prior to surgical intervention, sometimes employing a multimodal approach. Once dormancy has been achieved, chronic progressive etiologies can be treated using the same graduated surgical algorithm as with non-progressive disease. Surgical repair ranges from eyelid margin rotation procedures to more advanced eyelid margin reconstruction with mucous membrane grafts.

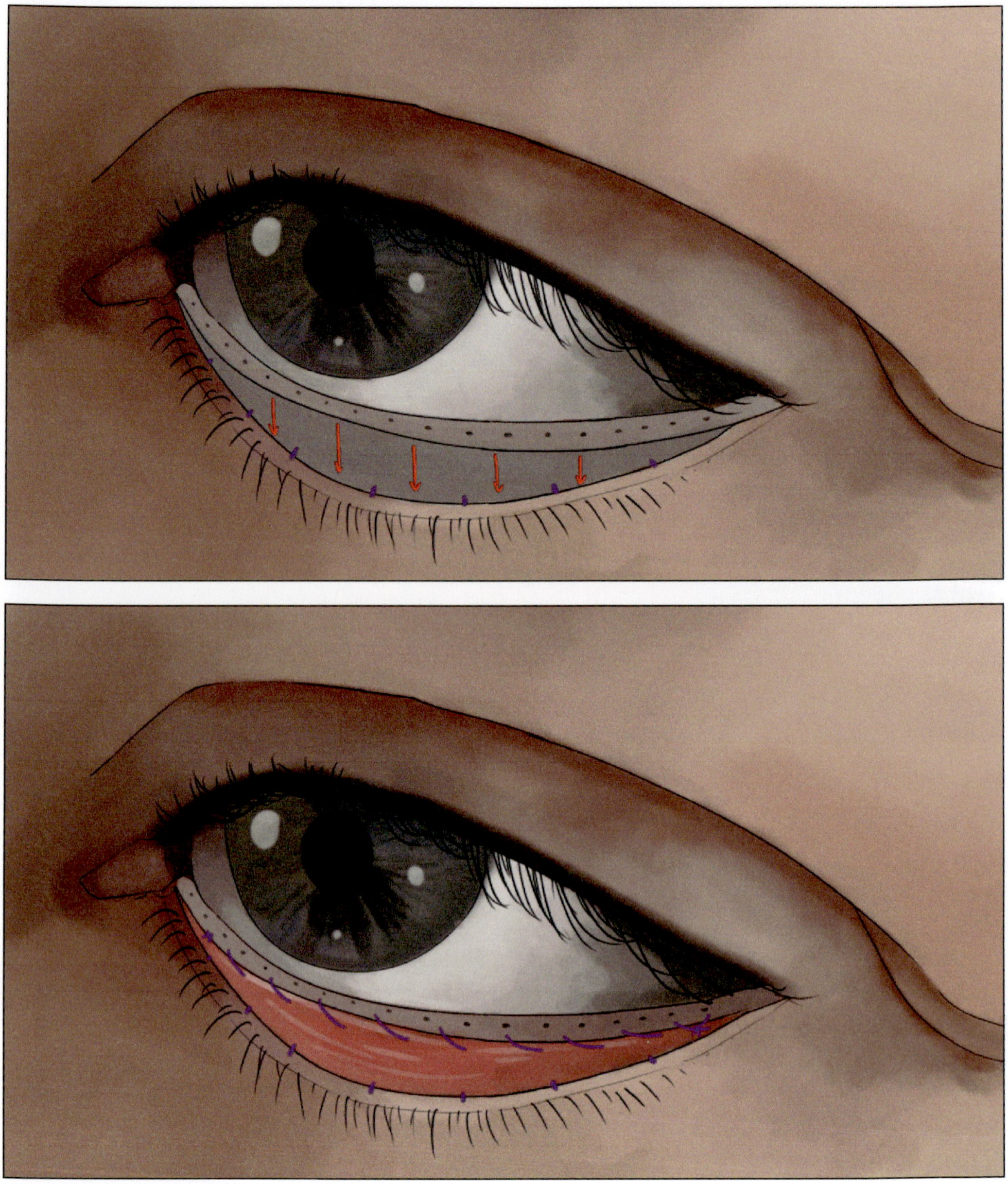

Fig. 10 Eyelid margin splitting, anterior lamella recession, and mucous membrane graft (illustration by Michael Han)

References

1. Heuer DK, Parrish RK, Gressel MG, Hodapp E, Palmberg PF, Anderson DR. 5-fluorouracil and glaucoma filtering surgery II. A pilot study. Ophthalmology. 1984;91(4):384–94. https://doi.org/10.1016/s0161-6420(84)34291-9.
2. Heuer DK, Parrish RK, Gressel MG, et al. 5-Fluorouracil and glaucoma filtering surgery. III. Intermediate follow-up of a pilot study. Ophthalmology. 1986;93(12):1537–46. https://doi.org/10.1016/s0161-6420(86)33542-5
3. Gupta R, Thomas R, Almukhtar F, Kiran A. Use of 5-fluorouracil injections in traumatic cicatricial malposition of eyelids. Plast Reconstr Surg. 2022;150(3):713e. https://doi.org/10.1097/PRS.0000000000009431.
4. Fitzpatrick RE. Treatment of inflamed hypertrophic scars using intralesional 5-FU. Dermatol Surg. 1999;25(3):224–32. https://doi.org/10.1046/j.1524-4725.1999.08165.x.
5. Yoo DB, Azizzadeh B, Massry GG. Injectable 5-FU with or without added steroid in periorbital skin grafting: Initial observations. Ophthal Plast Reconstr Surg. 2015;31(2):122–6. https://doi.org/10.1097/IOP.0000000000000214.
6. Branisteanu DC, Stoleriu G, Branisteanu DE, et al. Ocular cicatricial pemphigoid (review). Exp Ther Med. 2020;20(4):3379–82. https://doi.org/10.3892/etm.2020.8972.
7. Chan RY, Bhol K, Tesavibul N, et al. The role of antibody to human beta4 integrin in conjunctival basement membrane separation: possible in vitro model for ocular cicatricial pemphigoid. Invest Ophthalmol Vis Sci. 1999;40(10):2283–90.
8. Tyagi S, Bhol K, Natarajan K, Livir-Rallatos C, Foster CS, Ahmed AR. Ocular cicatricial pemphigoid antigen: partial sequence and biochemical characterization. Proc Natl Acad Sci U S A. 1996;93(25):14714–9.
9. Chang JH, McCluskey PJ. Ocular cicatricial pemphigoid: manifestations and management. Curr Allergy Asthma Rep. 2005;5(4):333–8. https://doi.org/10.1007/s11882-005-0078-9.
10. Long Q, Zuo YG, Yang X, Gao TT, Liu J, Li Y. Clinical features and in vivo confocal microscopy assessment in 12 patients with ocular cicatricial pemphigoid. Int J Ophthalmol. 2016;9(5):730–7. https://doi.org/10.18240/ijo.2016.05.17.
11. Foster CS. Cicatricial pemphigoid. Trans Am Ophthalmol Soc. 1986;84:527–663.
12. Mondino BJ, Brown SI. Ocular cicatricial pemphigoid. Ophthalmology. 1981;88(2):95–100. https://doi.org/10.1016/s0161-6420(81)35069-6.
13. Labowsky MT, Stinnett SS, Liss J, Daluvoy M, Hall RP, Shieh C. Clinical implications of direct immunofluorescence findings in patients with ocular mucous membrane pemphigoid. Am J Ophthalmol. 2017;183:48–55. https://doi.org/10.1016/j.ajo.2017.08.009.
14. Bernauer W, Elder MJ, Leonard JN, Wright P, Dart JK. The value of biopsies in the evaluation of chronic progressive conjunctival cicatrisation. Graefes Arch Clin Exp Ophthalmol Albrecht Von Graefes Arch Klin Exp Ophthalmol. 1994;232(9):533–7. https://doi.org/10.1007/BF00181996.
15. Chung WH, Wang CW, Dao RL. Severe cutaneous adverse drug reactions. J Dermatol. 2016;43(7):758–66. https://doi.org/10.1111/1346-8138.13430.
16. Morales ME, Purdue GF, Verity SM, Arnoldo BD, Blomquist PH. Ophthalmic manifestations of Stevens-Johnson syndrome and toxic epidermal necrolysis and relation to SCORTEN. Am J Ophthalmol. 2010;150(4):505–510.e1. https://doi.org/10.1016/j.ajo.2010.04.026.
17. Gueudry J, Roujeau JC, Binaghi M, Soubrane G, Muraine M. Risk factors for the development of ocular complications of Stevens-Johnson syndrome and toxic epidermal necrolysis. Arch Dermatol. 2009;145(2):157–62. https://doi.org/10.1001/archdermatol.2009.540.
18. Chang YS, Huang FC, Tseng SH, Hsu CK, Ho CL, Sheu HM. Erythema multiforme, Stevens-Johnson syndrome, and toxic epidermal necrolysis: acute ocular manifestations, causes, and management. Cornea. 2007;26(2):123–9. https://doi.org/10.1097/ICO.0b013e31802eb264.
19. De Rojas MV, Dart JKG, Saw VPJ. The natural history of Stevens Johnson syndrome: Patterns of chronic ocular disease and the role of systemic immunosuppressive therapy. Br J Ophthalmol. 2007;91(8):1048–53. https://doi.org/10.1136/bjo.2006.109124.
20. Trachoma. Accessed 1 Mar 2023. https://www.who.int/news-room/fact-sheets/detail/trachoma
21. Trachoma: global magnitude of a preventable cause of blindness. Br. J. Ophthalmol. Accessed 1 Mar 2023. https://bjo.bmj.com/content/93/5/563.long
22. Taylor HR, Burton MJ, Haddad D, West S, Wright H. Trachoma. Lancet. 2014;384(9960):2142–52. https://doi.org/10.1016/S0140-6736(13)62182-0.
23. Solomon AW, Burton MJ, Gower EW, et al. Trachoma. Nat Rev Dis Primer. 2022;8(1):1–20. https://doi.org/10.1038/s41572-022-00359-5.
24. Burton M, Habtamu E, Ho D, Gower EW. Interventions for trachoma trichiasis. Cochrane Database Syst Rev. 2015;2015(11):CD004008. https://doi.org/10.1002/14651858.CD004008.pub3
25. Burton MJ, Kinteh F, Jallow O, et al. A randomised controlled trial of azithromycin following surgery for trachomatous trichiasis in the Gambia. Br J Ophthalmol. 2005;89(10):1282–8. https://doi.org/10.1136/bjo.2004.062489.
26. Burton MJ, Bowman RJC, Faal H, et al. Long term outcome of trichiasis surgery in the Gambia. Br J Ophthalmol. 2005;89(5):575–9. https://doi.org/10.1136/bjo.2004.055996.

27. Hu VH, Holland MJ, Burton MJ. Trachoma: Protective and pathogenic ocular immune responses to chlamydia trachomatis. PLoS Negl Trop Dis. 2013;7(2): e2020. https://doi.org/10.1371/journal.pntd.0002020.
28. Rajak SN, Habtamu E, Weiss HA, et al. Absorbable versus silk sutures for surgical treatment of trachomatous trichiasis in Ethiopia: a randomised controlled trial. PLoS Med. 2011;8(12): e1001137. https://doi.org/10.1371/journal.pmed.1001137.
29. West SK, West ES, Alemayehu W, et al. Single-dose azithromycin prevents trichiasis recurrence following surgery: randomized trial in Ethiopia. Arch Ophthalmol. 2006;124(3):309–14. https://doi.org/10.1001/archopht.124.3.309.
30. Zhang H, Kandel RP, Atakari HK, Dean D. Impact of oral azithromycin on recurrence of trachomatous trichiasis in Nepal over 1 year. Br J Ophthalmol. 2006;90(8):943–8. https://doi.org/10.1136/bjo.2006.093104.
31. Mohebbi M, Mirghorbani M, Afshan A, Towfighi M. Lichen planus in ocular surface: major presentations and treatments. Ocul Immunol Inflamm. 2019;27(6):987–94.
32. Canavan TN, Mathes EF, Frieden I, Shinkai K. Mycoplasma pneumoniae–induced rash and mucositis as a syndrome distinct from Stevens-Johnson syndrome and erythema multiforme: A systematic review. J Am Acad Dermatol. 2015;72(2):239-245.e4. https://doi.org/10.1016/j.jaad.2014.06.026.
33. Gise R, Elhusseiny AM, Scelfo C, Mantagos IS. Ocular involvement in recurrent infectious mucocutaneous eruption (RIME): a variation on a theme. J Am Assoc Pediatr Ophthalmol Strabismus. 2021;25(1):62–4. https://doi.org/10.1016/j.jaapos.2020.10.003.
34. Correale CE, Walker C, Murphy L, Craig TJ. Atopic dermatitis: a review of diagnosis and treatment. Am Fam Phys. 1999;60(4):1191–8.
35. Guglielmetti S, Dart JK, Calder V. Atopic keratoconjunctivitis and atopic dermatitis. Curr Opin Allergy Clin Immunol. 2010;10(5):478–85. https://doi.org/10.1097/ACI.0b013e32833e16e4.
36. Garrity JA, Liesegang TJ. Ocular complications of atopic dermatitis. Can J Ophthalmol J Can Ophtalmol. 1984;19(1):21–4.
37. Bielory L, Delgado L, Katelaris CH, Leonardi A, Rosario N, Vichyanoud P. ICON: diagnosis and management of allergic conjunctivitis. Ann Allergy Asthma Immunol. 2020;124(2):118–34. https://doi.org/10.1016/j.anai.2019.11.014.
38. Chukwuma O, Saikaly SK, Montanez-Wiscovich M, Winslow C, Motaparthi K. Ocular pseudopemphigoid with concomitant eyelid dermatitis secondary to rosacea. JAAD Case Rep. 2020;7:62–4. https://doi.org/10.1016/j.jdcr.2020.11.007.
39. Ravage ZB, Beck AP, Macsai MS, Ching SST. Ocular rosacea can mimic trachoma: a case of cicatrizing conjunctivitis. Cornea. 2004;23(6):630–1. https://doi.org/10.1097/01.ico.0000126329.00100.9d.
40. Wladis EJ, Adam AP. Treatment of ocular rosacea. Surv Ophthalmol. 2018;63(3):340–6. https://doi.org/10.1016/j.survophthal.2017.07.005.
41. Awais M, Anwar MI, Iftikhar R, Iqbal Z, Shehzad N, Akbar B. Rosacea—the ophthalmic perspective. Cutan Ocul Toxicol. 2015;34(2):161–6. https://doi.org/10.3109/15569527.2014.930749.
42. Aultbrinker EA, Stark MB, Donnenfeld ED. Linear IgA disease: the ocular manifestations. Ophthalmology. 1988;95(3):340–3. https://doi.org/10.1016/S0161-6420(88)33188-X.
43. Balasubramaniam SC, Raja H, Nau CB, Shen JF, Schornack MM. Ocular graft-versus-host disease: a review. Eye Contact Lens. 2015;41(5):256–61. https://doi.org/10.1097/ICL.0000000000000150.
44. Malta JB, Soong HK, Shtein RM, et al. Treatment of ocular graft-versus-host disease with topical cyclosporine 0.05%. Cornea. 2010;29(12):1392–96. https://doi.org/10.1097/ICO.0b013e3181e456f0
45. Kim SK. Ocular graft versus host disease. Ocul Surf. 2005;3(4, Supplement):S-177. https://doi.org/10.1016/S1542-0124(12)70250-1
46. Singh S, Donthineni PR, Shanbhag SS, et al. Drug induced cicatrizing conjunctivitis: a case series with review of etiopathogenesis, diagnosis and management. Ocul Surf. 2022;24:83–92. https://doi.org/10.1016/j.jtos.2022.02.004.
47. External disease and cornea. Basic and clinical science course (BCSC). Vol external disease and cornea. American Academy of Ophthalmology; 2014.
48. Jovanovic N, Russell WW, Heisel CJ, Hood CT, Kahana A. Direct injection of 5-fluorouracil improves outcomes in cicatrizing conjunctival disorders secondary to systemic disease. Ophthal Plast Reconstr Surg. 2021;37(2):145–53. https://doi.org/10.1097/IOP.0000000000001717.
49. Collin J. A manual of systematic eyelid surgery. Churchill Livingstone; 1983.
50. Paus R, Burgoa I, Platt CI, Griffiths T, Poblet E, Izeta A. Biology of the eyelash hair follicle: an enigma in plain sight. Br J Dermatol. 2016;174(4):741–52. https://doi.org/10.1111/bjd.14217.
51. Johnson RL, Collin JR. Treatment of trichiasis with a lid cryoprobe. Br J Ophthalmol. 1985;69(4):267–70.
52. Wingfield DL, Fraunfelder FT. Possible complications secondary to cryotherapy. Ophthalmic Surg. 1979;10(8):47–55.
53. Collin JR, Coster DJ, Sullivan JH. Cryosurgery for trichiasis. Trans Ophthalmol Soc U K. 1978;98(1):81–3.
54. Wood JR, Anderson RL. Complications of cryosurgery. Arch Ophthalmol. 1981;99(3):460–3. https://doi.org/10.1001/archopht.1981.03930010462014.
55. Elder MJ, Bernauer W. Cryotherapy for trichiasis in ocular cicatricial pemphigoid. Br J Ophthalmol. 1994;78(10):769–71.

56. Reacher MH, Muñoz B, Alghassany A, Daar AS, Elbualy M, Taylor HR. A controlled trial of surgery for trachomatous trichiasis of the upper lid. Arch Ophthalmol. 1992;110(5):667–74. https://doi.org/10.1001/archopht.1992.01080170089030.
57. Lyon DB, Dortzbach RK. Entropion, trichiasis, and distichiasis. In: Ophthalmic plastic surgery: prevention and management of complications. Raven Press, Ltd.; 1994. p. 31–48.
58. Bartley GB, Lowry JC. Argon laser treatment of trichiasis. Am J Ophthalmol. 1992;113(1):71–4. https://doi.org/10.1016/s0002-9394(14)75756-3.
59. Huneke J. Argon laser treatment for trichiasis. Ophthalmic Plastic Reconstruct Surg. 1992;8(1):50–5.
60. Sharif KW, Arafat AF, Wykes WC. The treatment of recurrent trichiasis with argon laser photocoagulation. Eye Lond Engl. 1991;5(Pt 5):591–5. https://doi.org/10.1038/eye.1991.102.
61. A comparison of argon laser and radiofrequency in trichiasis treatment. Accessed 19 Oct 2022. https://oce-ovid-com.ucsf.idm.oclc.org/article/00002341-201109000-00002?relatedarticle=y
62. Gossman MD, Yung R, Berlin AJ, Brightwell JR. Prospective evaluation of the argon laser in the treatment of trichiasis. Ophthalmic Surg. 1992;23(3):183–7.
63. Kemp EG, Collin JR. Surgical management of upper lid entropion. Br J Ophthalmol. 1986;70(8):575–9.
64. Kersten RC, Kleiner FP, Kulwin DR. Tarsotomy for the treatment of cicatricial entropion with trichiasis. Arch Ophthalmol. 1992;110(5):714–7. https://doi.org/10.1001/archopht.1992.01080170136042.
65. Chi M, Kim HJ, Vagefi R, Kersten RC. Modified tarsotomy for the treatment of severe cicatricial entropion. Eye. 2016;30(7):992–7. https://doi.org/10.1038/eye.2016.77.
66. Wies F. Surgical treatment of entropion. J Int Surg. 1954;21:758–60.
67. Bleyen I, Dolman PJ. The Wies procedure for management of trichiasis or cicatricial entropion of either upper or lower eyelids. Br J Ophthalmol. 2009;93(12):1612–5. https://doi.org/10.1136/bjo.2008.142505.
68. El Toukhy E, Lewallen S, Courtright P. Routine bilamellar tarsal rotation surgery for trachomatous trichiasis: short-term outcome and factors associated with surgical failure. Ophthal Plast Reconstr Surg. 2006;22(2):109–12. https://doi.org/10.1097/01.iop.0000203494.49446.60.
69. Adamu Y, Alemayehu W. A randomized clinical trial of the success rates of bilamellar tarsal rotation and tarsotomy for upper eyelid trachomatous trichiasis. Ethiop Med J. 2002;40(2):107–14.
70. Seiff SR, Carter SR, Canales JLT y, Choo PH. Tarsal margin rotation with posterior lamella superadvancement for the management of cicatricial entropion of the upper eyelid. Am J Ophthalmol. 1999;127(1):67–71. https://doi.org/10.1016/S0002-9394(98)00277-3
71. Russell DJ, Seiff SR. Long-term results for entropion repair by tarsal margin rotation with posterior lamella superadvancement. Ophthal Plast Reconstr Surg. 2017;33(6):434–9. https://doi.org/10.1097/IOP.0000000000000815.
72. Fin A, De Biasio F, Lanzetta P, Mura S, Tarantini A, Parodi PC. Posterior lamellar reconstruction: a comprehensive review of the literature. Orbit Amst Neth. 2019;38(1):51–66. https://doi.org/10.1080/01676830.2018.1474236.
73. Gu J, Wang Z, Sun M, Yuan J, Chen J. Posterior lamellar eyelid reconstruction with acellular dermis allograft in severe cicatricial entropion. Ann Plast Surg. 2009;62(3):268–74. https://doi.org/10.1097/SAP.0b013e31817d8814.
74. Dutton JJ, Tawfik HA, DeBacker CM, Lipham WJ. Anterior tarsal v-wedge resection for cicatricial entropion. Ophthal Plast Reconstr Surg. 2000;16(2):126–30.
75. Aghai GH, Gordiz A, Falavarjani KG, Kashkouli MB. Anterior lamellar recession, blepharoplasty, and supratarsal fixation for cicatricial upper eyelid entropion without lagophthalmos. Eye. 2016;30(4):627–31. https://doi.org/10.1038/eye.2016.12.
76. Koreen IV, Taich A, Elner VM. Anterior lamellar recession with buccal mucous membrane grafting for cicatricial entropion. Ophthal Plast Reconstr Surg. 2009;25(3):180–4. https://doi.org/10.1097/IOP.0b013e3181a13f0e.
77. Elder MJ, Collin R. Anterior lamellar repositioning and grey line split for upper lid entropion in ocular cicatricial pemphigoid. Eye. 1996;10(4):439–42. https://doi.org/10.1038/eye.1996.96.

Involutional Entropion Repair

Teresa H. Chen, Maria Belen Camacho, Jenny N. Wang and Jeremiah P. Tao

Abstract

Involutional changes, most commonly due to aging, may cause in-turning of the lower eyelid. Eye irritation or ocular surface damage are indications for repair. Factors that contribute to this condition include vertical and horizontal eyelid laxities, as well as overriding of the preseptal orbicularis oculi muscle. Different surgical techniques address key variables in involutional entropion. This chapter details the surgical repair of involutional entropion according to clinical findings.

Keywords

Involutional lower eyelid entropion · Vertical laxity · Horizontal laxity · Overriding preseptal orbicularis oculi

Supplementary Information The online version contains supplementary material available at https://doi.org/10.1007/978-3-031-36175-3_16.

T. H. Chen (✉) · M. B. Camacho · J. N. Wang · J. P. Tao
Divison of Oculofacial Plastic and Orbital Surgery, University of California, Irvine, CA, USA
e-mail: teresahc@hs.uci.edu

1 Introduction

Involutional entropion is the most common cause of entropion in the lower eyelid. Its prevalence increases with age and may have a higher incidence in East Asians compared to non-East Asians [1, 2]. Patients often present with symptoms of foreign body sensation, redness, tearing, and discharge [3]. Several causes of involutional entropion have been described, including vertical and horizontal laxities of the lower eyelid, and overriding of the preseptal orbicularis oculi muscle (Fig. 1) [4, 5]. Surgical repair addresses these factors.

2 Anatomy

The lower eyelid derives stability from the position of the lower eyelid retractors, tightness of the canthal tendons, and tone of the preseptal orbicularis oculi muscle. These components maintain balanced anterior and posterior tension and keep the eyelid apposed to the globe.

2.1 Vertical Laxity

Normally, the lower eyelid retractors (LER) help keep the eyelid margin in normal position by stabilizing the tarsus inferiorly and posteriorly (Fig. 2). In patients with involutional entropion,

J. P. Tao (ed.), *Plastic Surgery of the Lower Eyelids*,
https://doi.org/10.1007/978-3-031-36175-3_16

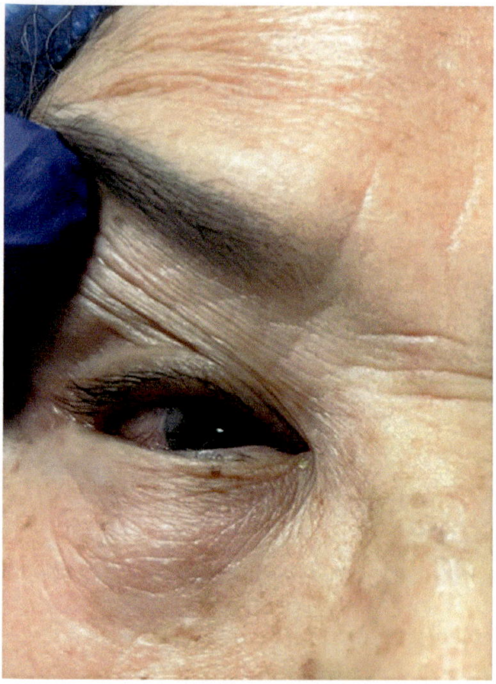

Fig. 1 Involutional entropion. Lax lower eyelid retractors and overriding preseptal orbicularis oculi muscle cause the eyelid margin to turn inward

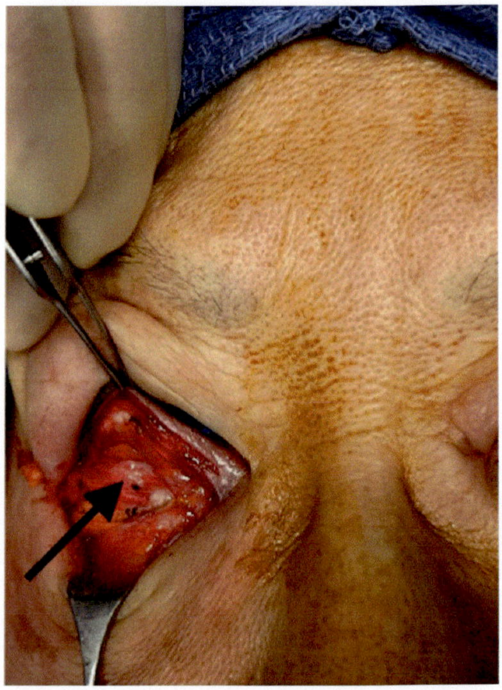

Fig. 2 Lower eyelid retractors (black arrow). The retractors achieve slight inferior and posterior tension on the inferior tarsus, thus stabilizing the eyelid

there is an average increased distance between the LER and the inferior border of the tarsus [6]. When there is laxity or dehiscence of the LER, the inferior edge of the tarsus rotates away from the eye, consequently inverting the eyelid margin. Similarly, as the LER relax with age, the position of the lower eyelid elevates and causes a concomitant reverse ptosis. Lower eyelid retractor function can be evaluated by measuring lower eyelid excursion in downgaze, which is normally around 3–4 mm. On slit lamp examination, a white line of LER that may be visible through the palpebral conjunctiva may signify disinsertion [7].

2.2 Horizontal Laxity

While laxity of the LER is the primary cause of involutional entropion, horizontal laxity is usually present as well. Tarsal plates are attached to the orbital rims by medial and lateral canthal tendons, which lengthen with age. Loosened canthal tendons are demonstrated in about 80% of patients with primary and recurrent involutional entropion [8]. Horizontal laxity can be evaluated with the eyelid distraction and snap-back tests. The eyelid distraction test is performed by pulling the eyelid away from the globe anteriorly, medially, and laterally; signs of excessive horizontal laxity are anterior distraction greater than 6–8 mm, medial displacement of the lower punctum beyond the caruncle, and lateral displacement of the lower punctum beyond the midpoint between the plica and medial corneal limbus [2, 9, 10]. The snap-back test is performed by pulling the lower eyelid inferiorly toward the inferior orbital rim. A normal eyelid returns to its natural position without any blinks, while a lax eyelid will remain away from the eye. The amount of laxity can be estimated with the number of blinks that are required to return the lid to the natural position [10].

2.3 Overriding of the Preseptal Orbicularis Oculi Muscle

The fine attachments of the LER to the orbicularis oculi muscle can also weaken with age, causing the preseptal orbicularis oculi muscle (OOM) to override the pretarsal OOM and rotate the eyelid margin. Overriding of the preseptal OOM has been demonstrated in cadavers and botulinum toxin injections in the preseptal OOM have been shown to be temporarily effective in treating involutional entropion [11, 12]. To elicit override of the preseptal OOM, the patient is instructed to look down while the examiner pinches the central lower eyelid and roll the skin over the superior tarsal border, pressing it against the globe then releasing. With the patient in downgaze, the entropion persists with eye movements and blinking for at least three minutes [13].

3 Surgical Techniques

The aim for surgical treatment is to reestablish the normal position of the LER, restore the tension of the canthal structures, and correct the tone of the preseptal OOM. The approach depends on the patient's anatomy and specifically addressing the contributing factors lead to lower recurrence rates of involutional entropion.

3.1 Correction of Vertical Laxity

Lower Eyelid Retractor Reinsertion

Internal (Transconjunctival) Approach

A 4-0 silk traction suture is placed through the eyelid margin and the eyelid is everted. An incision in the conjunctiva below the inferior tarsal border is made from lateral to the punctum to the lateral canthus. Dissection is continued toward the inferior orbital rim and orbital fat is dissected to expose the LER. The LER are dissected free from the conjunctiva and sutured to the anterior, inferior border of the tarsus with 5-0 or 6-0 polyglactin buried sutures. The conjunctival edges remain in close apposition and no closure is necessary.

External (Subciliary) Approach (Video 1)

A 4-0 silk traction suture is placed through the eyelid margin and a subciliary incision is made, extending from the punctum medially to the lateral canthus laterally (Figs. 3A, 4A). Dissection is continued between the orbicularis and orbital septum toward the inferior orbital rim (Fig. 3B). The orbital septum is opened, and the central lower fat pad is dissected to expose the LER (Fig. 4B). The LER are dissected free from the conjunctiva and sutured to the anterior, inferior border of the tarsus with 6-0 polyglactin

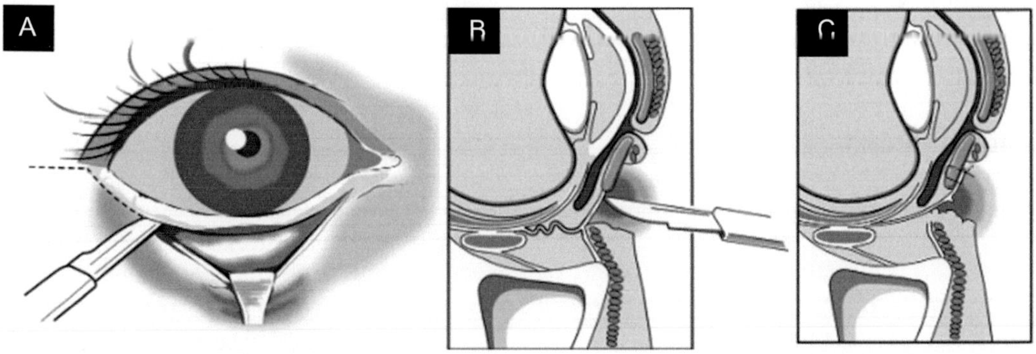

Fig. 3 Retractor reinsertion operation. (A) Subciliary incision with a no. 15 blade. (B) The orbital septum is opened expose the lower eyelid retractors. (C) Lateral view of the lower eyelid retractors advanced and reattached to the anterior, inferior tarsus

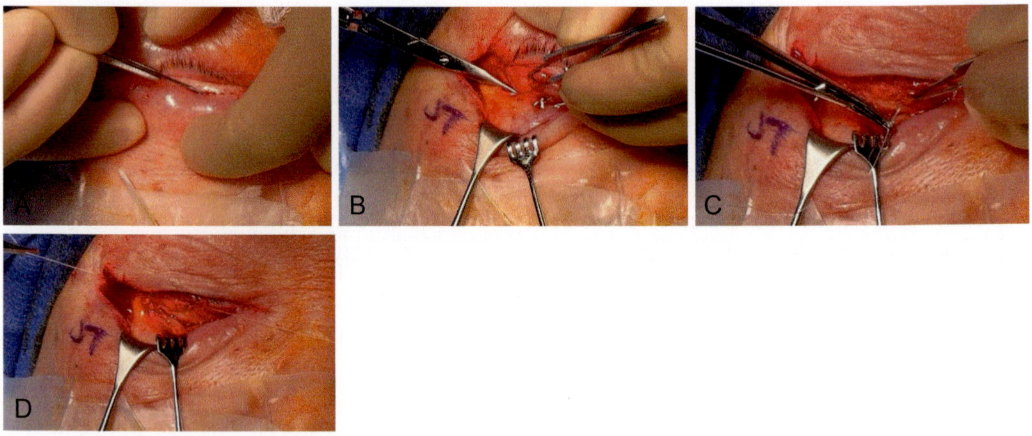

Fig. 4 Retractor reinsertion operation. (A) Subciliary incision with a no. 15 blade. (B) The septum is opened to expose the lower eyelid retractors found posterior to the orbital fat (C-D) The lower eyelid retractors are sutured to the anterior, inferior border of the tarsus with 6-0 polyglactin or 7-0 silk sutures

buried sutures (Figs. 3C, 4C). Three to four of such sutures are placed. The subciliary incision is closed with absorbing suture (e.g. 6-0 plain or 6-0 polyglactin) and the traction suture is removed.

While tightening of the LER is essentially the same whether approached internally or externally, the latter affords the ability to resect redundant anterior lamella tissues including orbicularis. External approaches, thus may be associated with a lower recurrence rate and yet there may be a greater risk for post-operative ectropion due to overcorrection or anterior lamellar scarring [14]. Adding a horizontal tightening procedure such as a lateral tarsal strip, may improve the success rate and durability [15].

Quickert sutures

Described in 1971, Quickert sutures are a quick, in-office procedure consisting of full-thickness eyelid everting sutures [16]. Double-armed 4-0 or 5-0 chromic or polyglactin sutures are placed in the inferior fornix below the inferior tarsal border, through the LER, then through the skin superior to the level of insertion; a more superior exit through the skin near the lash follicles causes more eyelid eversion. Two or three separate double armed sutures are placed and then tied. (Fig. 5) Recurrence is common, with 20% recurrence at 6 months and 50% by two years [17, 18].

When Quickert rotation sutures are combined with lateral tarsal strip, there is a statistically significant decrease in recurrence compared to Quickert sutures alone; the recurrence rate of the combined approach is 2% at 9 months and 12% at 2 years [19–21]. The Quickert sutures procedure alone is usually inadequate in providing long-term resolution of entropion, but it may be an appropriate procedure for patients with higher operative risk or with other procedures that address horizontal laxity. Quickert sutures may also be performed efficiently at the bedside or in the office and thus fill a void of patients who are unstable for more definitive, open surgical repair.

3.2 Correction of Horizontal Laxity

There exist several variations of canthoplasty or horizontal eyelid tightening. These are typically combined with other vertical tightening procedures, described above, to achieve durable entropion repair. These are also described in Chapter "Ectropion Repair and Lateral Canthal Anchoring".

Lateral Tarsal Strip

A lateral canthotomy and inferior cantholysis is performed to release the lower eyelid. Sharp dissection along the gray line separates the anterior and posterior lamella. The mucocutaneous

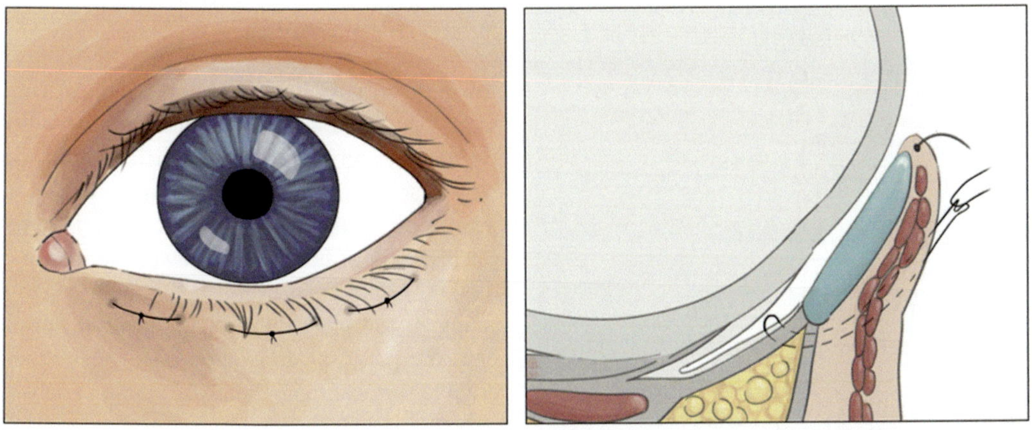

Fig. 5 Eyelid rotation (Quickert) sutures. Double arm sutures are passed from the fornix to the exit externally just inferior to the lashes. Sutures are tied externally to achieve rotation of the eyelid margin. *(illustration by Michael Han)*

junction is excised with Westcott scissors along the length of the strip. Conjunctival epithelium is debrided from the posterior surface with a blade. A horizontal incision is made through the tarsus to create the tarsal strip and shortened with Westcott scissors, usually between 3 and 5 mm depending on the laxity of the eyelid. The tarsal strip is attached to the periosteum with double-armed 4-0 or 5-0 braided polyester or polyglactin suture posterior to the lateral orbital rim approximately 2 mm superior to the medial canthus (Fig. 6). Once satisfactory lateral canthus placement and lower eyelid contour are achieved, the second suture is placed in the same manner and the sutures are tied and cut. The lash follicles of the anterior lamella of the tarsal strip are excised. The lateral canthal angle is formed by suturing the anterior lamella to the strip medial to the lateral orbital rim with 6-0 plain suture. The lateral canthotomy is closed with interrupted fast absorbing suture.

Bick Type Procedure

A lateral canthotomy and inferior cantholysis is performed to release the lower eyelid. The lower eyelid is distracted laterally to the desired position and the triangle of lower lid tissue overlapping the upper eyelid is excised [22]. The lateral upper and lower eyelid margins posterior to the gray line are denuded for 2-3 mm. A 4-0 or 5-0 braided polyester or polyglactin suture is passed through the lateral cut edge of tarsus and sutured to the lateral orbital rim. The lateral canthal angle is reformed with buried 6-0 plain sutures through the cut edges of the upper and lower eyelid margins. The lateral canthotomy is then closed. When combined with Quickert sutures, there was no recurrence of entropion with a median follow up of 29 months [23].

Canthopexy

Transblepharoplasty canthopexy can be performed in patients who are undergoing upper eyelid surgery and need very mild lower eyelid tightening. Through the blepharoplasty incision, dissection is carried out between the orbicularis and orbital septum to expose the superolateral orbital rim. A double-armed 4–0 or 5–0 polypropylene or other permanent suture is introduced through the blepharoplasty incision and exits at the level of the meibomian glands of the lateral lower eyelid. The needle is then placed adjacent to this exit wound and directed posteriorly to engage the periosteum of the superior orbital rim and pulled through the blepharoplasty incision. The suture is pulled to demonstrate the tightening effect of the canthopexy, and once satisfactory lower eyelid contour is achieved, the suture is tied. The blepharoplasty incision is then closed.

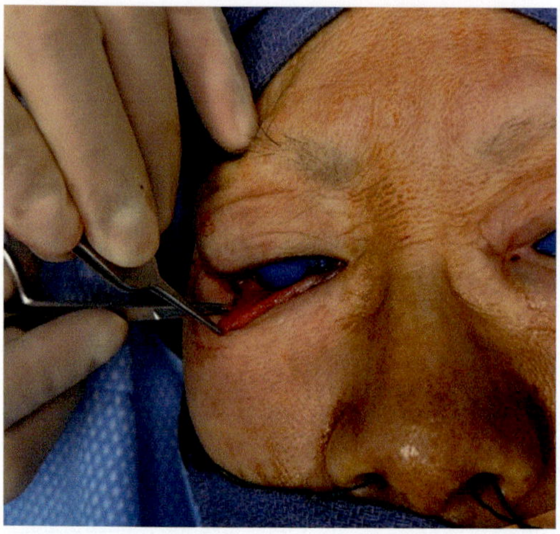

Fig. 6 Lateral tarsal strip. The tarsal strip is attached to the periosteum with double-armed 4-0 Braided polyester or 5-0 polyglactin suture posterior to the lateral orbital rim

Transcanthal canthopexy can also be performed in conjunction with LER reinsertion with successful results and no reported lateral canthal deformity [24]. An 8–10 mm skin incision is made along the lateral canthal rhytids, anterior to the lateral orbital rim. A stab incision is made at the lateral commissure or on the eyelid margin medial to the lateral commissure. A double-armed 4-0 or 5-0 polypropylene is inserted into the stab incision, passed through the periosteum of the lateral orbital rim, and pulled out the skin incision. The skin incision is then closed.

3.3 Correction of Overriding of Preseptal Orbicularis Oculi Muscle

During LER reinsertion procedures, a strip of orbicularis may be excised or ablated inferior to the tarsus to reduce preseptal orbicularis override. Anterior lamella resection is a component of epiblepharon repair (described in another chapter).

4 Conclusions

Involutional entropion is one of the most common functional conditions seen in the aging population and may cause eye irritation or ocular surface damage. Three factors contribute to involutional entropion: (1) vertical eyelid laxity (disinsertion or laxity of the lower eyelid retractors), (2) horizontal eyelid laxity, and (3) overriding of the preseptal orbicularis oculi muscle onto the pretarsal orbicularis oculi. Proper and durable surgical repair addresses these variables.

References

1. Carter SR, Chang J, Aguilar GL, Rathbun JE, Seiff SR. Involutional entropion and ectropion of the Asian lower eyelid. Ophthalmic Plast Reconstr Surg. 2000;16:45–9.
2. Nishimoto H, Takahashi Y, Kakizaki H. Relationship of horizontal lower eyelid laxity, involutional entropion occurrence, and age of Asian patients. Ophthalmic Plast Reconstr Surg. 2013;29:492–6.
3. Damasceno RW, Osaki MH, Dantas PEC, Belfort R. Involutional entropion and ectropion of the lower eyelid: prevalence and associated risk factors in the elderly population. Ophthalmic Plast Reconstr Surg. 2011;27:317–20.
4. Michels KS, Czyz CN, Cahill KV, Foster JA, Burns JA, Everman KR. Age-matched, case-controlled comparison of clinical indicators for development of entropion and ectropion. J Ophthalmol. 2014;2014:231487.
5. Benger RS, Musch DC. A comparative study of eyelid parameters in involutional entropion. Ophthalmic Plast Reconstr Surg. 1989;5:281–7.
6. Hawes MJ, Dortzbach RK. The microscopic anatomy of the lower eyelid retractors. Arch Ophthalmol. 1982;100:1313–8.
7. Nowinski TE. Color Atlas of oculoplastic surgery, 2nd ed. Lippincott Williams & Wilkins; 2011. p. 44–53.
8. Olver JM, Barnes JA. Effective small-incision surgery for involutional lower eyelid entropion. Ophthalmology. 2000;107:1982–8.
9. Lin P, Kitaguchi Y, Mupas-Uy J, Sabundayo MS, Takahashi Y, Kakizaki H. Involutional lower eyelid entropion: causative factors and therapeutic management. Int Ophthalmol. 2019;39:1895–907.

10. Nerad JA. Techniques in ophthalmic plastic surgery: a personal tutorial. Philadelphia: Saunders Elsevier; 2010.
11. Kakizaki H, Chan WO, Takahashi Y, Selva D. Overriding of the preseptal orbicularis oculi muscle in Caucasian cadavers. Clin Ophthalmol. 2009;3:243–6.
12. Clarke JR, Spalton DJ. Treatment of senile entropion with botulinum toxin. Br J Ophthalmol. 1988;72:361–2.
13. Faria-E-Sousa SJ, de Paula Gomes Vieira M, Silva JV. Uncovering intermittent entropion. Clin Ophthalmol. 2013;7:385–8.
14. Ben Simon GJ, Molina M, Schwarcz RM, McCann JD, Goldberg RA. External (subciliary) vs internal (transconjunctival) involutional entropion repair. Am J Ophthalmol. 2005;139:482–7.
15. Erb MH, Uzcategui N, Dresner SC. Efficacy and complications of the transconjunctival entropion repair for lower eyelid involutional entropion. Ophthalmology. 2006;113:2351–6.
16. Quickert MH, Rathbun E. Suture repair of entropion. Arch Ophthalmol. 1971;85:304–5.
17. Jang SY, Choi SR, Jang JW, Kim SJ, Choi HS. Long-term surgical outcomes of Quickert sutures for involutional lower eyelid entropion. J Craniomaxillofac Surg. 2014;42:1629–31.
18. Tsang S, Yau GSK, Lee JWY, Chu ATK, Yuen CYF. Surgical outcome of involutional lower eyelid entropion correction using transcutaneous everting sutures in Chinese patients. Int Ophthalmol. 2014;34:865–8.
19. Scheepers MA, Singh R, Ng J, Zuercher D, Gibson A, Bunce C, et al. A randomized controlled trial comparing everting sutures with everting sutures and a lateral tarsal strip for involutional entropion. Ophthalmology. 2010;117:352–5.
20. Ho SF, Pherwani A, Elsherbiny SM, Reuser T. Lateral tarsal strip and Quickert sutures for lower eyelid entropion. Ophthalmic Plast Reconstr Surg. 2005;21:345–8.
21. Barnes JA, Bunce C, Olver JM. Simple effective surgery for involutional entropion suitable for the general ophthalmologist. Ophthalmology. 2006;113:92–6.
22. Barrett RV, Meyer DR. The modified Bick quick strip procedure for surgical treatment of eyelid malposition. Ophthalmic Plast Reconstr Surg. 2012;28:294–9.
23. Golan S, Lelli GJ. Involutional entropion repair combining the modified Bick quick strip procedure with Quickert rotational sutures. Orbit. 2019;38:130–2.
24. Ishida Y, Takahashi Y, Kakizaki H. Posterior layer advancement of lower eyelid retractors with transcanthal canthopexy for involutional lower eyelid entropion. Eye (Lond). 2016;30:1469–74.

Lower Eyelid Repair with Hard Palate and other Spacer Grafts

Mariana Dias Gumiero
and Allan C. Pieroni Gonçalves

Abstract

Certain forms of lower eyelid retraction require a spacer graft to lengthen the posterior lamella and elevate the central lower eyelid where there exists minimal anatomic support. Rejection or resorption are concerns with allografts or xenografts. Hard palate may be ideal owing to the rigidity and thickness characteristics. The chief limitation is the second surgical site morbidity including pain. This chapter details surgical eyelid retraction repair with the use of a hard palate and alternatives such as ear cartilage and donor sclera.

Keywords

Lower eyelid retraction · Hard palate graft · Posterior lamella spacer · Ear cartilage graft

Supplementary Information The online version contains supplementary material available at https://doi.org/10.1007/978-3-031-36175-3_17.

M. D. Gumiero · A. C. Pieroni Gonçalves (✉)
University of São Paulo, São Paulo, Brazil
e-mail: allan.pieroni@hc.fm.usp.br

1 Introduction

Lower eyelid retraction is a malposition of the lower eyelid, in which the eyelid margin is displaced inferiorly, resulting in increased exposure of the surface of the eye also known as scleral show. This condition poses both functional and aesthetic concerns. It may cause dry eye symptoms and lead to exposure keratitis, corneal ulcer, and corneal scarring.

The position of the lower eyelid depends on the balance among a set of factors, including position and tension of the horizontal canthal ligaments, lower eyelid length and tonicity, the distensibility of the vertical lower eyelid retractors, the sufficiency of the fornix and palpebral conjunctivae, the tightness of the orbicularis oculi and the degree of eye prominence [1].

Prominent eyes or negative vector increase the risk of complications associated with lower eyelid blepharoplasty. There exist limited structures supporting lower eyelid position. As such, even small amounts of fibrosis, laxity, or muscle tone can induce inferior scleral show [2].

Lower eyelid malposition after cosmetic surgery may be due to the combination of inadequate skin (anterior lamellar insufficiency) and/or middle lamellar inflammation and subsequent scarring. Commonly, lower eyelid laxity is also contributory. Adjuncts to lower blepharoplasty such as fat redraping if not performed correctly can compromise the middle lamellae [3].

J. P. Tao (ed.), *Plastic Surgery of the Lower Eyelids*,
https://doi.org/10.1007/978-3-031-36175-3_17

Another common cause of LER is thyroid eye disease (TED). Retractor band contracture as well as exophthalmos cause the central lower eyelid to displace inferiorly. The retractors may be altered by fibrosis of the capsulopalpebral itself or indirect tension from connections with a hypertrophied inferior rectus muscle [2].

Lastly, normal aging and involutional changes can cause lower eyelid retraction. The midface relaxes, orbital and facial bones remodel, malar fat pad descends secondary to gravity, as well as fat atrophy, which result in lower eyelid descent and malposition [4].

Understanding of anatomic changes and pathophysiology of lower eyelid retraction is key in surgical treatment. Surgical interventions span a broad array of procedures aimed to treat horizontal laxity and vertical inadequacy of the anterior, middle, or posterior lamella. This chapter highlights spacer graft placement to the posterior lamella to treat eyelid retraction.

2 Treatment Approach

While minimal lower eyelid retraction can be corrected without grafts, many cases need further interventions such as midface lifting or grafting to the eyelid [5–7]. In general, when retraction exceeds 1.5 mm due to middle lamella shortening, spacer grafts are required to push the lower eyelid margin upwards. These grafts require mild rigidity to achieve sufficient eyelid support.

A variety of homologous, autologous, alloplastic, or xenoplastic options have been used to improve the stability of the middle and posterior lamella. Examples of homologous grafts that are preserved tissues obtained from cadavers, are eye bank sclera, fascia lata and tarsus. Banked sclera may have ideal geometric and rigidity characteristics. Moreover, whole donor shells provide sufficient material that can be sized to the desired configurations. However, rejection and infectious disease transmission remain concerns. Autogenous grafts include hard palate mucosa, auricular or nasal septal cartilage, tarsus, and dermis [8]. The use of autologous grafts decreases concerns for rejection or transmission of disease; however, it is relatively more time-consuming and associated with donor site morbidity. Lower eyelid grafting can be approached anteriorly through the skin or posteriorly through the conjunctiva. To avoid manipulation of skin, orbicularis muscle and the anterior septum, the posterior approach is often ideal. However, in cases when skin incisions are already in use (e.g. concomitant skin muscle lift), anterior approaches may be appropriate.

3 Surgical Technique

3.1 Posterior Approach (Video 1)

Silk retraction sutures are placed in the eyelid margin to evert the lower eyelid over a Desmarres retractor. The conjunctiva is infiltrated with local anesthetic. The conjunctiva is incised across the entire inferior border of the tarsus. The conjunctiva is dissected from the inferior tarsal muscle to the fornix. The fused lower eyelid retractors and orbital septum are transected at the lower aspect of the tarsus and dissected anteriorly and inferiorly. Middle lamellar scarring, if present, should be released with dissection. Next, the graft is inserted between the tarsus and the superior edge of the lower eyelid retractors. The size of the graft is determined based on on the amount of scleral show. The graft usually has a 15–20 mm length with variable height (see below). The graft is sutured in the lower border of the tarsus place with three buried 6-0 polyglactin or plain sutures. Lastly, the inferior border of the graft is then sutured to the retractor. A postoperative Frost suture may be placed to achieve vertical traction for several days.

3.2 Anterior Approach

Through a skin incision (usually subciliary and in the context of external blepharoplasty or midface lifting) the CPF can be identified posterior to the orbicularis and septum. The inferior border of tarsus is exposed and a posterior lamella spacer is inserted between the tarsus and recessed retractor band.

Through either a posterior or anterior approach and in most patients, horizontal tightening and lateral canthal anchoring is required to further support the eyelid [9].

Through either a posterior or anterior approach and in most patients, horizontal tightening and lateral canthal anchoring is required to further support the eyelid [9].

Hard palate mucosa is considered the gold standard because its similarity to lower eyelid tarsus contour, thickness, and stiffness. It has a mucosal surface, easily vascularized, and rejection or shrinkage are uncommon. The hard plate generally measures at 4–5 mm × 20–25 mm. For every 1 mm of desired vertical lower eyelid lift, using 2–3 mm of hard palate graft is recommended. Therefore, it is not suitable as a standalone for moderate to severe cases.

Harvesting of palatal mucosa poses some challenges owing to the tight surgical confines of the oral cavity (Fig. 1). A sweetheart retractor is useful to improve exposure through distraction of the cheeks and tongue. There exist variations in the size and shape of palatal vaults, which affect the available harvest of donor tissue; with similar horizontal palatal width, tissue availability is greater in high arched palates [10].

Hard palate harvesting causes donor-site discomfort and other complications such as bleeding. These may be minimized by meticulous surgical technique and appropriate postoperative care. Use of a custom-molded oral retainer may reduce donor site discomfort in the early postoperative period. In addition to bleeding, other complications include bone necrosis due to excessive diathermy, oro-nasal fistula and compromised healing due to pathogenic process including oral candidiasis [11, 12].

Autologous alternatives to hard palate include autogenous dermal graft or auricular cartilage grafts. Dermis fat may be a good alternative in special situations of lower eyelid retraction with concomitant inferior periorbital volume loss [13, 14]. The use of these grafts are detailed in another chapter.

Ear cartilage provides good support to the retracted eyelid due to stiffness and firmness, particularly to moderate to severe scleral show. Ear cartilage may be harvested from the antihelix or concha through a postauricular skin incision (Figs. 2, 3, 4 and 5). They may be associated with less shrinkage or resorption than other tissue grafts.

Disadvantages are the rigidity, memory, and thickness, that may create bulk to the eyelid (Fig. 7). Also, the edges of the graft may be more prone to show. Postsurgical sequelae of the donor site are minimal, some mild chronic pain and rare conspicuous deformity of the ear [15].

4 Conclusion

A posterior lamella spacer graft is an excellent choice for lower eyelid retraction repair. (Figs. 8, 9, 10 and 11) Hard palate is widely considered the gold standard but is associated with second surgical site morbidity. Autologous ear cartilage or donor sclera may be useful, as well.

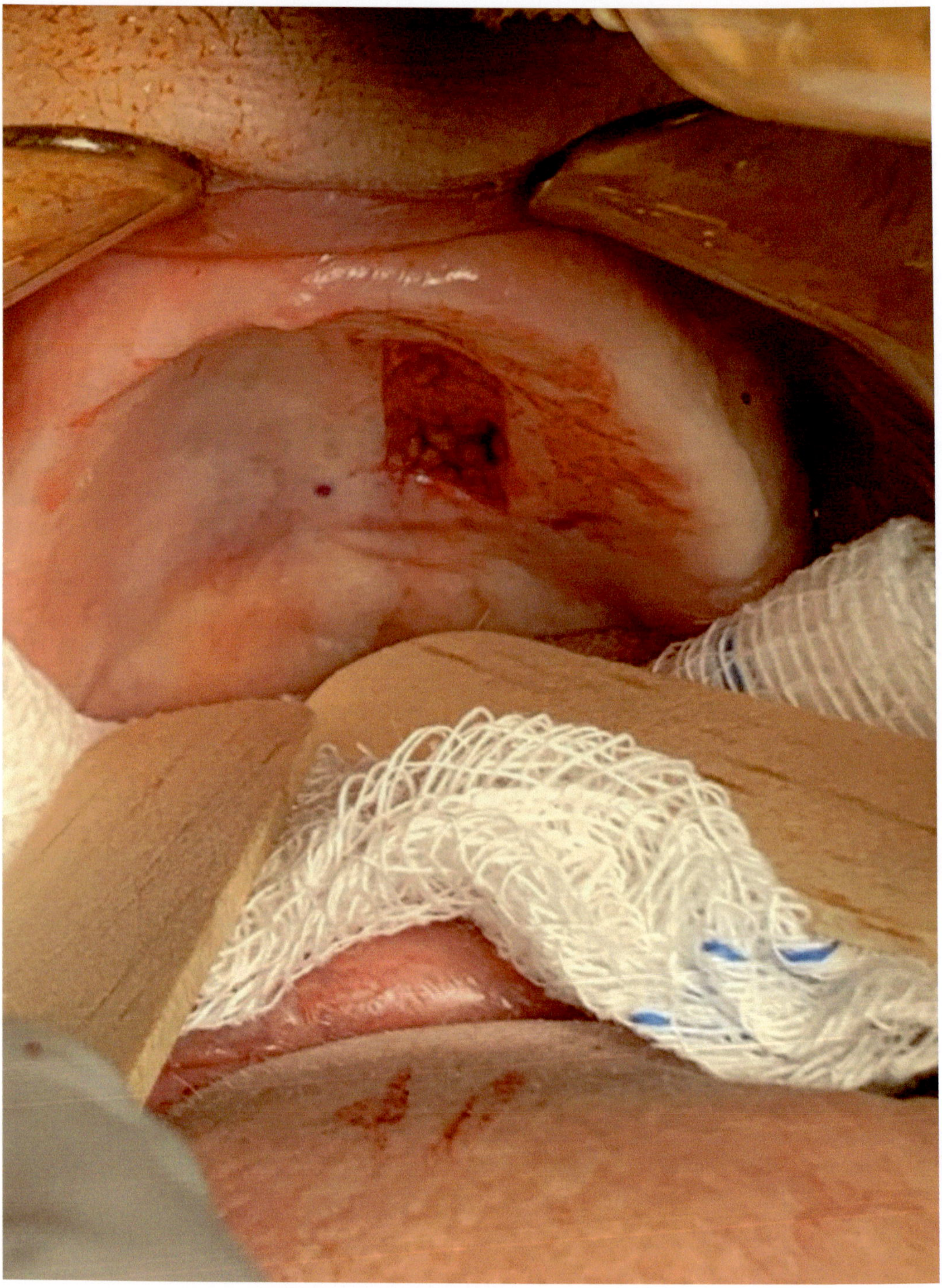

Fig. 1 Hard palate post graft resection. The wound is left to heal by second intention

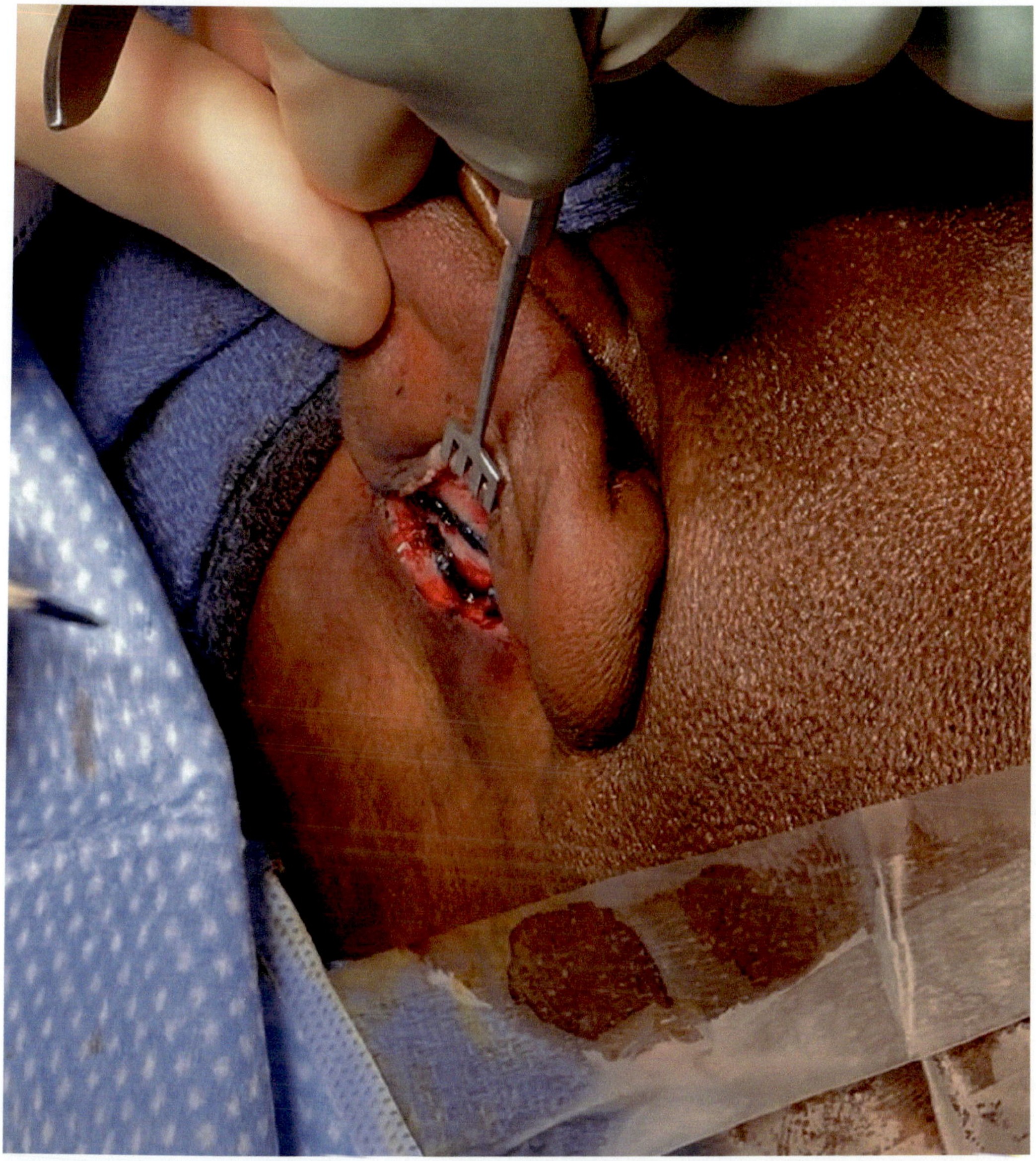

Fig. 2 Postauricular skin incision reflected to expose conchal cartilage

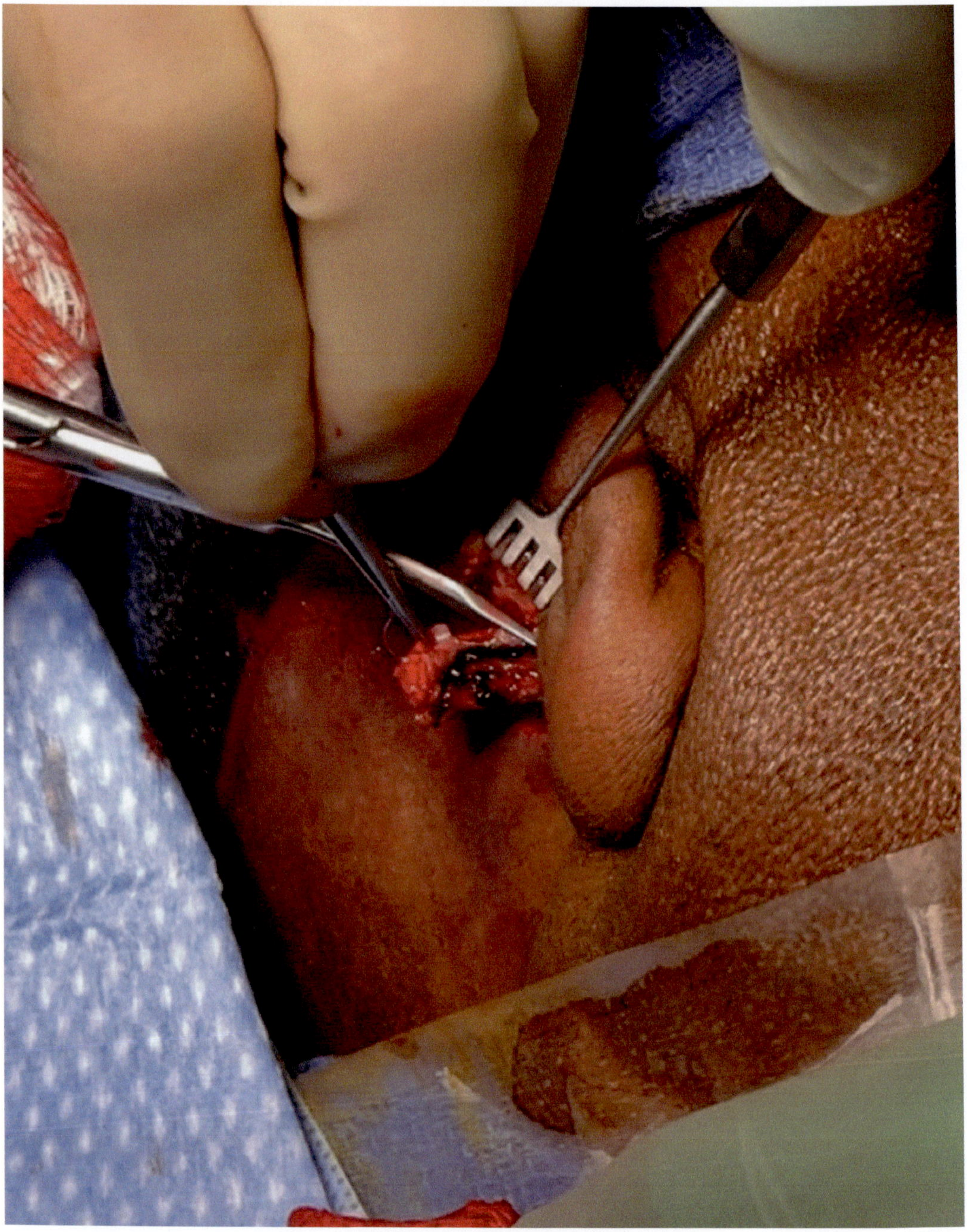

Fig. 3 Ear cartilage harvested with sharp dissection

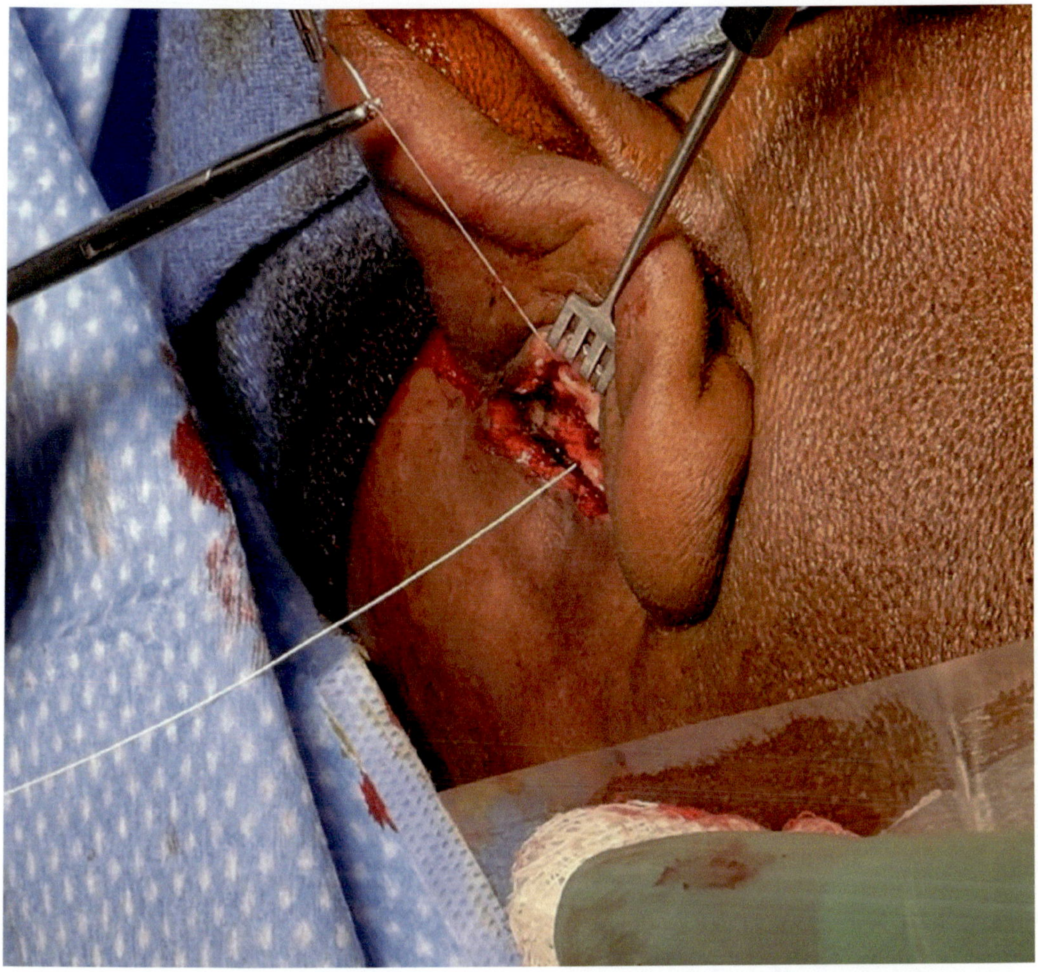

Fig. 4 Wound closed with or without sutures to the cartilage defect

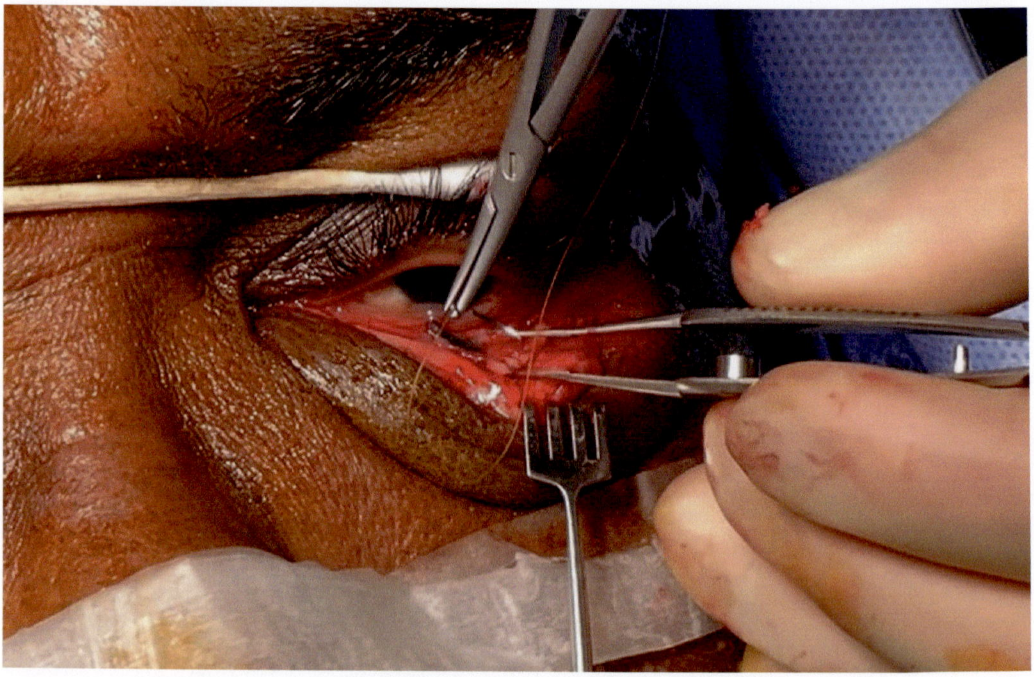

Fig. 5 Ear cartilage sewn into posterior eyelid lamella between the infratarsal border and recessed retractor band

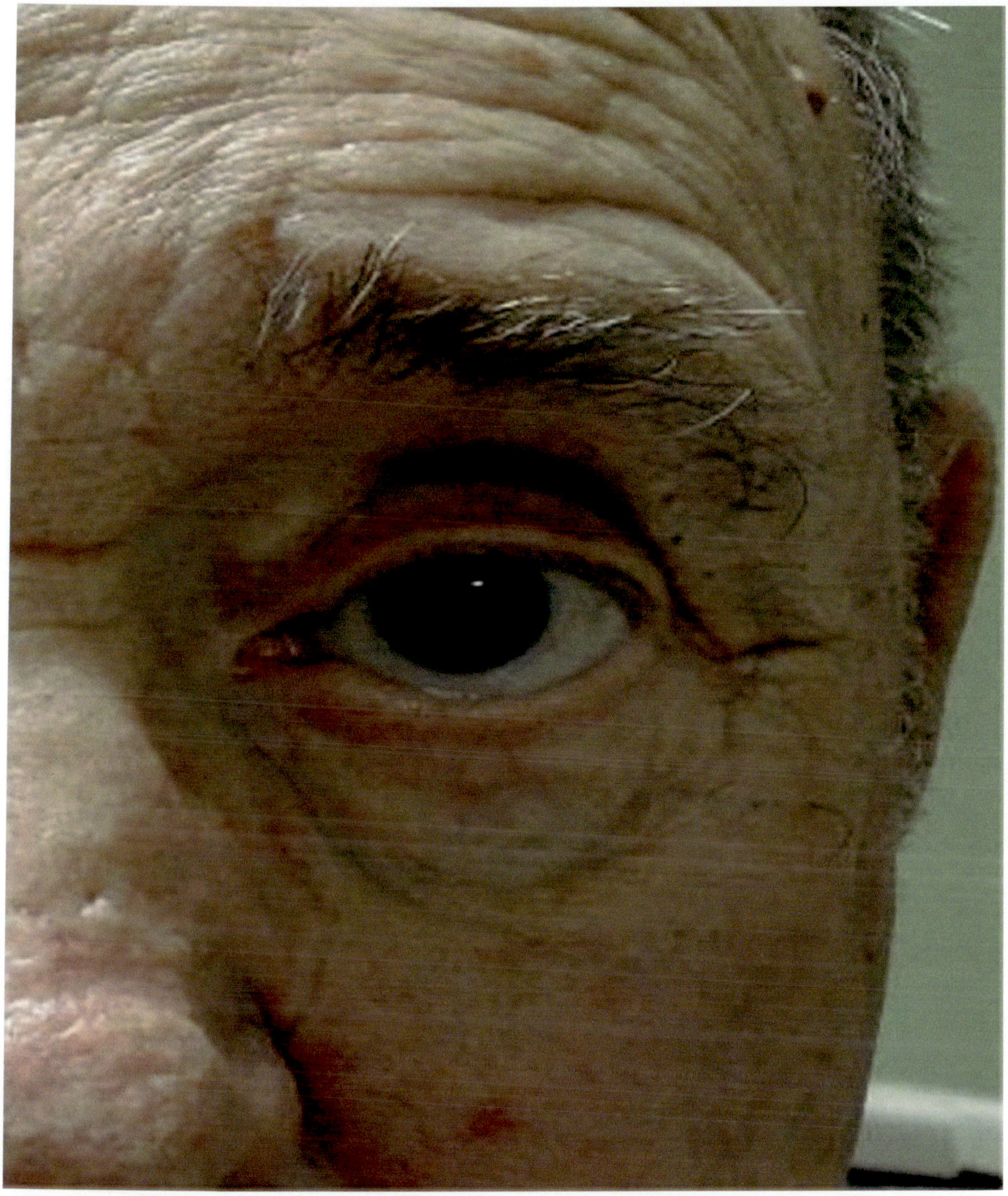

Fig. 6 Lower eyelid retraction and inferior scleral show

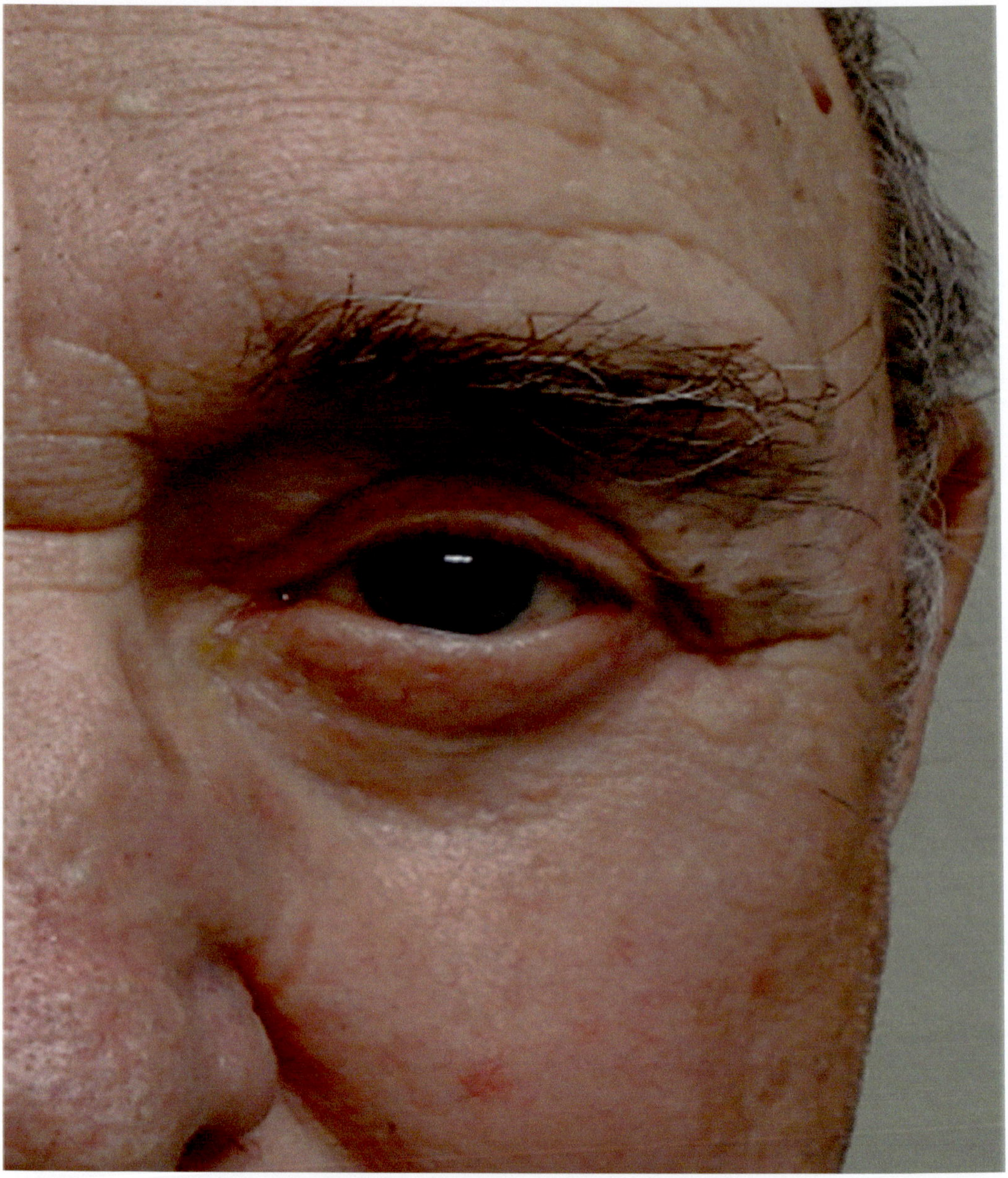

Fig. 7 Patient in Fig. 6 after ear cartilage spacer graft with concomitant cheek lift. Inferior scleral show is absent postoperatively. Note slight thickening of lower eyelid due to the bulky ear cartilage graft

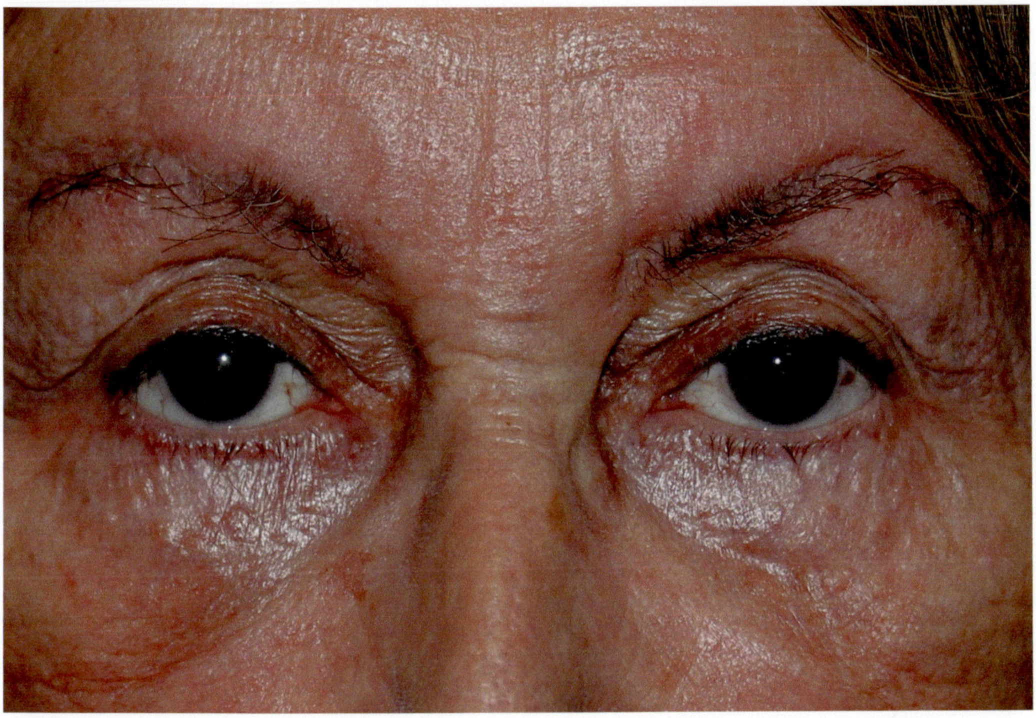

Fig. 8 Moderate bilateral cicatricial lower eyelid retraction after lower blepharoplasty

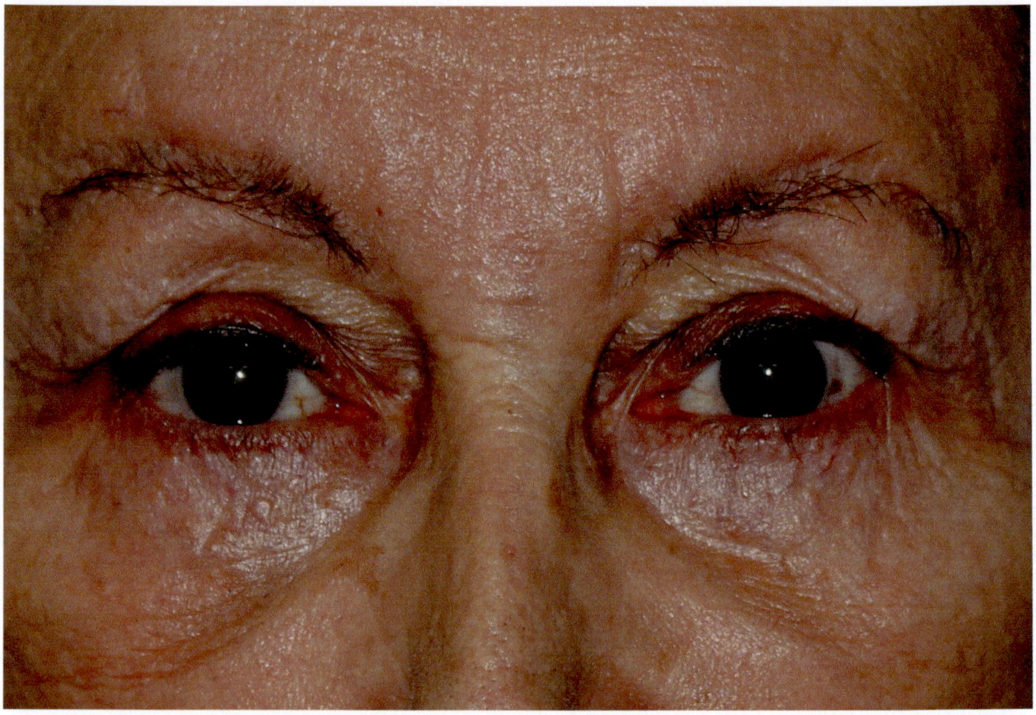

Fig. 9 Patient in Fig. 8 6 months after canthopexy and lower eyelid correction with hard palate graft bilaterally (she also underwent upper eyelid ptosis repair)

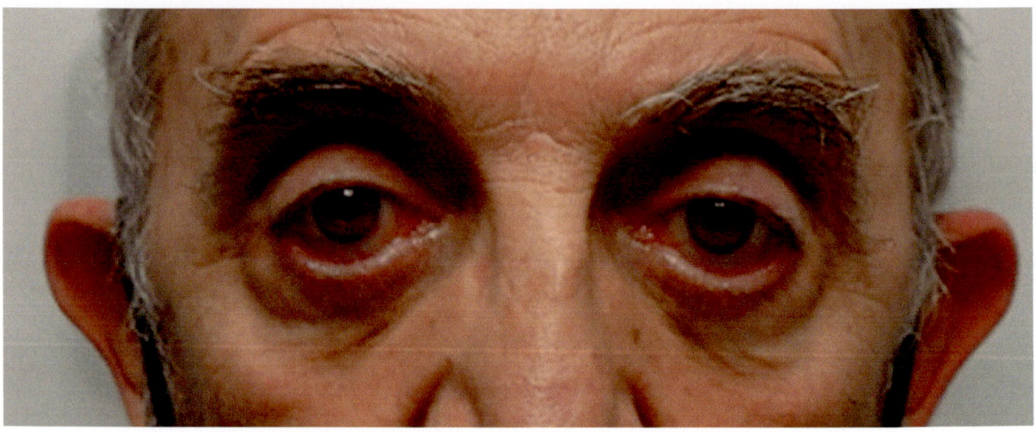

Fig. 10 Bilateral lower eyelid retraction due to involutional and negative vectors

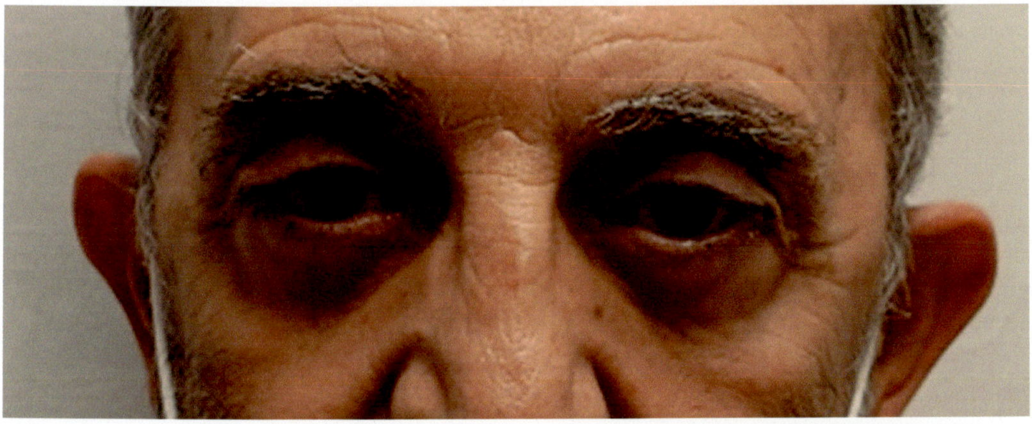

Fig. 11 Patient in Fig. 10 six months after bilateral lower eyelid retraction repair with canthoplasty and hard palate graft

Implanted to the posterior lamella, these grafts push up and support the central eyelid as well as create a barrier to forestall contracture of eyelid retractor bands.

References

1. Kim KH, et al. Causes and surgical outcomes of lower eyelid retraction. Korean J Ophthalmol. 2017;31(4):290–8.
2. Pieroni Goncalves AC, de Rezende JS Lower Eyelid retraction: correction using orbital decompression. In Hartstein ME, Burkat CN, Ramesh S, Holds JB, editors. Avoiding and managing complications in cosmetic oculofacial surgery. Cham: Springer; 2020.
3. Patipa M. The evaluation and management of lower eyelid retraction following cosmetic surgery. Plast Reconstr Surg. 2000;106(2):438–53; discussion 454–439.
4. Fezza JP, Massry G. Lower eyelid length. Plast Reconstr Surg. 2015;136(2):152e–9e.
5. Scawn RL, Joshi N. Commentary on: lower eye lid retraction surgery without internal spacer graft. Aesthet Surg J. 2017;37(2):140–2.
6. Taban MR. Lower eyelid retraction surgery without internal spacer graft. Aesthet Surg J. 2017;37(2):133–6.
7. Pascali M, Botti C, Cervelli V, et al. Vertical midface lifting with periorbital anchoring in the management of lower eyelid retraction: a 10-year clinical retrospective study. Plast Reconstr Surg. 2017;140(1):33–45.
8. Olver JM, Rose GE, Khaw PT, Collin JR. Correction of lower eyelid retraction in thyroid eye disease: a randomised controlled trial of retractor tenotomy with adjuvant antimetabolite versus scleral graft. Br J Ophthalmol. 1998;82(2):174–80.
9. Wang Y, Holds JB, Douglas RS, Massry GG. The spectrum of aesthetic canthal suspension. Facial Plast Surg Clin North Am. 2021;29(2):275–289. https://doi.org/10.1016/j.fsc.2021.01.005. Epub 2021 Apr 24. PMID: 33,906,760
10. Reiser GM, Bruno JF, Mahan PE, et al. The subepithelial connective tissue graft palatal donor site: anatomic considerations for surgeons. Int J Periodon Rest Dent. 1996;16:130–7.
11. Kim JW, Kikkawa DO, Lemke BN. Donor site complications of hard palate mucosal grafting. Ophthalmic Plast Reconstr Surg. 1997;13(1):36–9.
12. Wearne MJ, Sandy C, Rose GE, Pitts J, Collin JR. Autogenous hard palate mucosa: the ideal lower eyelid spacer? Br J Ophthalmol. 2001;85(10):1183–7.
13. Brock WD, Bearden W, Tann T 3rd, Long JA. Autogenous dermis skin grafts in lower eyelid reconstruction. Ophthalmic Plast Reconstr Surg. 2003;19(5):394–7.
14. Ding Y, Huang X, Lu L, Jin R, Sun D, Yang J, Luo X. A systematic review of the treatment of lower eyelid retraction and our attempt of a dermal-orbicularis oculi suspension flap. Chin J Plast Reconstr Surg. 2022;4(1):38–43. ISSN 2096–6911
15. Baylis HI, Perman KI, Fett DR, Sutcliffe RT. Autogenous auricular cartilage grafting for lower eyelid retraction. Ophthalmic Plast Reconstr Surg. 1985;1(1):23–7.

Lower Eyelid Retraction Repair with Dermis Fat Graft

Nicole Topilow, Niloofar Radgoudarzi, Catherine Liu, Don Kikkawa and Bobby S. Korn

Abstract

In cases of lower eyelid retraction caused by middle and posterior lamellar deficiencies associated with volume loss, dermis fat grafts are an excellent option for retraction repair. Benefits of dermis fat grafting include abundant harvestable tissue, volume supplementation, and low donor site morbidity. This chapter describes lower eyelid retraction repair and volumization with an autologous dermis fat graft.

Keywords

Lower eyelid retraction · Lower eyelid retraction · Dermis fat graft · Eyelid spacer · Eyelid volumization

N. Topilow · N. Radgoudarzi · C. Liu · D. Kikkawa · B. S. Korn (✉)
Viterbi Family Department of Ophthalmology, Division of Oculofacial Plastic and Reconstructive Surgery, University of California, San Diego, USA
e-mail: bkorn@ucsd.edu

1 Introduction

Lower eyelid retraction has many etiologies. Anterior lamellar deficiency due to actinic changes, trauma, and surgical removal of lower eyelid skin as in lower eyelid blepharoplasty is a common cause lower eyelid retraction [1–3]. Poor orbicularis muscle tone due to facial nerve palsy, and scarring of the orbital septum from trauma, lower eyelid blepharoplasty, and orbital surgery can also lead to lower eyelid retraction [1–3]. Fibrosis of posterior lamella structures such as the capsulopalpebral fascia in thyroid eye disease reduces lower eyelid retractor distensibility and is yet another cause [1–3]. Regardless of etiology, lower eyelid retraction can result in poor cosmesis, dry eye symptoms, and exposure keratopathy with corneal ulceration and perforation. When aggressive ocular lubrication for mild lower eyelid retraction is insufficient, or in moderate to severe cases of lower eyelid retraction, surgical correction of eyelid position is necessary.

The clinical examination of the retracted lower eyelid is essential because the repair is directed towards the underlying pathophysiology. In the case of anterior lamellar deficiency, pedicle-based skin flaps or full thickness skin grafting can be employed. To preserve cosmesis, anterior lamellar recruitment can be obtained from lifting of the midface. Scarring of the middle lamella can

J. P. Tao (ed.), *Plastic Surgery of the Lower Eyelids*,
https://doi.org/10.1007/978-3-031-36175-3_18

be identified by digital elevation of the lower eyelid. If there is resistance to elevation, middle lamellar scarring is likely present and anterior lamellar supplementation will not be sufficient. Correction of middle lamellar scarring consists of lysis of the cicatrix followed by placement of a suitable spacer graft.

Historically, dermis fat grafts (DFG) have been used for orbital volume augmentation as primary implants at the time of enucleation, in cases of superior sulcus deformity, and in contracted sockets [4]. DFG have also been used with success in cases of lower eyelid retraction caused by middle and posterior lamellar deficiencies associated with volume loss (Fig. 4) [3, 5, 6]. One benefit of DFG over more traditional spacer grafts such as hard palate and allografts is that they simultaneously provide volume and posterior lamellar supplementation [3, 7]. A common scenario is lower eyelid retraction after blepharoplasty in which skin and fat were over resected.

The amount of volume provided by the graft is customizable, and the available harvestable tissue is abundant (e.g., hip, abdomen, post-auricular) [3, 6, 7]. Additional benefits of DFG over allografts include the non-immunogenicity of tissue and lack of concern for disease transmission [3, 7]. Compared to hard palate grafts, the donor site may have less pain and it may obviate risks of infection from the oronasal flora [3, 8]. Lower eyelid tightening procedures and midface lifting can be simultaneously performed to augment results.

2 Surgical Technique

An ellipse measuring approximately 25 × 50 mm is marked on the skin of the hip inferior & posterior to superior iliac crest. A #15 blade or diamond burr rotating at 20,000 rpm is used to denude the epithelium down to the level of the deep dermis. Alternatively, the epidermis and adnexal appendages can be removed with direct lamellar excision with a scalpel. The graft, composed of the deep dermis tissue and underlying fat, is harvested using sharp dissection. The wound is closed in deep and superficial layers using absorbable sutures (Fig. 1).

A lateral canthotomy and inferior cantholysis are performed. A transconjunctival incision is made beneath the inferior tarsal border. Scar tissue in the middle lamella is lysed. The graft is placed deep in the inferior fornix with the dermis side facing the ocular surface (Fig. 2).

Two 6-0 polypropylene sutures are passed in a horizontal mattress fashion through the lower eyelid margin, upper eyelid margin, and brow and tied with foam bolsters to achieve vertical tension. To minimize corneal irritation, a large diameter contact lens can be placed. The sutures are removed 1 week after surgery (Figs. 3 and 4).

3 Potential Complications

Potential complications associated with the use of DFG in lower eyelid retraction repair include graft contracture with recurrent eyelid retraction, keratinization or hair growth on the dermal side, and corneal epithelial defects [3].

4 Conclusion

Dermis fat grafting is an effective tool for the correction of lower eyelid retraction repair with benefits including abundant harvestable tissue, volume supplementation, and low donor site morbidity. The described technique can be considered over more traditional spacer grafts, especially in cases of lower eyelid retraction associated with volume loss.

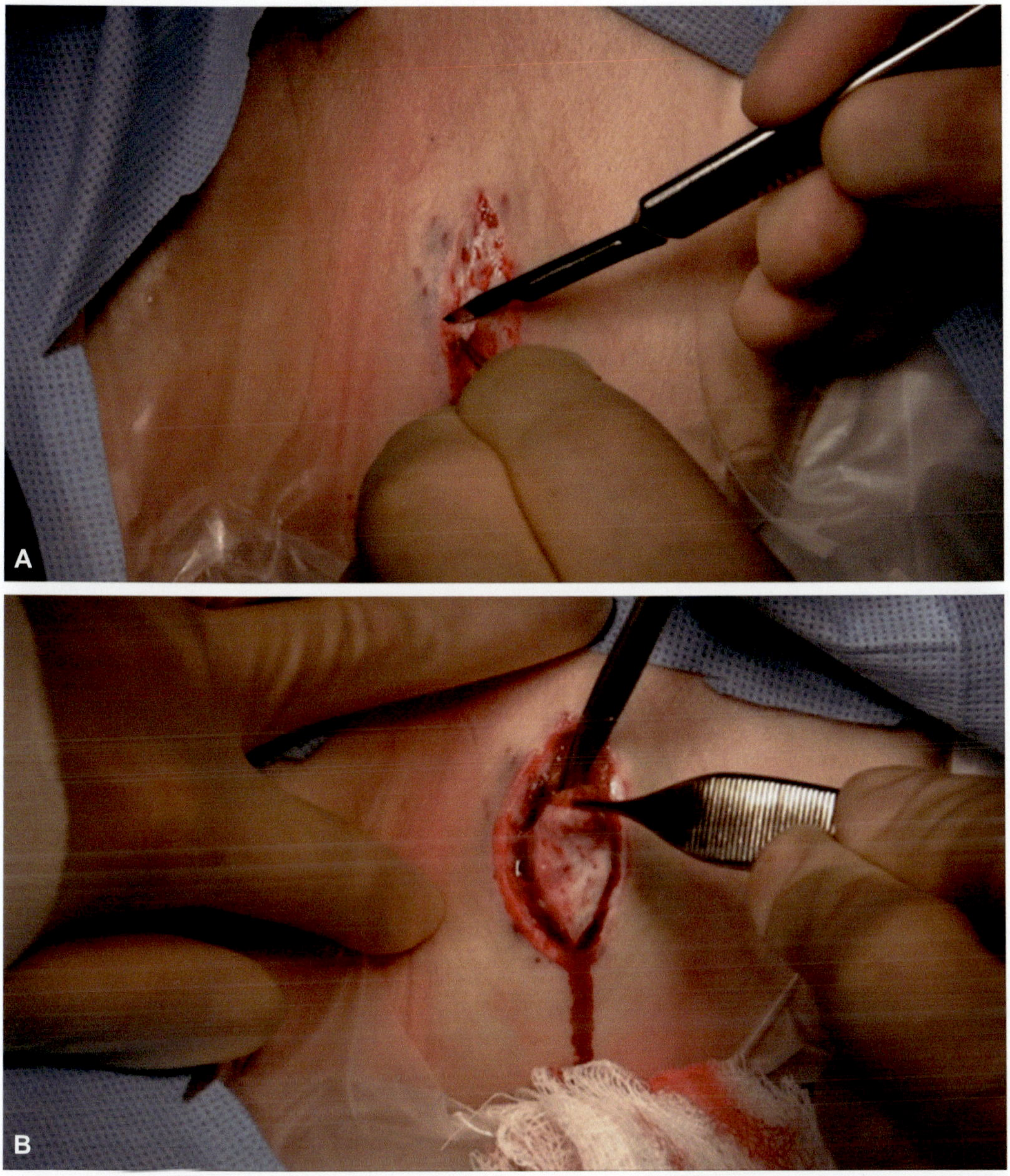

Fig. 1 Dermis fat graft harvesting

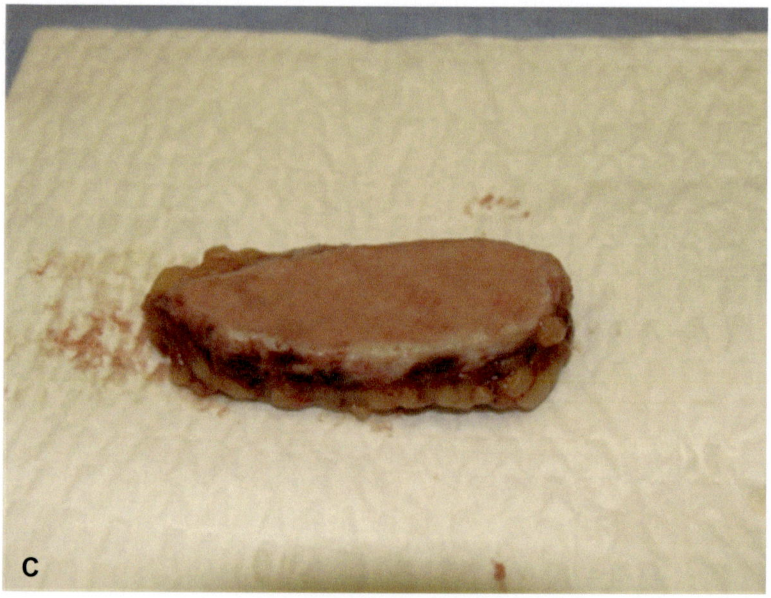

Fig. 1 (continued)

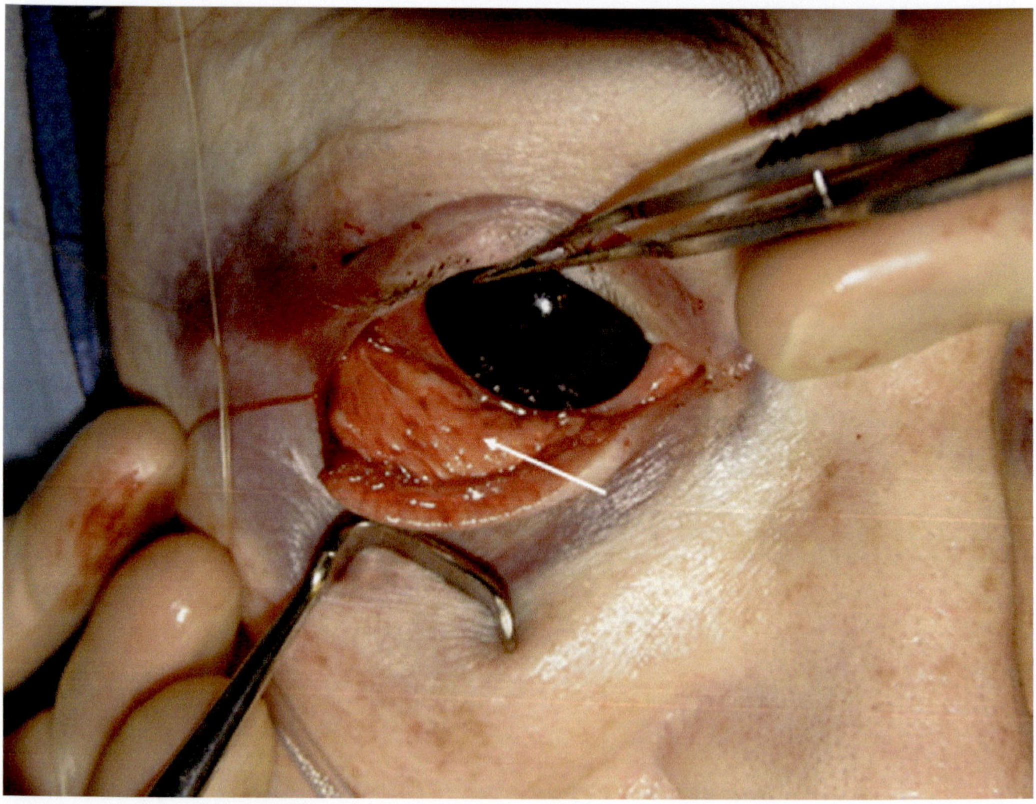

Fig. 2 Placement of dermis fat graft (white arrow) and the fat side facing anteriorly. The edges of the graft are meticulously affixed to the surrounding conjunctiva with 6-0 rapid absorbing gut suture to allow for post-operative conjunctival epithelial cell migration over the DFG

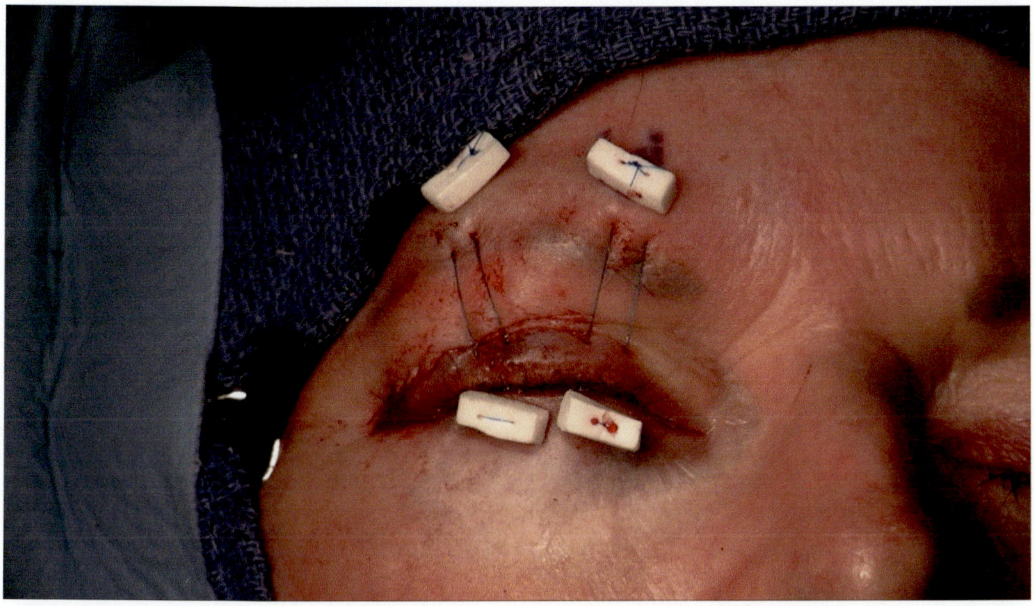

Fig. 3 Placement of suspension (Frost) sutures to stretch the lower eyelid post-operatively

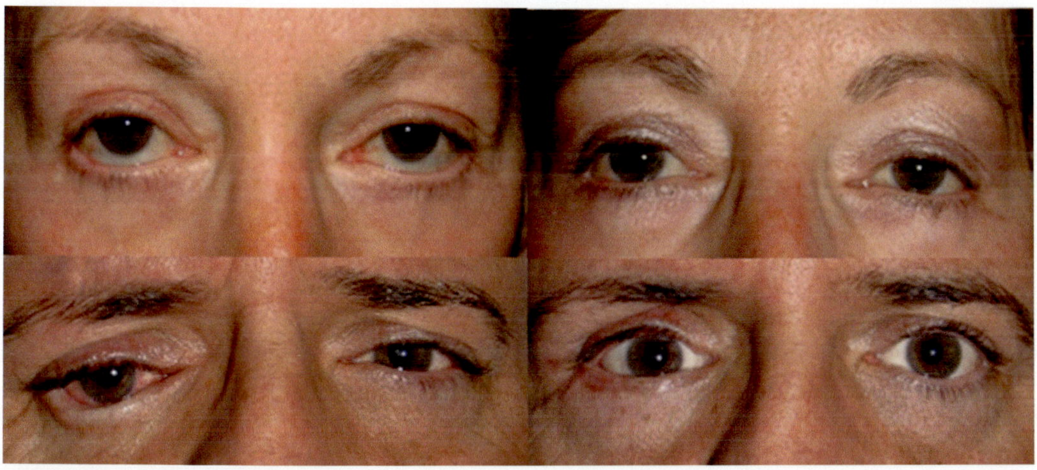

Fig. 4 **Left**: Pre-operative clinical photographs demonstrating bilateral lower eyelid (top) and right lower eyelid retraction (bottom) in two middle aged patients. **Right**: Post-operative clinical photographs demonstrating significant improvement in the lower eyelid position in both patients following dermis fat grafting

References

1. Kim KH, Baek JS, Lee S, Lee JH, Choi HS, Kim SJ, et al. Causes and surgical outcomes of lower eyelid retraction. Korean J Ophthalmol. 2017;31(4):290–8.
2. Patipa M. The evaluation and management of lower eyelid retraction following cosmetic surgery. Plast Reconstr Surg. 2000;106(2):438–53; discussion 54–9.
3. Korn BS, Kikkawa DO, Cohen SR, Hartstein M, Annunziata CC. Treatment of lower eyelid malposition with dermis fat grafting. Ophthalmology. 2008;115(4):744-51.e2.
4. Smith B, Bosniak S, Nesi F, Lisman R. Dermis-fat orbital implantation: 118 cases. Ophthalmic Surg. 1983;14(11):941–3.
5. Godfrey KJ, Tooley AA, Kazim M. Bipedicle dermis fat graft for orbital volume augmentation and repair

of lower eyelid retraction in an anophthalmic socket with prior orbital implant placement. Ophthalmic Plast Reconstr Surg. 2019;35(2):e39–41.

6. Chang HS, Lee D, Taban M, Douglas RS, Goldberg RA. "En-glove" lysis of lower eyelid retractors with AlloDerm and dermis-fat grafts in lower eyelid retraction surgery. Ophthalmic Plast Reconstr Surg. 2011;27(2):137–41.
7. Elabjer BK, Miletić D, Bušić M, Tvrdi AB, Bosnar D, Bjeloš M. Dermis-fat graft for correction of recurrent severe upper eyelid retraction in Graves' orbitopathy. Acta Clin Croat. 2018;57(1):173.
8. Park E, Lewis K, Alghoul MS. Comparison of efficacy and complications among various spacer grafts in the treatment of lower eyelid retraction: a systematic review. Aesthet Surg J. 2017;37(7):743–54.

Lower Eyelid Retraction Repair with Acellular Dermal Matrix (Allograft or Xenografts)

Anne Barmettler and Tiffany Cheng

Abstract

The goal of an acellular dermal matrix graft repair of lower eyelid retraction is to restore the position of the lower eyelid to a normal anatomic height, thus treating the symptoms of ocular irritation and discomfort, as well as improving cosmesis and facial symmetry. Acellular dermal matrix grafts are a biologic framework of collagen, elastin, proteoglycans, and other extracellular matrix components that serve as a scaffold, to reinforce the host tissue. These grafts may be derived from human cadaveric tissue (AlloDerm, Biohorizons, Birmingham, AL, USA), human noncadaveric tissue (BellaDerm, Musculoskeletal Transplant Foundation, Edison, NJ), porcine tissue (Enduragen, Stryker, Kalamazoo, MI, USA), or bovine tissue (Surgimend, Integra, Plainsboro, NJ, USA). Acellular dermal matrix grafts have become increasingly popular due to their off-the-shelf availability, decreasing surgical time and risk from a second surgical site. Additionally, they have similar clinical outcomes to their autologous graft counterparts. This chapter details use of these spacer grafts for lower eyelid retraction, often implanted in conjunction with canthoplasty.

Keywords

Lower eyelid retraction · Spacer graft · Acellular dermal matrix · Allograft · Xenograft · Lateral tarsal strip

1 Introduction

Lower eyelid retraction repair with an acellular dermal matrix graft is a surgical technique that elevates an inferiorly malpositioned lower eyelid to restore its normal anatomic height and position. While the use of various spacer grafts has been described in the literature, acellular dermal matrix grafts have gained popularity due to their off-the-shelf availability, predictable rigidity profile, flexibility in size and configuration, and their relative ease of application. Furthermore, their use may enhance the wound healing process, as the graft's collagenous framework theoretically attracts glycosaminoglycans, fibronectin and other wound healing components to the surgical site. The use of acellular dermal matrices may also confer a lower rejection or reaction risk compared to other traditional grafts, as the

Supplementary Information The online version contains supplementary material available at https://doi.org/10.1007/978-3-031-36175-3_19.

A. Barmettler (✉) · T. Cheng
Albert Einstein College of Medicine/Montefiore Medical Center, Bronx, NY, USA
e-mail: annebarmettler@gmail.com

J. P. Tao (ed.), *Plastic Surgery of the Lower Eyelids*,
https://doi.org/10.1007/978-3-031-36175-3_19

matrices are cell-free. Most importantly, these spacer grafts do not require a donor site and the associated morbidity. However, acellular dermal matrix grafts have an upfront cost (~ $850 for 2 cm × 5 cm porcine graft vs. ~ $250 for 3 cm × 3 cm bovine graft) compared to autologous grafts, whose cost is in the form of longer operating times and a second surgical site. Other spacer grafts commonly used for lower eyelid retraction repair include autologous hard palate, auricular cartilage, dermis fat, or tarsus. These grafts' size, thickness, shape, pliability, and structural composition may limit their use, along with the need for a second surgical site [3].

Acellular dermal matrix grafts may be warranted in scenarios where autologous graft options are inadequate or when donor site morbidity precludes their use. The surgeon may opt to use human cadaveric or human noncadaveric tissue, porcine tissue, or bovine tissue. Each of these acellular dermal matrix grafts has their own advantages and disadvantages. Human cadaveric grafts exhibit directionality that complicates placement; the basement membrane must be oriented towards the globe. Additionally, human cadaveric and bovine tissue must be soaked in room temperature saline solution prior to use, increasing its operating time [2]. While the choice of the spacer graft is at the surgeon's discretion, the surgical technique employed is very similar. This procedure is achieved by first performing a lateral canthotomy and inferior cantholysis to facilitate access to the lower eyelid retractors. A traction suture through the lower eyelid margin allows excellent visualization of the conjunctival tarsus, where a horizontal transconjunctival incision is made inferior to the tarsus. Next, an elliptical spacer graft is sutured into the newly created incision, inferior to the tarsus. The lateral tarsal strip is fixated to the lateral orbital rim and the canthal angle is then carefully recreated. Lastly, the traction suture is sutured to the forehead above the brow, as a Frost suture. This technique results in restoration of the lower eyelid position to its normal height with excellent cosmesis and durability.

1.1 Advantages

- Correction of lower eyelid retraction with ready-to-use bioengineered acellular dermal matrix graft
- Excellent cosmesis (the visibility of the acellular dermal matrix graft contour through the skin is typically less than that of autologous grafts)
- Reduced operative time, exposure to anesthesia, facility use/fees, and faster patient recovery time associated with not needing a second harvest site
- Enhanced wound healing, as acellular dermal matrix grafts contain collagen, glycosaminoglycans, fibronectin, and other wound-healing components
- Low risk of graft rejection or inflammatory reaction, as acellular dermal matrices are devoid of cells.

1.2 Disadvantages

- Higher potential of post-operative graft contracture compared to hard palate graft [4, 5]
- Potential risk of transmission of disease through use of allograft/xenograft
- Cost and availability (the different acellular dermal matrices have different price points and availability internationally).

1.3 Indications

Lower eyelid retraction can be congenital or acquired, but most often occurs secondary to thyroid eye disease, over-aggressive blepharoplasty, facial nerve paralysis, extraocular muscle surgery or injury, or weakening of the orbicularis oculi [6]. Acellular dermal matrix grafts offer structural support inferior to the tarsus, allowing elevation of the lower eyelid margin. Indications for their use include severe lower eyelid retraction and/or failure of conservative treatments (i.e. artificial tears, topical ointments) to relieve ocular symptoms. They may also be indicated in scenarios in which autologous graft options are inadequate or donor site morbidity is unacceptable. Some alternative non-surgical modalities include hyaluronic acid fillers, steroid injections, and botulinum toxin type A [7]. While these non-surgical modalities provide only a temporary correction, they may be appropriate for poor surgical candidates or those with potentially temporary pathologies (e.g. Bell palsy).

1.4 Soft Contraindications

- Patients with ocular cicatricial pemphigoid (consider intra- and post-operative steroids)
- Patients with coexisting severe or unstable medical conditions
- Patients with liver disease/cirrhosis, bleeding diathesis or coagulopathies.

1.5 Considerations

- Aesthetic surgery patients with unrealistic expectations or psychological instability
- Patients who may oppose the use of allografts or xenografts
- Ipsilateral monocular patients may need to avoid patching post-operatively (the Frost suture can be placed more temporally and potentially for a shorter post-operative period).

2 Preoperative Preparation

- ***Patient Discussion***: As there are several etiologies of lower eyelid retraction, a thorough pre-operative history and examination to determine underlying cause and aid in surgical planning. The following components of the pre-operative visit should be obtained:
  - A complete medical and surgical history, including previous surgical attempts at correcting the lower eyelid malposition or fillers to the area
  - Review of systems
  - Family history and social history
  - History of bleeding and use of blood thinners or aspirin-containing products (Patients should be counseled to consult with their prescribing physician to determine when the medications should be discontinued.)
  - Old photographs (To monitor progression of the lower eyelid retraction or to serve as a 'before" picture for comparison with results).
- ***Risks/Benefits/Alternatives & Post-operative Course:*** The risks and benefits of surgery should be discussed, including bleeding, infection, need for additional surgery, as well as:
  - Under- or overcorrection
  - Thickening or visibility of graft contour through the skin
  - Corneal abrasion.

The post-operative course should also be explained, including nausea, headaches, and other side effects from anesthesia, local pain and discomfort at the operative site, avoidance of heavy lifting, contact lens, and make-up application, incision care, and signs of infection (i.e. fever, chills, redness, or discharge from the incision) prompting immediate return.

3 Examination

Eyelid position, eyelid laxity, and the presence of scarring or contraction of the anterior, middle, or posterior lamellae should be noted. Lower eyelid retraction can be quantified by measuring the amount of sclera visible between the corneal limbus and the lower eyelid margin in millimeters. Alternatively, the margin reflex distance 2 (MRD2), or the distance between the corneal light reflex to the lower eyelid in primary gaze, can be measured in millimeters (Fig. 1). While any distance greater than 5.5 mm should raise suspicion for lower eyelid retraction, symptoms can still arise in patients with MRD2 less than 5.5 mm. Eyelid laxity can be assessed by the eyelid distraction test, where the distance between the globe and manually distracted lower eyelid is measured, or the snap-back test, where the examiner pulls the lower eyelid away from the globe, releases, and measures the time to return to original position. A distraction test exceeding 6 mm or delay in snap-back indicates eyelid laxity, which would indicate a need for lateral canthal tendon tightening.

Additional pre-operative concerns include malar fat pad positioning and the presence of a negative vector, where a prominent globe or depressed cheeks can lead to poorer outcomes. In these cases, additional treatments, such as orbital decompression or preperiosteal malar fat pad elevation may be helpful.

Determination of spacer graft requirement is often guided by experience but can be as follows [8]:

- The examiner places a finger at the lateral canthus and pushes upward and laterally. If this maneuver restores the normal position of the lower eyelid, lateral canthal tendon tightening likely will be sufficient. (Fig. 2A, B).
- If this maneuver does not restore the position of the lower eyelid margin to above the inferior limbus, a finger is placed at the central lower eyelid margin to lift it superiorly. If this successfully repositions the lower eyelid, a spacer graft can be considered in conjunction with the lateral canthal tendon tightening.
- If a finger at the lower eyelid margin pushing upwards fails to lift the lower eyelid margin to the superior limbus, additional surgery is likely required, such as a full thickness skin graft or midface elevation.

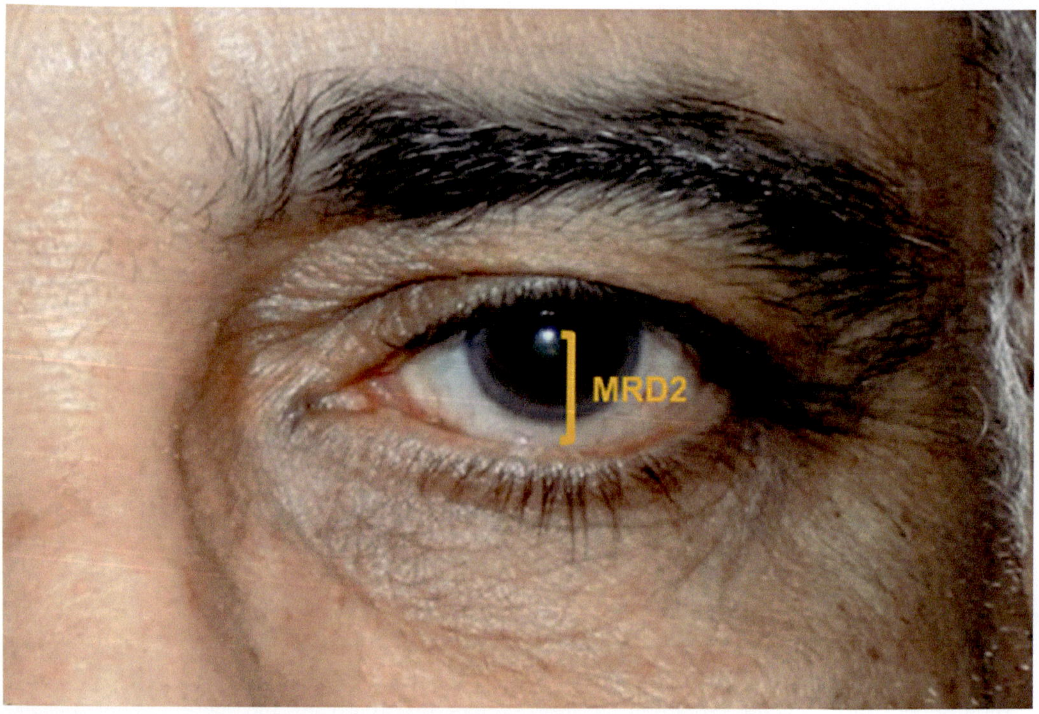

Fig. 1 MRD2 of 7 mm in this patient, measured with the patient looking into the light source in primary gaze, indicates severe lower eyelid retraction

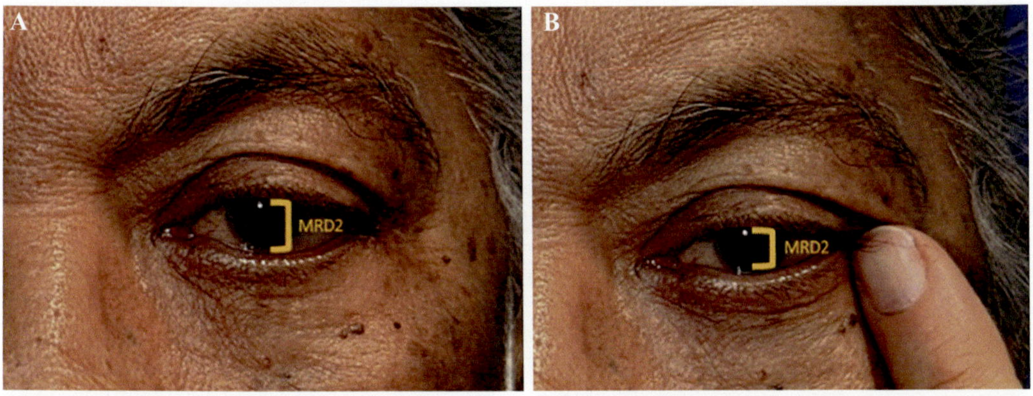

Fig. 2 **A, B**. Examiner demonstrating a method to determine surgical approach. (A) shows a patient with an MRD2 of 6 mm. (B) A finger gently lifts the lateral canthal angle to bring the MRD2 from 6 mm to an acceptable height of 4 mm. This patient most likely will do well with solely a lateral canthoplasty

Symptoms of exposure keratopathy should also be assessed and an anterior slit lamp examination to evaluate the tear film should be conducted. Presence and quantification of lagophthalmos (in millimeters), including corneal show (in millimeters), should be documented. Additionally, frontal and profile photographs of the non-smiling face in primary gaze should be obtained at the pre-operative visit.

4 Operative Technique

- ***Anesthesia***

Local anesthesia with or without intravenous sedation is commonly used for this procedure. Local anesthesia is made with 2% lidocaine with 1:100,000 epinephrine in a 50/50 mixture with 0.5% Marcaine with 1:100,000 epinephrine. This is administered to the lower eyelid, lateral canthus, as well as the area superior to the temporal brow tail.

- ***Surgical Technique***

(1) ***Lower eyelid retractor release***

First, a lateral canthotomy and inferior cantholysis is fashioned to facilitate access to the lower eyelid retractors and to address any aspect of horizontal laxity. A 4-0 traction suture is placed through the lower eyelid margin at the level of the meibomian glands. The authors prefer a double armed braided polyester suture on a pre-placed bolster, but silk sutures may be used. The lower eyelid is then everted over a cotton-tip applicator to expose the posterior aspect of the lower eyelid and a conjunctival incision is made approximately 1–2 mm below the inferior border of the tarsus (See Fig. 3). This incision typically extends from inferior to the punctum to 20 mm laterally. The depth of this incision involves releasing lower eyelid retractors or upon reaching the orbicularis oculi. Hemostasis can be achieved using high temperature cautery.

(2) ***Placement of the acellular dermal matrix graft***

Next, the acellular dermal matrix graft is prepped prior to its placement. If the graft of choice is a porcine acellular dermal matrix, a pre-hydrated 1.0 mm thick graft may be used. If a bovine acellular dermal matrix is used, the thickness of the product may vary between 0.75 and1.54 mm due the natural variation of the product. The bovine acellular dermal matrix must be soaked for approximately 5 min in room temperature saline solution until it is softened. Human cadaveric acellular dermal matrix grafts must also be soaked in saline solution for up to 30 min prior to its use.

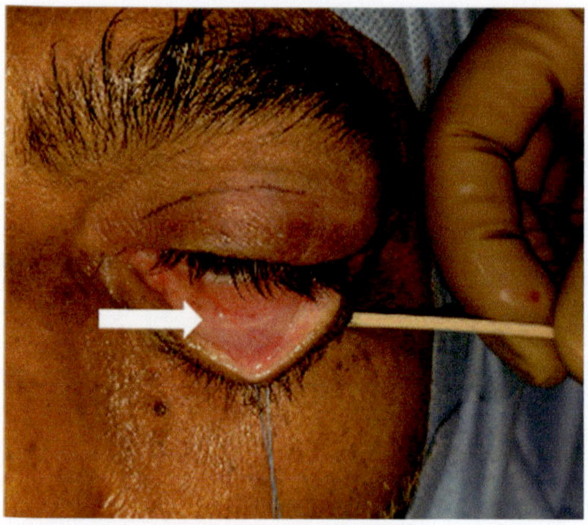

Fig. 3 A 4-0 braided polyester suture traction suture through the lower eyelid margin is pulled inferiorly over a cotton tipped applicator to expose the desired location of the horizontal conjunctival incision inferior to the tarsus (arrow)

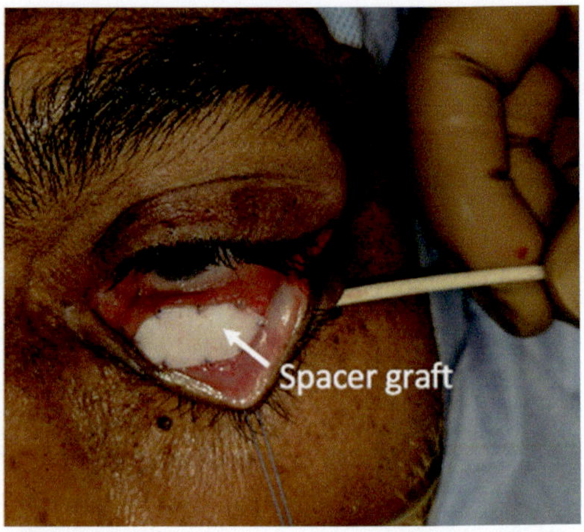

Fig. 4 After the horizontal conjunctival incision is made inferior to the tarsus, eight interrupted, buried sutures are used to fixate the spacer graft, which can be an acellular dermal matrix graft or other materials, such as hard palate or auricular cartilage

The acellular dermal matrix graft can then be trimmed into an elliptical shape to the desired size for each patient depending on the extent of retraction, negative canthal angle, and symptomatic exposure present. In the author's experience, the average graft height was most often between 7 and 8 mm with a length of 20 mm.

Next, the graft can then be placed onto the lower eyelid conjunctival defect and sutured into the posterior lamellar bed using interrupted, buried 6-0 polyglactin sutures (see Fig. 4). The authors typically put in eight sutures. Of note, if human cadaveric tissue is utilized, attention must be paid to ensure that the basement membrane side is facing the globe.

(3) ***Lateral canthoplasty***

Attention can then be turned to the lateral canthus, where a lateral tarsal strip or similar lateral tarsal anchoring is performed. The anterior lamella is dissected from the tarsus with Westcott scissors and the tarsus can be shortened to the appropriate length. A double-armed 4-0 or 5-0 non-absorbable suture is then passed posteriorly to anteriorly through the lateral tarsal strip. Each arm is passed through the periosteum of the lateral orbital rim at the level of the lateral orbital tubercle and tied into place. The lateral canthus is reformed with a circular 6-0 plain gut suture. The skin of the lateral canthus is then reapproximated using a 6-0 plain gut suture.

(4) ***Frost suture***

Lastly, a Frost suture is used to put the eyelid on stretch. Each arm of the double-armed 4-0 traction is passed through the skin and subcutaneous tissue and sutured to the area superior to the temporal brow (Fig. 5). The Frost suture may be removed at postoperative week 1.

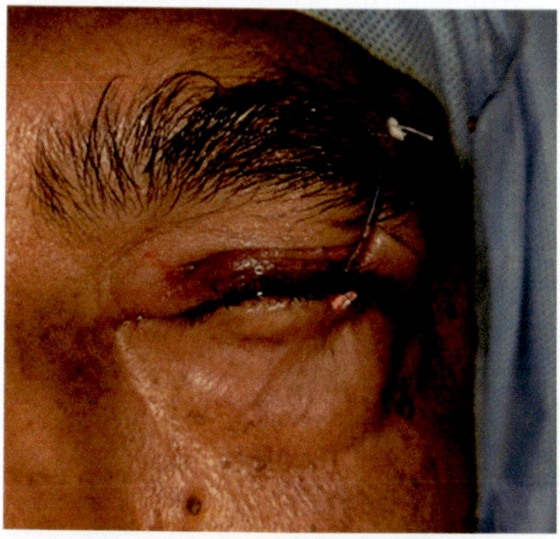

Fig. 5 Suspension (Frost) suture

5 Tips and Pearls

- It is better to procure a graft 1–2 mm larger than the conjunctival defect to address graft contraction.
- When suturing the graft into place, cut sutures on the knot and ensure the knot is buried to avoid causing ocular irritation. Post-operatively, if patients complain of excessive pain, tearing, and redness, they should be examined to rule out corneal abrasion. Patients with corneal abrasions or significant ocular discomfort may require a bandage contact lens and topical antibiotic drops.

6 *Complications* [4]

- Infection
- Hematoma/edema of eyelid
- Graft necrosis/dehiscence
- Graft contracture
- Corneal abrasion
- Conjunctival granuloma.

7 Postoperative Care

- The authors place two eye pads over the eye and Frost suture to prevent accidental pulling on the Frost suture during the healing period. The Frost suture is removed in the office four to 10 days later.
- Severe post-operative pain and infections are rare. For prevention of surgical site infection and inflammation, topical antibiotic-steroid ointment may be used twice daily upon removal of the eye patch four to 10 days post-operatively.

8 Alternative Technique of Middle Lamella Placement and Lateral Rim Fixation to Splint a Severely Lax Eyelid

While posterior lamella placement as described above is the most common, an acellular dermal matrix may also be placed in the middle lamella to support and splint the eyelid in cases of severe eyelid laxity (Fig. 6). In severe floppy eyelid syndrome or eyelid profound laxity, lateral fixation of the matrix implant may further support the eyelid. Through a subciliary

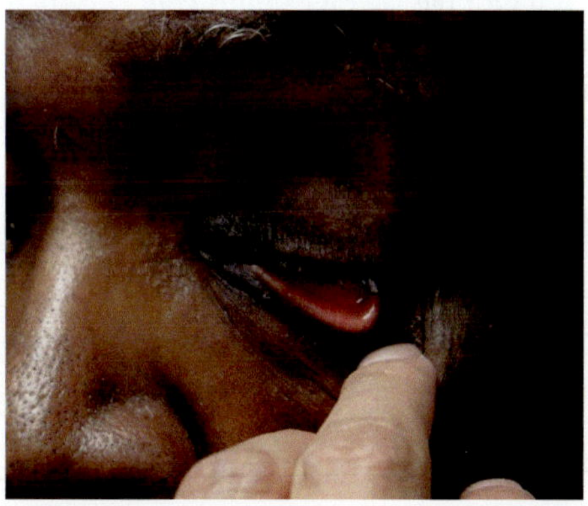

Fig. 6 Severe laxity in an anophthalmic socket causing non retention of an ocular prosthesis

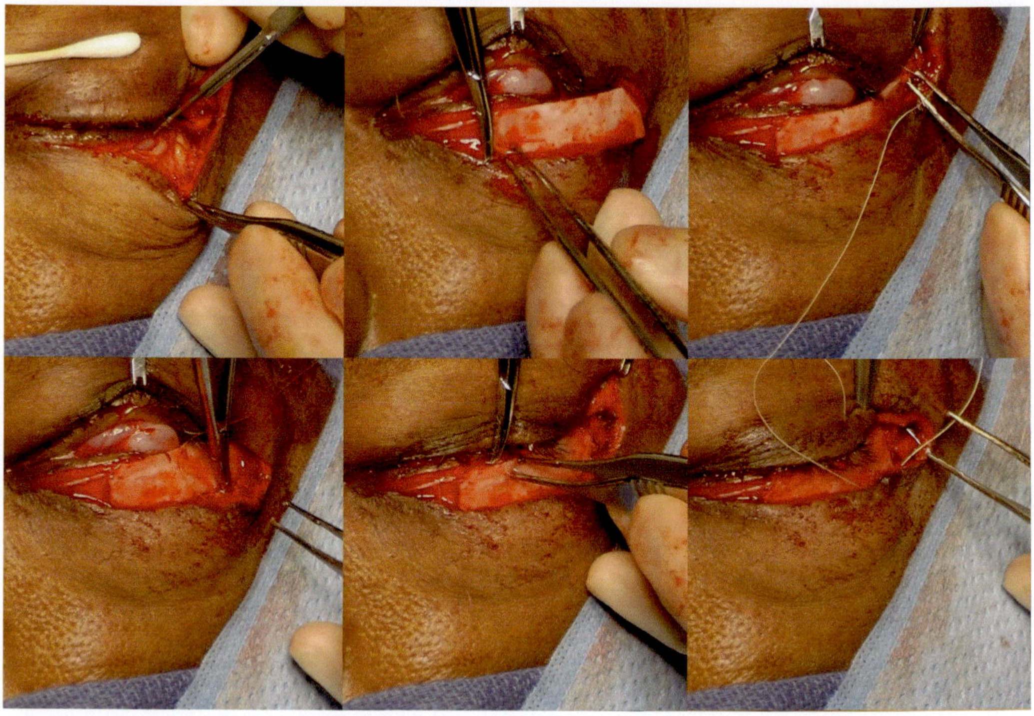

Fig. 7 Sequence of a porcine acellular dermal matrix implant secured to the middle lamella and secured to laterally to the orbital rim using 5–0 polyglactin suture

incision, a matrix sheet (approximately 1.0 by 3.0 cm) is secured to the middle lamella, inferior to the tarsus and secured to the lateral rim periosteum past the lateral canthus (Fig. 7, Video 1). A skin and muscle flap midface lift is performed anteriorly. In this method, the implant that is attached laterally secures the lower eyelid and adds some rigidity as well (Fig. 8A and B).

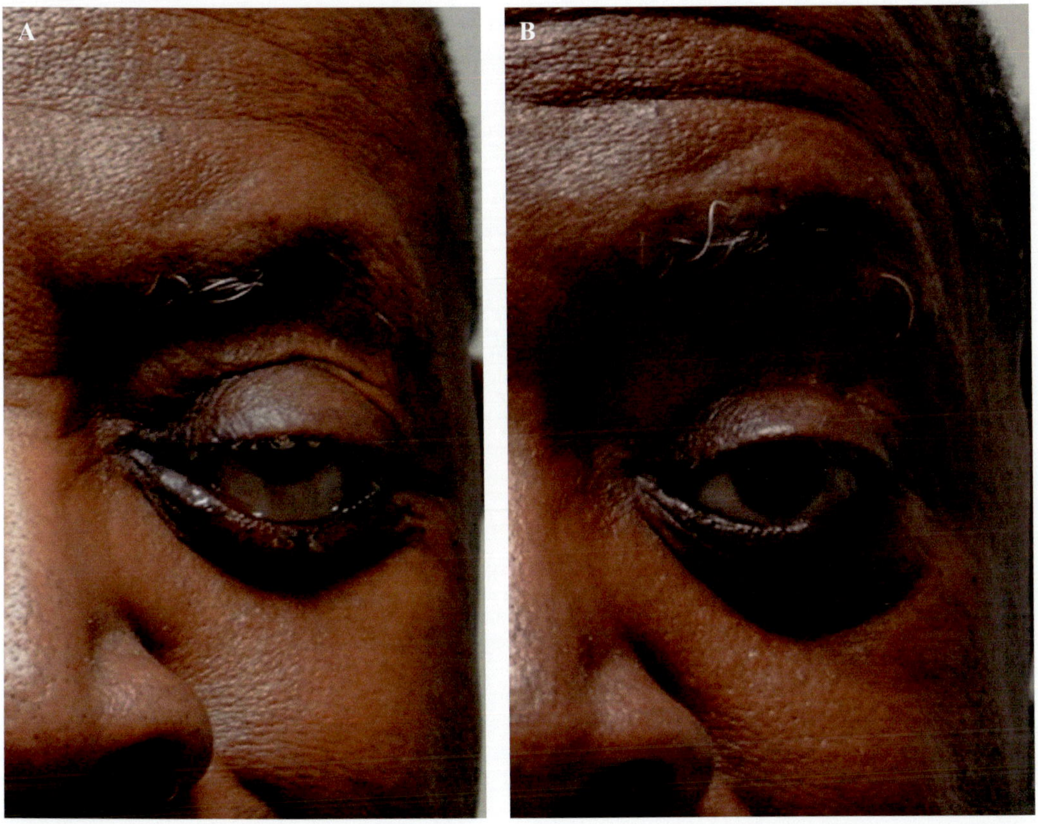

Fig. 8 **A** Profound lower eyelid retraction due to laxity and mechanical vectors (prosthesis stretching eyelid). **B** Patient in Fig. 8A 6 months after a porcine acellular dermal matrix implant secured to the middle lamella and secured to laterally to the orbital rim with improved lower eyelid retraction, tone, and ability to retain an ocular prosthesis

9 Conclusions

Acellular dermal matrix offers an off the shelf spacer graft repair of lower eyelid retraction.

Their use may decrease surgical time and risk from a second surgical site. Complications include reaction, contracture, or resorption but they may compare favorably to other spacers such as autologous or donor grafts.

References

1. Macadam SA, Lennox PA. Acellular dermal matrices: use in reconstructive and aesthetic breast surgery. Can J Plast Surg. 2012;20(2):75–89. https://doi.org/10.1177/229255031202000201.
2. Barmettler A, Heo M. A prospective, randomized comparison of lower eyelid retraction repair with autologous auricular cartilage, bovine acellular dermal matrix (Surgimend), and porcine acellular dermal matrix (Enduragen) spacer grafts. Ophthalmic Plast Reconstr Surg. 2018;34(3):266–73. https://doi.org/10.1097/iop.0000000000000946.
3. Tao JP, Aakalu VK, Wladis EJ, et al. bioengineered acellular dermal matrix spacer grafts for lower eyelid retraction repair: a report by the American Academy of Ophthalmology. Ophthalmology. 2020;127(5):689–95. https://doi.org/10.1016/j.ophtha.2019.11.011.
4. Park E, Lewis K, Alghoul MS. Comparison of efficacy and complications among various spacer grafts in the treatment of lower eyelid retraction: a systematic review. Aesthetic Surg J. 2017;37(7):743–54. https://doi.org/10.1093/asj/sjx003.
5. Sullivan SA, Dailey RA. Graft contraction: a comparison of acellular dermis versus hard palate mucosa in lower eyelid surgery. Ophthalmic Plast Reconstr Surg. 2003;19(1):14–24. https://doi.org/10.1097/01.Iop.0000040678.19893.F7.
6. Kim KH, Baek JS, Lee S, et al. Causes and surgical outcomes of lower eyelid retraction. Korean J Ophthalmol. 2017;31(4):290–8. https://doi.org/10.3341/kjo.2016.0059.

7. Grisolia ABD, Couso RC, Matayoshi S, Douglas RS, Briceño CA. Non-surgical treatment for eyelid retraction in thyroid eye disease (TED). Br J Ophthalmol. 2017. https://doi.org/10.1136/bjophthalmol-2017-310695.
8. Patipa M. The evaluation and management of lower eyelid retraction following cosmetic surgery. Plast Reconstr Surg. 2000;106(2):438–53; discussion 454–9. https://doi.org/10.1097/00006534-200008000-00033.

Tarsal Graft to the Lower Eyelid

Amy P. Jain, Julia L. Kerolus and Swapna Vemuri

Abstract

Free tarsal grafts can be used to reconstruct full-thickness lower eyelid defects or address lower eyelid retraction. Tarsal grafts are not only autologous but offer perhaps the best match for lower eyelid repair since they are harvested form another eyelid. The chief risk is donor site morbidity, namely elevation of the upper eyelid margin. This chapter describes relevant anatomy and surgical techniques for free tarsal graft harvest and placement into a recipient lower eyelid.

Keywords

Free tarsal graft · Lower eyelid tarsal graft · Lower eyelid retraction · Eyelid spacer graft

A. P. Jain (✉)
Private Practice, Newport Beach, CA, USA
e-mail: amypatel09@gmail.com

J. L. Kerolus
Private Practice, Atlanta, GA, USA
S. Vemuri Henry Ford Health, Detroit, MI, USA

1 Introduction

First described in 1918 by Blasovic, tarsal grafts have been successfully used to help restore lower eyelid anatomy and function [1]. They have been used to address full-thickness lower eyelid defects, lower eyelid retraction, and other eyelid pathology [2]. Traditional teaching emphasizes the importance of bilamellar reconstruction of the lower eyelid and the need for a vascular supply to at least either the anterior or posterior lamella to ensure adequate tissue survival [3]. With a flap to reconstruct the anterior lamella, a free tarsal graft may be an excellent choice for the posterior lamella [4, 5]. Free tarsal grafts can also be used in lower eyelid retraction repair by lengthening and supporting the posterior lamella.

2 Lower Eyelid Anatomy

The lower eyelid is divided anatomically into lamellae. The anterior lamella of the lower eyelid consists of the skin and orbicularis oculi muscle, which is subdivided into the orbital and palpebral regions. The palpebral region of the orbicularis oculi muscle is organized into preseptal and pretarsal segments. The pretarsal component covers the tarsus and produces involuntary blinking and aides in tear flow. The preseptal segment is more inferior and covers the orbital septum. It helps with involuntary blinking. The middle lamella

J. P. Tao (ed.), *Plastic Surgery of the Lower Eyelids*,
https://doi.org/10.1007/978-3-031-36175-3_20

is composed of the orbital septum. The posterior lamella consists of the tarsus and conjunctiva. The tarsal plate is the main structural component of the eyelid and is 25 mm long, approximately 1 mm thick, and 5 mm in height in the lower eyelid. It is made of dense connective tissue and merges with the canthal tendons medially and laterally as well as the capsulopalpebral fascia inferiorly [6].

3 Lower Eyelid Reconstruction

For large defects in the lower eyelid, the posterior lamella is commonly reconstructed from a tarsoconjunctival flap raised centrally from the upper eyelid [7–9]. A skin graft or flap forms the anterior lamella [2]. Advantages of the tarsoconjunctival flap include a maintained blood supply via the pedicle which theoretically optimizes survivability and mitigates risk of necrosis as well as inherent upward traction which can help support the lower eyelid and mitigate lower eyelid retraction. The main disadvantages of the tarsoconjunctival flap include visual obstruction for approximately 2–6 weeks and morbidity associated with a second procedure involving flap takedown.

A small myocutaneous advancement or rotational flap may sometimes be left bare posteriorly. Alternatively a tarsal graft may be used to rebuild the posterior lamella [2, 3, 5, 10]. This obviates visual obstruction during the healing process with tarsoconjunctival flaps and the need for a second flap division surgery [11–13].

Disadvantages include donor site morbidity including eyelid retraction or peaking, ocular discomfort, and keratopathy. Subsequent procedures that may be required to alter the position of the donor eyelid may be less predictable after tarsal graft harvest [14].

4 Lower Eyelid Spacer in Lower Eyelid Retraction

Numerous spacer graft materials have been described in the literature to address lower eyelid retraction caused by posterior lamellar deficiency. These include autologous hard palate or ear cartilage, and acellular dermal allografts or xenografts (described in other chapters) [15–19]. Free autologous tarsal grafts have also been used as a biological spacer [15]. Simultaneous midface lifting is often required to provide additional support to the lower eyelid. The graft is often required to be oversized to account for tissue contraction with wound healing. Limitations of a tarsal graft as a biological spacer include an upper vertical height limit to the graft size due to the need to preserve at least 4 mm vertical height of tarsus at the harvest site. Advantages are minimal donor site morbidity and tissue that is most biocompatible. Disadvantages include donor site morbidity including keratopathy and upper eyelid malposition changes—both of which may exacerbate any underlying pathology related to lower eyelid retraction [19].

5 Surgical Technique for Tarsal Graft Harvesting

The procedure can be performed under local anesthesia or with sedation if required. The amount of tarsal graft to be harvested is predetermined based on the defect size or the reconstructive needs. It is important to consider the graft limitations where 4 mm of vertical tarsus must be preserved on the host eyelid to maintain adequate stability.

A 4-0 traction suture is placed through the upper eyelid margin. The upper eyelid is everted over a Desmarres retractor. A caliper is used to measure 4 mm vertically from the superior eyelid margin and marked to ensure adequate tarsus remains in the upper eyelid. The required horizontal graft size is noted by the surgeon and marked on the upper eyelid tarsus. Local anesthetic is infiltrated into the supratarsal subconjunctival plane and anterior to the tarsus. A horizontal incision is made along the length of the previously marked tarsus with a number 15 blade. The graft is raised centrally, where the tarsal plate has the greatest vertical dimension. Wescott scissors are used to dissect the levator aponeurosis and pretarsal orbicularis oculi muscle from tarsal surface thus completing the graft harvest. (Fig. 1) If the tarsal graft is being using to reconstruct the lower eyelid margin, a small cuff of conjunctiva should be left attached to the tarsal graft at the superior border. Hemostasis at the donor site is achieved with gentle pressure and cautery. The donor site does not require repair and can be left to heal by second intention. The harvested free tarsal graft can then be sutured to the recipient lower eyelid posterior lamella.

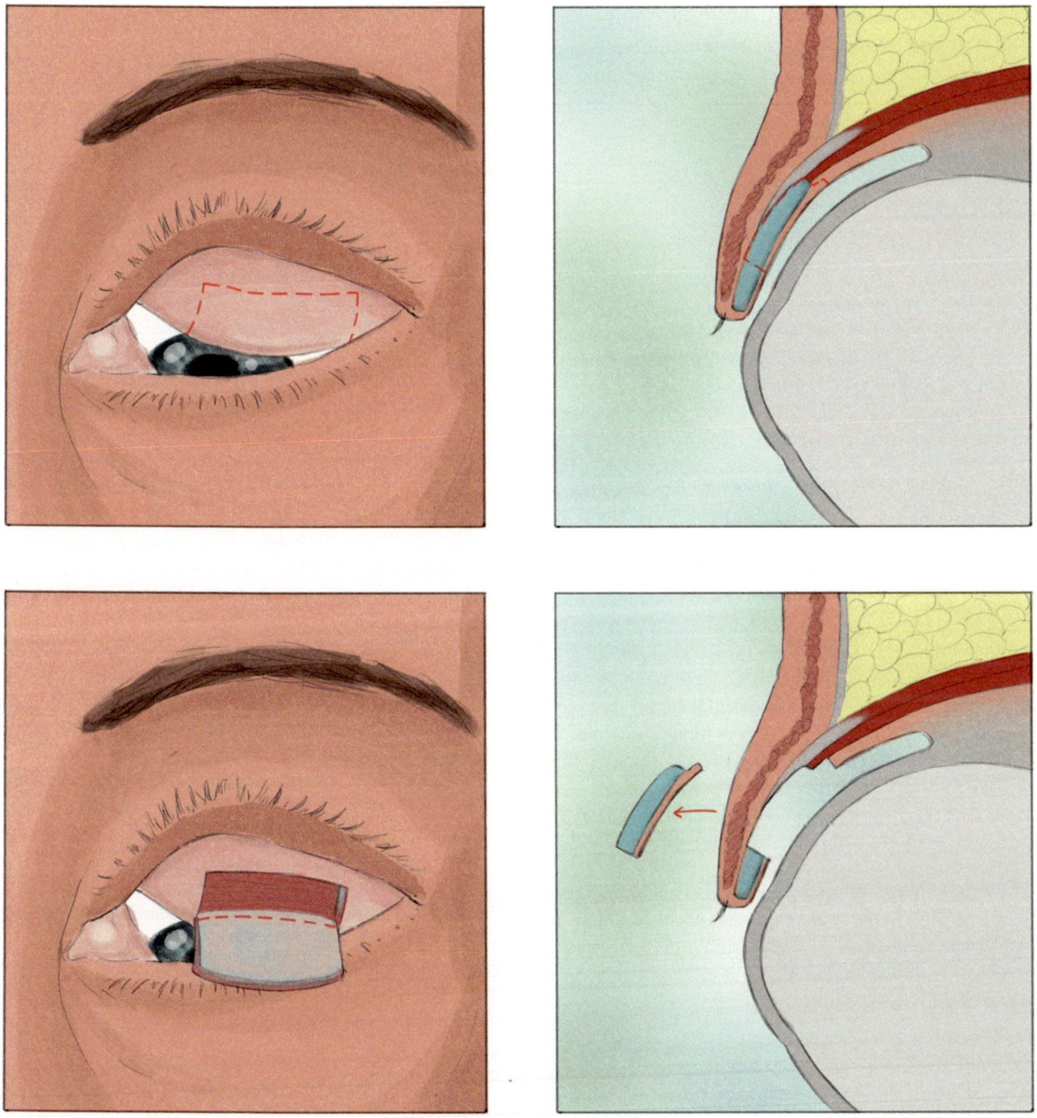

Fig. 1 The upper eyelid is everted and the tarsus is marked for resection. The horizontal incision should be 4 mm superior to the eyelid margin to maintain stability of the host upper eyelid. The graft is harvested with sharp dissection preserving pretarsal orbicularis oculi muscle and skin anteriorly. Illustrations by *Michael Han*

6 Conclusion

Tarsal grafts may be useful for variety of lower eyelid defects [2]. Tarsal grafts play an important role in reconstruction of the lower eyelid as they both line and stabilize the eyelid. They may also be used as a spacer graft material to help recess the capsulopalpebral fascia in lower eyelid retraction repair. Their autologous and especially upper eyelid source, make them an ideal graft for the lower eyelid except that they are limited in size.

References

1. Blaskovics L. Über Totalplastik des unteren Lideyelides. Bildung einer hinteren Lideyelidplatte durch Transplantation eines Tarsus und Bindehautstreifens aus dem Oberlide. Ophthalmologica 1918;40: 222–7.
2. Stephenson CM, MD, Brown BZ, MD. The use of tarsus as a free autogenous graft in eyelid surgery. Ophthalmic Plast Reconstr Surg. 1985;1(1):43–50.
3. Bartley GB, Messenger MM. The dehiscent Hughes flap: outcomes and implications. Trans Am Ophthalmol Soc. 2002;100:61–65; discussion 65–66.
4. Bortz JG, Al-Shweiki S. Free tarsal graft and free skin graft for lower eyelid reconstruction. Ophthalmic Plast Reconstr Surg. 2020;36(6):605–9. https://doi.org/10.1097/IOP.0000000000001680.
5. Memarzadeh K, Gustafsson L, Blohme J, Malmsjö M. Evaluation of the microvascular blood flow, oxygenation, and survival of tarsoconjunctival flaps following the modified Hughes procedure. Ophthalmic Plast Reconstr Surg. 2016;32:468–72.
6. A, Massry G. Eyelid and periorbital anatomy, in The art of aesthetic surgery: principles and techniques, 3rd ed. 2019.
7. Hughes WL. A new method for rebuilding a lower lid: report of a case. Arch Ophthalmol. 1937;17:1008–17. https://doi.org/10.1001/archopht.1937.00850060064005.
8. Rohrich RJ, Zbar RI. The evolution of the Hughes tarsoconjunctival flap for the lower eyelid reconstruction. Plast Reconstr Surg. 1999;104(2):518–22; quiz 523; discussion 524–6. https://doi.org/10.1097/00006534-199908000-00033. PMID: 10654700.
9. Leibovitch I, Selva D. Modified Hughes flap: division at 7 days. Ophthalmology. 2004;111:2164–7.
10. Hawes MJ. Free autogenous grafts in eyelid tarsoconjunctival reconstruction. Ophthalmic Surg. 1986;18:37–41.
11. Bortz JG, Al-Shweiki S. Free tarsal graft and free skin graft for lower eyelid reconstruction. Ophthalmic Plast Reconstr Surg. 2020;36(6):605–9. https://doi.org/10.1097/IOP.0000000000001680. PMID: 32732536.
12. Zinkernagel MS, Catalano E, Ammann-Rauch D. Free tarsal graft combined with skin transposition flap for full-thickness lower eyelid reconstruction. Ophthalmic Plast Reconstr Surg. 2007;23(3):228–31. doi: https://doi.org/10.1097/IOP.0b013e318057797d. PMID: 17519664.
13. Collin JRO. A manual of systematic eyelid surgery. 3rd ed. Philadelphia, PA: Elsevier Inc.; 2006.
14. Leibovitch I, Selva D, Davis G, Ghabrial R. Donor site morbidity in free tarsal grafts. Am J Ophthalmol. 2004;138:430–3.
15. Baylis HI, Nelson ER, Goldberg RA. Lower eyelid retraction following blepharoplasty. Ophthal Plast Reconstr Surg. 1992;8:170–5.
16. Brock WD, Bearden W, Tann T 3rd, et al. Autogenous dermis skin grafts in lower eyelid reconstruction. Ophthal Plast Reconstr Surg. 2003;19:394–7.
17. Korn BS, Kikkawa DO, Cohen SR, et al. Treatment of lower eyelid malposition with dermis fat grafting. Ophthalmology. 2008;115:744-751.e2.
18. Yoon MK, McCulley TJ. Autologous dermal grafts as posterior lamellar spacers in the management of lower eyelid retraction. Ophthal Plast Reconstr Surg. 2014;30:64–8.
19. Leibovitch I, Malhotra R, Selva D. Hard palate and free tarsal grafts as posterior lamella substitutes in upper lid surgery. Ophthalmology. 2006;113(3):489–96. https://doi.org/10.1016/j.ophtha.2005.11.017. PMID: 16513464.

Lower Eyelid Surgery in Facial Paralysis

Suzana Matayoshi

Abstract

Facial paralysis and loss of orbicularis oculi muscle tone causes lower eyelid malposition. Ectropion and eyelid retraction are common, as is lagophthalmos. The ocular surface exposure can cause epiphora due to reflex hyper lacrimation. In this chapter, common surgical techniques to rehabilitate the paretic lower eyelid are described. These include horizontal tightening as well as eyelid retraction repair.

Keywords

Facial paralysis · Lagophthalmos · Lower eyelid retraction · Bell palsy · Facial paresis · Paralytic ectropion

1 Introduction

Facial nerve palsy can cause disfigurement and functional deficit. Immediate therapy should aim for corneal protection. Both short and long-term facial rehabilitation may be indicated.

Supplementary Information The online version contains supplementary material available at https://doi.org/10.1007/978-3-031-36175-3_21.

S. Matayoshi (✉)
University of São Paolo, São Paolo, Brazil
e-mail: suzana.matayoshi@gmail.com

The most frequent and benign etiology of facial nerve paralysis is Bell Palsy, which has an abrupt onset but recovers in most cases [1]. Trauma is another cause of facial paralysis, accounting for 10–23% of cases. It can be iatrogenenic, during otologic or parotid surgery, or acoustic neuroma resection. In these cases, whether there was total or partial involvement of the nerve will determine the prognosis. If the nerve was transected or resected completely, spontaneous resolution is not likely [2]. Infections and neoplasms of the facial nerve are other causes of facial paralysis. Cerebrovascular accidents are a central nervous system etiology.

Clinically, the patient presents with brow ptosis, labial commissure deviation, nasal ala collapse, and attenuation of frontal expression wrinkles. In the periocular region, the changes are related to paralysis of the orbicularis muscle, responsible for eyelid occlusion, and may vary in severity and presentation, depending on the patient's age and degree of paralysis. Exposure keratitis is a serious problem and the urgency of treatment may depend on the severity [3, 4]. In patients with eyelid laxity, generally the elderly, paralytic ectropion and eyelid retraction may be more profound due to loss of the lower eyelid tone (Fig. 1).

Exposure of the tarsus and tarsal conjunctiva causes a progressive congestive process, leading to hyperemia, epiphora, and conjunctival secretion. In some cases, upper eyelid movement may

J. P. Tao (ed.), *Plastic Surgery of the Lower Eyelids*,
https://doi.org/10.1007/978-3-031-36175-3_21

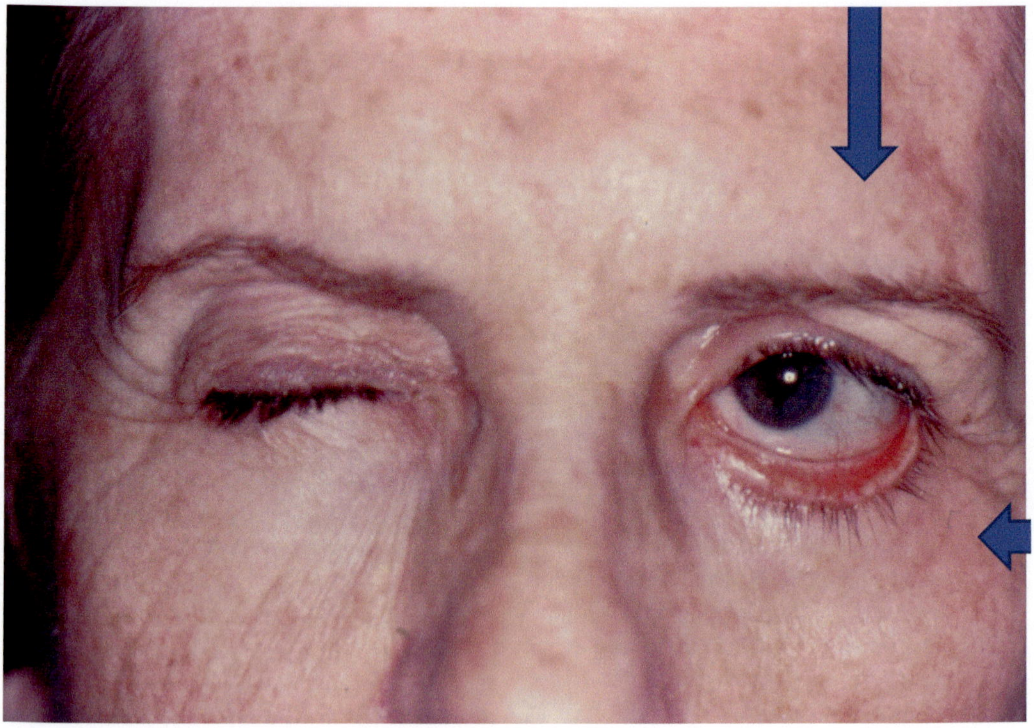

Fig. 1 Elderly patient presenting paralytic ectropion, lagophthalmos, and eyelid retraction

be impaired without significant loss of lower eyelid tone, causing lagophthalmos and incomplete blink reflex (Fig. 2).

This chapter will focus on corrective surgical techniques involving the lower eyelid. There exist two general goals: (1) horizontal eyelid tightening and (2) lower retraction correction.

2 Horizontal Tightening Procedures

These procedures reinforce tension of the lateral eyelid, such as the tarsal strip or canthoplasty. In the tarsal strip technique, a lateral canthotomy and inferior cantholysis are performed and a lateral strip of the tarsus fashioned by sharp dissection. The strip is shortened and anchored to the inner aspect of the orbital rim periosteum (Fig. 3) (see Chap. "Ectropion Repair and Lateral Canthal Anchoring"). If medial lower eyelid sagging occurs a medial ligament tuck may be required [5] (see Chap. "Medial Canthal Surgery").

3 Correction of Lower Eyelid Retraction

Even with good horizontal tension of the lower eyelid, lower retraction can contribute to exposure and disfigurement. There exist several approaches to correct lower eyelid retraction: graft interposition, midface lift, and upper to lower eyelid connection bands.

4 Lower Eyelid Grafts

Grafts typically aid in lower eyelid retraction through treating cicatricial or negative vectors. Their role in treating isolated paralytic vectors

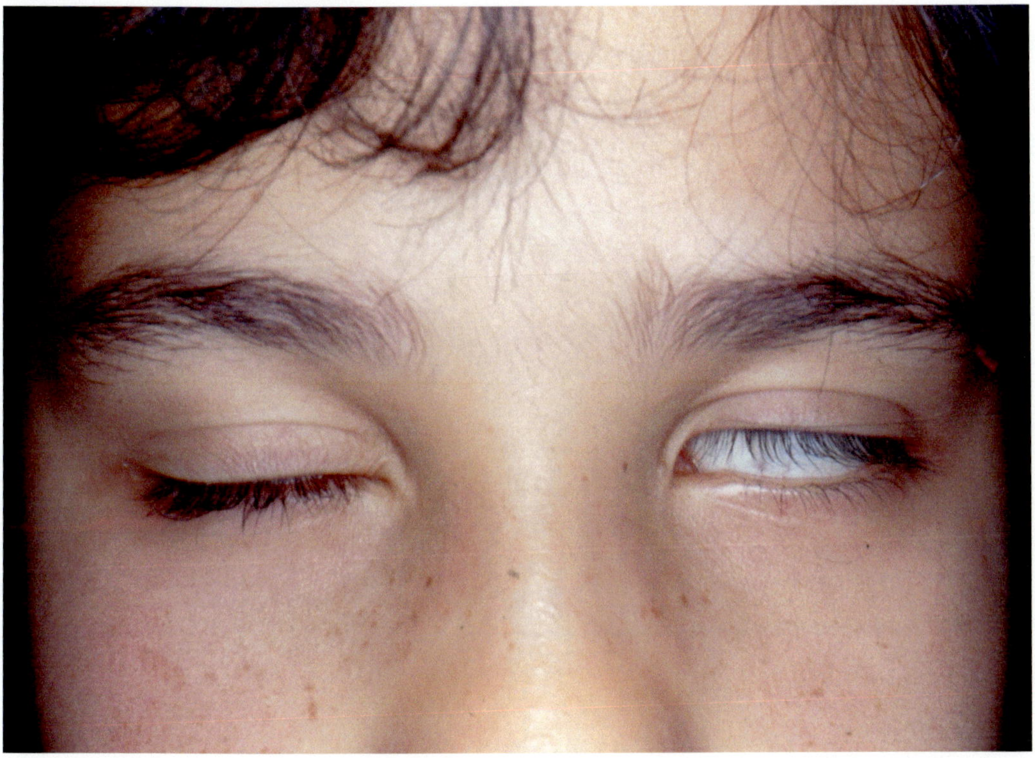

Fig. 2 A younger patient presented left lagophthalmos, lower eyelid in a good position and tone

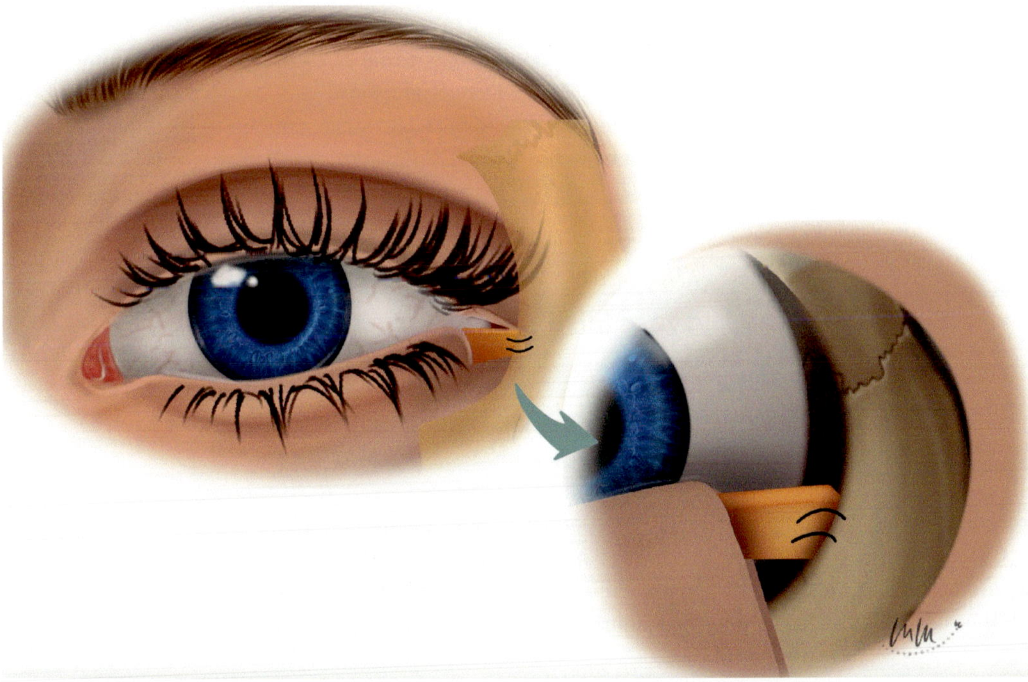

Fig. 3 Standard lateral tarsal strip – the detail shows tarsal sutures at the orbital periosteum

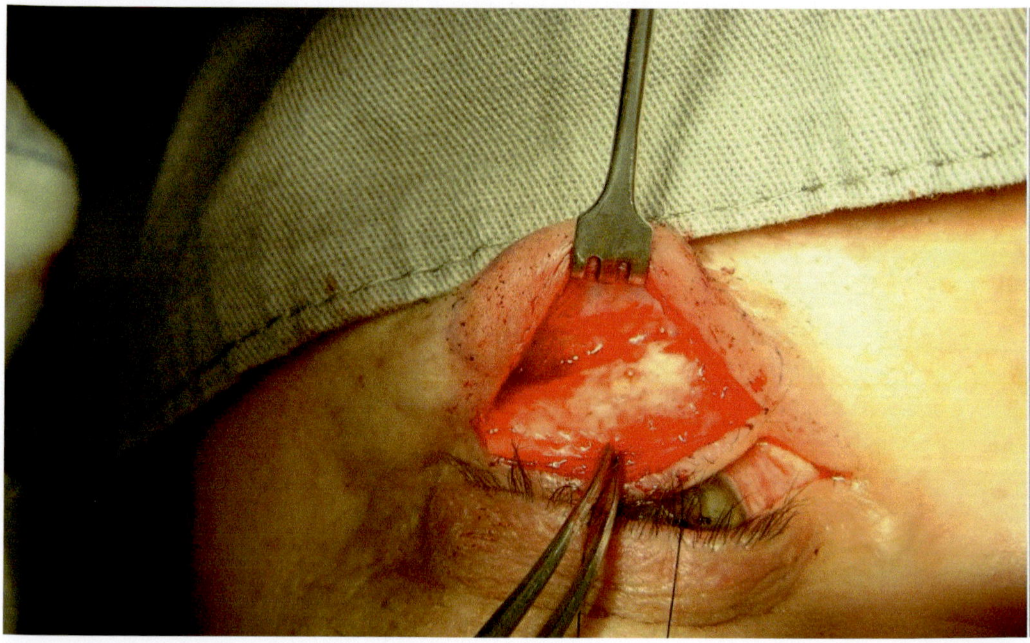

Fig. 4 Ear cartilage graft

is very limited. When supporting or lengthening the posterior lamella is desired, autologous materials such as ear cartilage (Fig. 4), hard palate, and dermis can be interposed for vertical support of the lower eyelid [5–7]. Acellular dermal matrix or donor sclera are are options that obviate a second surgical site. These grafts and interposition techniques are described in other chapters but are sometimes used in patients with multi-vector, including paralytic, lower eyelid retraction.

5 Elevation of the Mid Face (also see Chap. "Midface Lift")

Dissection and elevation of the midface, often described as a suborbicular oculi fat (SOOF) lift can be used alone or together with other procedures. The technique is described in detail in Chap. "Midface Lift". In short, it can be performed via a cutaneous or transconjunctival approach. The steps in both procedures are releasing the orbitomalar ligament, reaching the suborbicular fat, and its fixation in the lateral orbital rim. Lifting the midface is included in larger facial sling procedures that utilize fascia or other grafts to lift the sagging cheeks and lower face, including the oral commissure. Details of these are beyond the scope if this chapter but since patients with facial paralysis usually have midface ptosis, midface lifts also help improve facial symmetry (Fig. 5). In facial paralysis, the durability of midface lifting is limited, and regression of effect is expected in most patients.

6 Upper Eyelid Support Techniques for the Lower Eyelid

Upper eyelid retractors can be used to pull the lower eyelid superiorly. The authors highlight three techniques for this purpose: (1) lateral intermarginal adhesion tarsorrhaphy, (2)

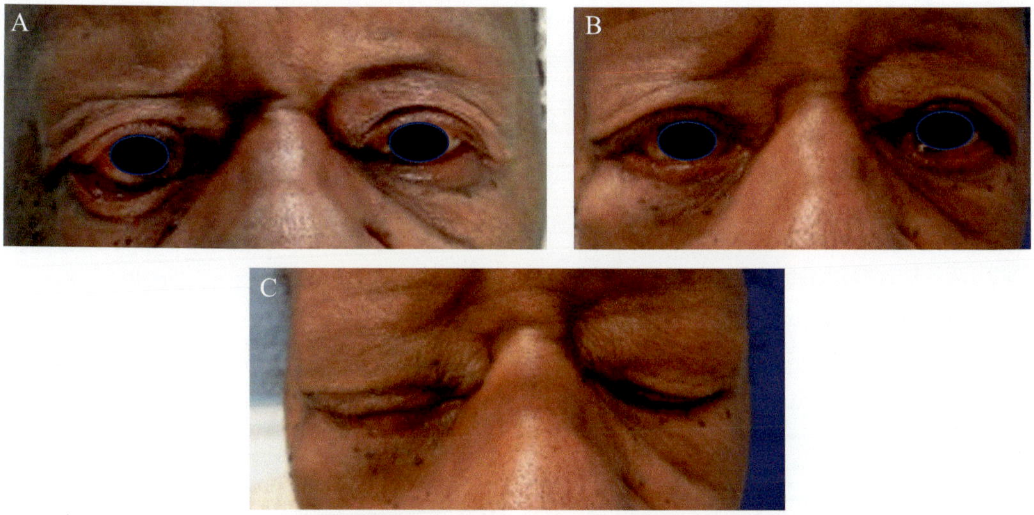

Fig. 5 Elderly patient with longstanding paralytic ectropium and cheek sagging. A. Before surgery. B. One month after right tarsal strip and SOOF elevation. C. Improved eyelid occlusion after surgery

tarsoconjuntival onlay flap, and (3) medial tarsorrhaphy with or without canaliculopalsty.

6.1 Lateral Intermarginal Adhesion Tarsorrhaphy Technique

An incision is made in the lower eyelid along the gray line (depending on the desired tension, between 5 and 8 mm). The skin and orbicularis are resected laterally to the lateral commissure (Fig. 6) with a reduction of the palpebral fissure horizontally. In the upper eyelid, an incision is made along the gray line (half the size of the lower eyelid), and a tarsoconjunctival triangle is resected. The lower posterior lamella is elevated and sutured to the upper eyelid. This technique is functionally excellent because it corrects the component of horizontal and vertical eyelid closure; however, patients often complain of facial asymmetry.

6.2 Lateral Tarsoconjunctival Onlay Flap (Video 1).

This technique uses an upper tarsoconjunctival flap (as described for reconstruction of large lower eyelid defects). The flap, 4–8 mm in horizontal extension, is dissected to 4 mm from the upper margin. A horizontal incision extended from the lateral fornix medially for 4–8 mm, depending on the desired amount of eyelid fissure closure. In the lower eyelid, in the same horizontal extension, a thin layer of posterior margin is resected. The upper eyelid flap is sutured to lower posterior lamella using interrupted stitches. The flap elevates the lower eyelid using upper eyelid strength (Fig. 7) [8]. The flap is usually concealed under the upper eyelid (Fig. 8) and is relatively inconspicuous. Owing to the attachment sight of the lower eyelid margin superior to the lateral (and posterior to) upper eyelid, the lower eyelid can be raised

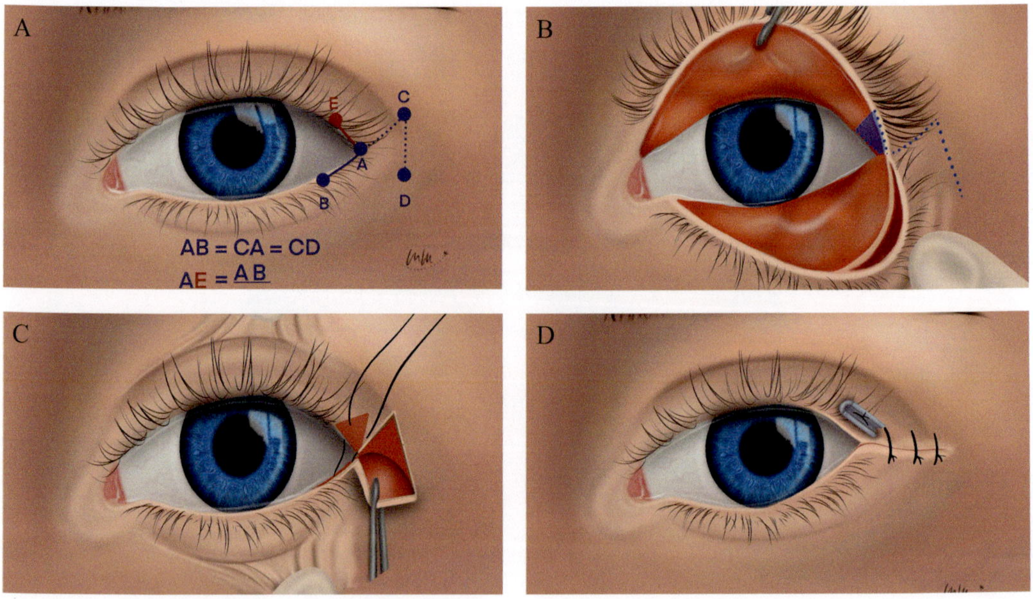

Fig. 6 Tessier canthoplasty: A- Drawing lines; B-Preparing triangles; C- lower posterior lamella sutured to upper eyelid; D- horizontal and vertical eyelid dimensions reduced

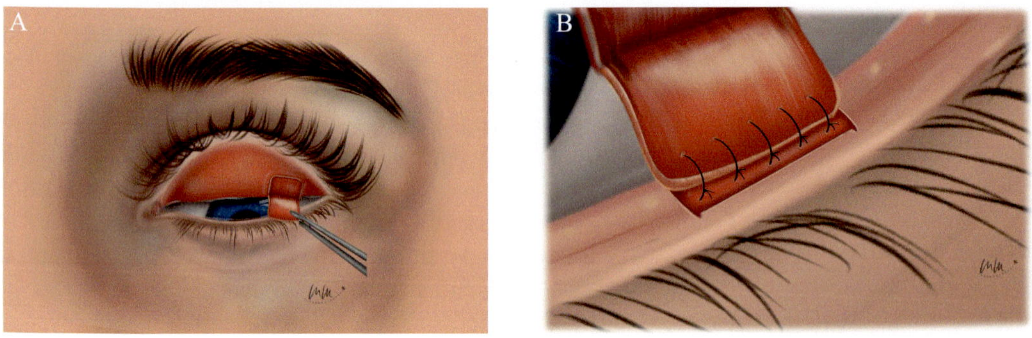

Fig. 7 Tarsoconjunctival onlay flap: A- upper lamella flap; B- flap is sutured to lower margin

higher than with an intermarginal adhesion tarsorrhaphy. In more profound lower eyelid paralytic retraction and lagophthalmos, flaps often require adjunctive procedures to elevate the medial lower eyelid.

Medial tarsorrhaphy with or without canaliculoplasty (Video 2).

The medial eyelid margin is deepithelialized with care to preserve the underlying canaliculus. A Bowman wire can aid in identifying the

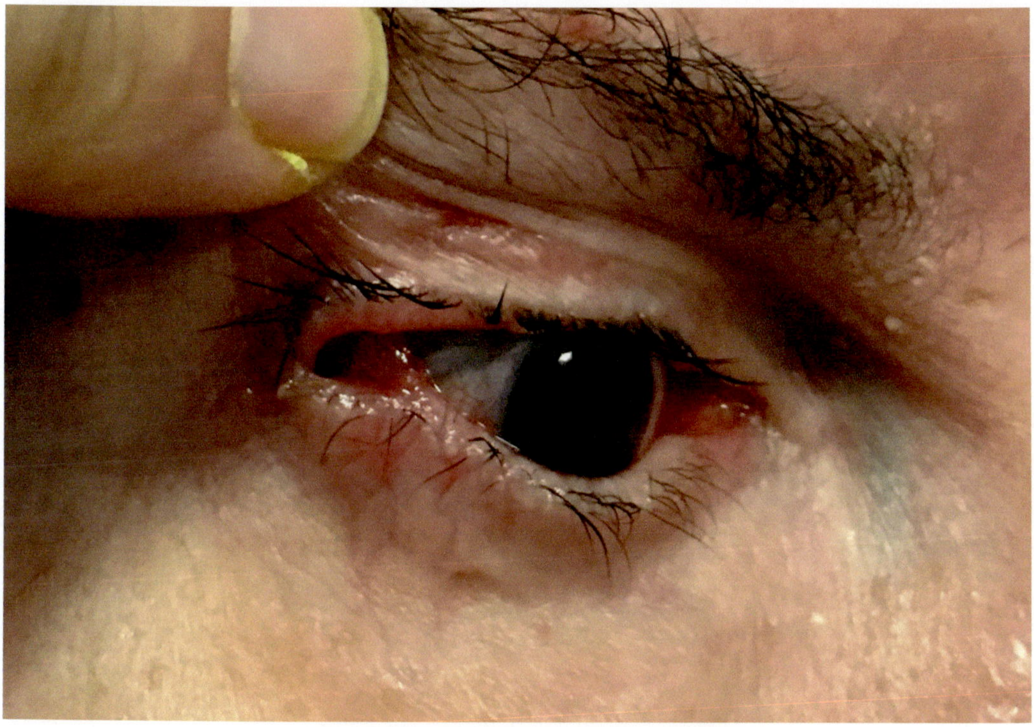

Fig. 8 The flap is concealed laterally by the upper eyelid

canaliculus. Absorbable sutures are used to fuse the medial eyelids. A temporary suture tarsorrhaphy can be placed to prevent dehiscence.

A modification is to incise the upper and lower canaliculus horizontally. The anterior cut edge of the canaliculi of the upper and lower eyelid are united yet maintain a posterior tear outflow entrance into the canalicular systems (Fig. 9). This technique provides medial closure and maintains a tear outflow channel to the lacrimal drainage apparatus (Fig. 10).

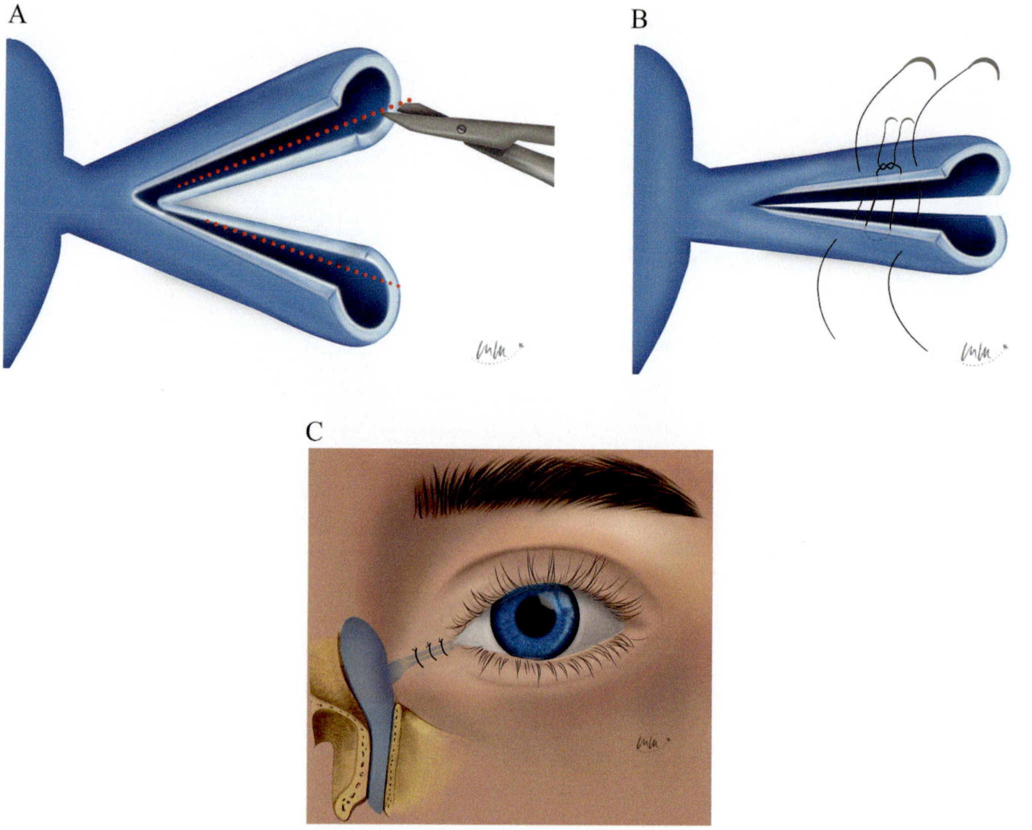

Fig. 9 Modified canaliculoplasty. A- Horizontal longitudinal incision of the upper and lower canaliculi; B- The upper and lower canaliculi are fused anteriorly to provide medial closure; C- Final appearance

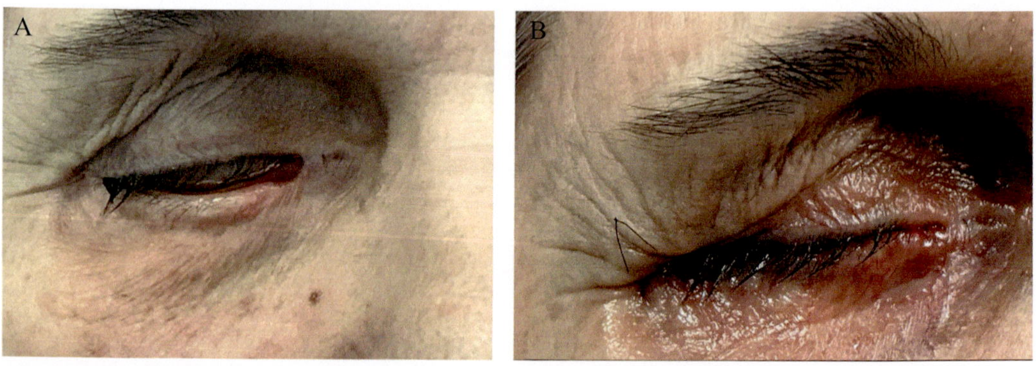

Fig. 10 Modified lacorphaphy. A-Partial eyelid fissure occlusion. B- After surgery

7 Conclusions

Several surgical techniques are available for correction of lower eyelid malposition in facial paralysis. The aims are to reposition the eyelid margin, correct horizontal sagging, and lower retraction. Concomitant vectors may be present and should be treated accordingly.

References

1. Zhang WXL, Luo T, Wu F, Zhao B, Li X. The etiology of Bell's palsy: a review. J Neurol. 2020;267(7):1896–905.
2. Spencer CR, Irving RM. Causes and management of facial nerve palsy. Br J Hosp Med (Lond). 2016;77(12):686–91.
3. Joseph SS, Joseph AW, Douglas RS, Massry GG. Periocular reconstruction in patients with facial paralysis. Otolaryngol Clin North Am. 2016;49(2):475–87.
4. Bergeron CM, Moe KS. The evaluation and treatment of lower eyelid paralysis. Facial Plast Surg. 2008;24(2):231–41.
5. Chang L, Olver J. A useful augmented lateral tarsal strip tarsorrhaphy for paralytic ectropion. Ophthalmology. 2006;113(1):84–91.
6. Allen RC. Controversies in periocular reconstruction for facial nerve palsy. Curr Opin Ophthalmol. 2018;29(5):423–7.
7. Ibrahim AM, Rabie AN, Kim PS, Medina M, Upton J, Lee BT, et al. Static treatment modalities in facial paralysis: a review. J Reconstr Microsurg. 2013;29(4):223–32.
8. Tao JP, Vemuri S, Patel AD, Compton C, Nunery WR. Lateral tarsoconjunctival onlay flap lower eyelid suspension in facial nerve paresis. Ophthalmic Plast Reconstr Surg. 2014;30(4):342–5.

Tarsoconjunctival Flap Lower Eyelid Suspension

Michael C. Yang, Seanna R. Grob and Jeremiah P. Tao

Abstract

A lateral tarsoconjunctival flap is an effective and minimally invasive treatment for lower eyelid retraction. In the technique, a lateral upper eyelid posterior lamella-based flap is used to suspend the lower eyelid. This narrows the palpebral fissure in a less conspicuous manner than the traditional intermarginal adhesion tarsorrhaphy. The far lateral placement of the flap is well camouflaged. The resultant canthal tilt and slightly dominant lateral upper eyelid margin conform to aesthetic ideals. It may be an adjunct or a standalone procedure that obviates incomplete retraction correction or disfigurement associated with other procedures. The flap can be augmented or reversed with relative ease. This chapter describes the indications and techniques for a tarsoconjunctival suspension flap.

Keywords

Lower eyelid retraction · Lateral tarsoconjunctival onlay flap · Lower eyelid suspension · Ectropion · Paralytic lagophthalmos

1 Introduction

Lower eyelid retraction can be due to involutional, paralytic, negative, or cicatricial vectors [1]. Lower eyelid retraction can cause unsatisfactory aesthetics or contribute to ocular irritation. In serious forms, permanent vision loss can ensue from ocular surface exposure.

In cicatricial lower eyelid retraction, the anterior, middle, and posterior lamella may be scarred [2]. Involutional or paralytic vectors may also cause lower eyelid retraction. In some patients, a negative vector due to a prominent globe or recessed midface or both may present additional challenges. Repairing lower eyelid retraction is often challenging due to these multiple variables that often coexist in the same eyelid.

Many individual procedures do not adequately treat lower eyelid retraction. For example, canthoplasty (e.g., lateral tarsal strip)

Illustrations by Michael Han

Supplementary Information The online version contains supplementary material available at https://doi.org/10.1007/978-3-031-36175-3_22.

S. R. Grob (✉)
Oculofacial Plastic and Orbital Surgery, Department of Ophthalmology, University of California, San Francisco, San Francisco, CA, USA
e-mail: seanna.grob@ucsf.edu

M. C. Yang · J. P. Tao
Gavin Herbert Eye Institute, University of California, Irvine, Irvine, CA, USA
e-mail: mcyang@hs.uci.edu

J. P. Tao (ed.), *Plastic Surgery of the Lower Eyelids*,
https://doi.org/10.1007/978-3-031-36175-3_22

addresses horizontal laxity but fails to improve vertical vectors [3]. On the other hand, utilizing skin, other grafts, or pillar tarsorrhaphies to support the eyelid vertically can result in conspicuous scars or disfiguring tissue bands [4, 5].

The use of a lateral tarsoconjunctival flap may obviate many problems with other approaches. A tarsoconjunctival suspension (a.k.a. tarsoconjunctival onlay) flap has been utilized to treat lower eyelid retraction in patients with paralytic, cicatricial and multi-vector factors [6–8] (Figs. 1, and 2). By joining the superior posterior lamella of the lateral upper eyelid to the lower eyelid margin, the lower eyelid is held up akin to how suspenders hold up pants. As it is connected to both the upper and lower eyelid, it can also assist in bringing the two eyelids together with blinking or eyelid closure to treat lagophthalmos or ocular exposure. The conjunctival band is well tolerated on the lateral ocular surface. It may act as a third eyelid or akin to a nictitating membrane seen in other species such as birds or reptiles.

While addressing functional issues, the flap maintains good cosmesis, which is especially important in cosmetic surgery patients. The tarsoconjunctival onlay flap is minimally invasive and does not require extensive surgery or the use of implants or grafts and can be reversible. The authors believe the lateral tarsoconjunctival suspension/onlay flap is one of the most powerful mechanisms to treat lower eyelid retraction.

Lastly, the small flap is also titratable, meaning a larger flap can address more severe lagophthalmos and ocular surface exposure. Like intermarginal adhesions though, larger tarsoconjunctival onlay flaps will lead to a smaller palpebral fissure and may impair the peripheral visual field.

2 Preoperative Evaluation

A history with particular attention to risk factors for lower eyelid retraction is important. These include prior ocular or facial surgeries, thyroid eye disease, facial nerve disorders, radiation therapy, trauma history and skin cancers. Symptoms of ocular exposure should also be assessed, including foreign body sensation, epiphora, and associated blurred vision.

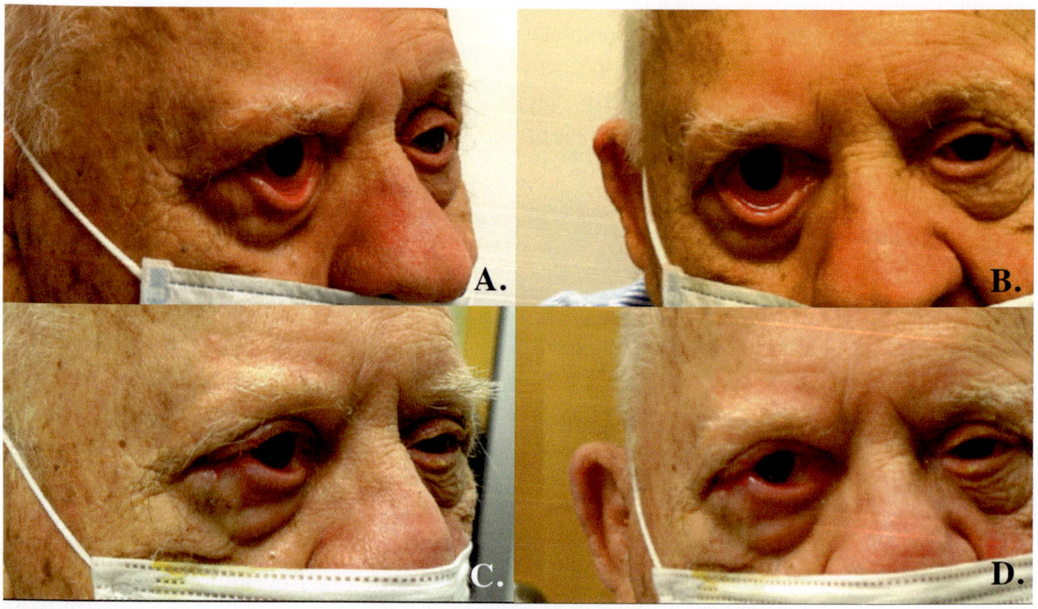

Fig. 1 **A, B.** Preoperative photographs of paralytic ectropion of the right lower eyelid from prior skull base infection. **C, D.** Postoperative photographs after a tarsoconjunctival suspension flap

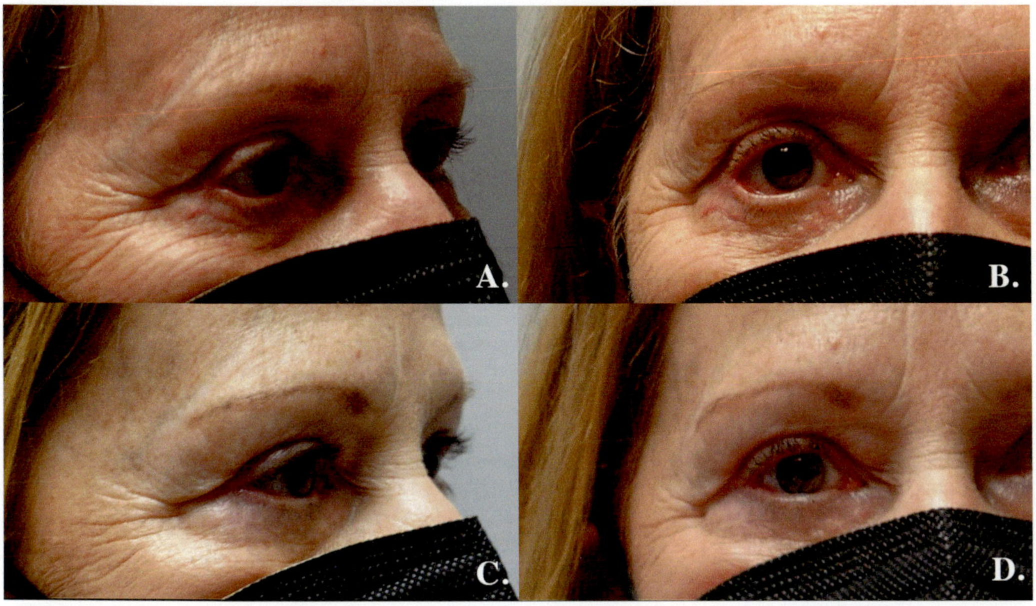

Fig. 2 **A, B.** Preoperative photographs of cicatricial ectropion of the right lower eyelid that failed multiple canthoplasties. **C, D.** Postoperative photographs, post-op month 4 after tarsoconjunctival suspension flap showing significantly improved lower eyelid position

Examination of the lower eyelid should include assessment for lagophthalmos, horizontal eyelid laxity, cicatricial changes, globe position in relation to orbital rim, as well as the rest of the midface. In the setting of facial nerve paralysis, facial muscle strength, especially the orbicularis oculi muscle, should be assessed. This includes blink excursion and eyelid closure. Assessing for blink weakness or blink lagophthalmos is key in many patients with exposure symptoms yet no frank ectropion or lower eyelid malposition in static assessment. Horizontal eyelid laxity can be evaluated with the eyelid distraction or snapback test. On the midface, malar fat pad descent and fat atrophy should be examined as additional negative vectors. Similarly, assessment for a prominent globe mechanically pushing the lower eyelid margin inferiorly is important. The cornea and ocular surface should be evaluated for exposure signs. Fluorescein or rose bengal dye may help highlight specific areas where the eye is exposed. In patients with lagophthalmos or an incomplete blink, the cornea may exhibit linear staining in the area that the eyelids fail to provide coverage.

3 Surgical Technique

The lateral tarsoconjunctival suspension/onlay flap is accomplished by creating a posterior lamella (conjunctiva with or without tarsus) flap from the lateral upper eyelid fornix. The leading edge of the flap is secured to the lateral lower eyelid margin.

Local anesthesia is injected into the upper and lower eyelid and lateral canthus. The procedure is well tolerated under local anesthesia but systemic anesthesia is sometimes indicated if more invasive procedures are performed concomitantly or if the patient is intolerant to local-only anesthesia. The periocular area is then prepped in the usual fashion for ophthalmic plastic surgery.

The four main stages of the procedure (Fig. 3A–E and Video 1):

1. Evert the lateral upper eyelid and expose posterior lamella (Fig. 3A).
2. Create the tarsoconjunctival flap in the upper eyelid lateral fornix with sharp dissection (Fig. 3B–C).

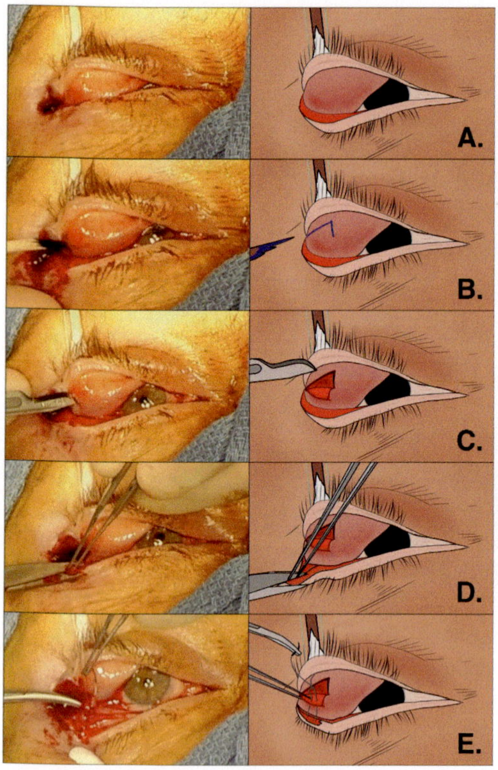

Fig. 3 Key surgical steps of the tarsoconjunctival suspension flap; intraoperative photos and corresponding illustrations. **A.** The upper eyelid is everted with a 4-0 silk or 5-0 polyglactin traction suture over a cotton-tipped applicator. **B.** The tarsoconjunctival flap is marked with methylene blue or a surgical marking pen. The horizontal length determines the width of the flap and is approximately 2–4 mm superior to the eyelid margin. **C.** The tarsoconjunctival flap is developed with at 15-blade followed by scissors. **D.** Westcott scissors or a 15-blade is used to create an incision along the gray line of the lower eyelid and denude the epithelium from the posterior lamella at the margin. The eyelashes are untouched. **E.** The leading edge of the tarsoconjunctival flap is sewn to the denuded posterior margin of the lower eyelid using a 5-0 polyglactin suture in an interrupted mattress fashion

3. De-epithelialize the lower eyelid margin to receive the flap (Fig. 3D).
4. Suture the leading edge of the tarsoconjunctival flap to the margin of the lower eyelid (Fig. 3E).

In the first stage, a temporary suture (the authors often use 5-0 polyglactin or 4-0 silk but the choice is inconsequential except that the suture needs to withstand the tension from eversion) is passed through the upper eyelid margin and the upper eyelid is everted over cotton-tipped applicators or a Desmarres retractor (Fig. 3A).

In the second stage, ink (methylene blue or marker) is used to delineate the tarsoconjunctival flap. Typically, a horizontal line is marked 2–4 mm superior to the upper eyelid margin from the far lateral canthus to the length of the flap. The medial aspect of the flap is demarcated with a vertical line (Fig. 3B). The horizontal width of the flap ranges 3–10 mm depending on the degree of desired palpebral fissure closure. In rare instances that complete ocular surface coverage is needed, the flap may be wider (20+ mm). With smaller flaps, minimal or no tarsus may be included. The amount of vertical dissection is dependent on the amount of lower eyelid elevation desired; less dissection is associated with a greater lift. A vertical incision and dissection of 2–5 mm is usually sufficient. Using a 15-blade, the flap is developed along the desired markings (Fig. 3C). The flap may be further developed with the 15-blade or Westcott scissors. Hemostasis can be achieved with electrocautery.

In the third stage, a 15-blade is used to create an incision at the gray line of the lower eyelid—the length of which corresponds with the size of the flap (Fig. 3D). In some cases, the attachment site of the flap on the lower eyelid margin is placed slightly medial to the sagittal plane of the medial aspect of the flap origin to achieve some lower eyelid horizontal tightening. This denuded area should also extend to the most lateral extent of the eyelid margin at the lateral canthus. The epithelium of the posterior lip of the lower eyelid margin is denuded with 15-blade or Westcott scissors and the lash line is left undisturbed.

In the fourth stage, the leading edge of the tarsoconjunctival flap is sewn to the denuded margin of the lower eyelid using a 5-0 polyglactin suture in an interrupted mattress fashion (Fig. 3E). The raw anterior aspect of the flap epithelializes as conjunctiva and appears as a pink band that is only visible with manual eyelid distraction (Fig. 4).

The flap may be used in isolation or with other procedures. Most commonly, a lateral

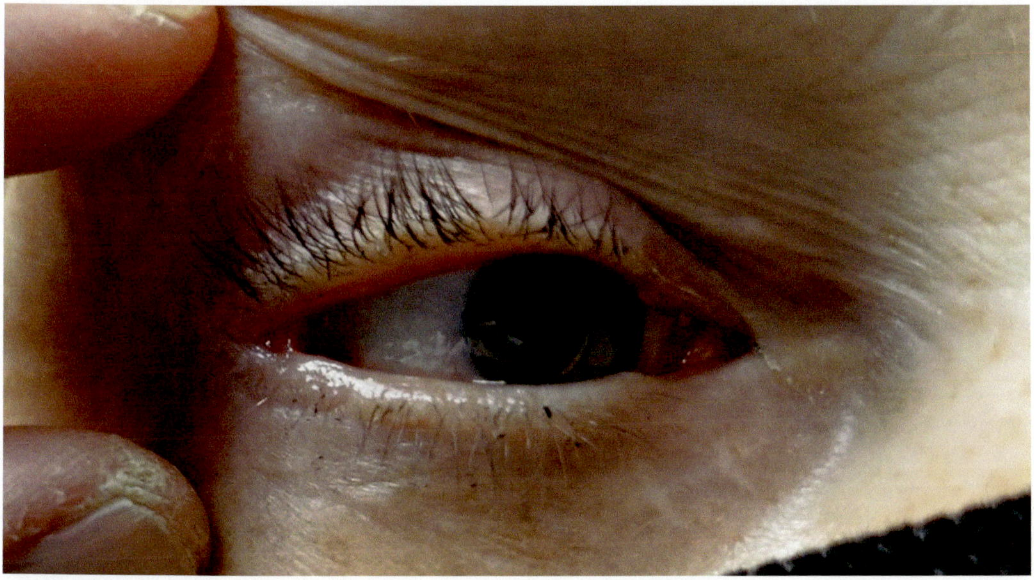

Fig. 4 Postoperative photograph. Post-op month 4 after tarsoconjunctival suspension flap. The lateral flap is normally camouflaged under the upper eyelid margin. It is only visible with manual eyelid distraction and appears as a pink/red conjunctival band epithelialized as palpebral conjunctiva

tarsal strip or any canthoplasty can be performed in conjunction to treat horizontal eyelid laxity (Figs. 5 and 6). Other treatments for lower eyelid malposition such as spacer grafts, skin grafts, or cheek flaps can also be performed concomitantly. If additional medial eyelid closure is needed, a medial tarsorrhaphy can be added (see Chaps. "Medial Canthal Surgery" and "Lower Eyelid Surgery in Facial Paralysis").

4 Discussion

The lateral tarsoconjunctival onlay flap has been successful to treat paretic, cicatricial and complex multi-vector mechanisms of lower eyelid retraction [6–8]. The benefits of the lateral tarsoconjunctival onlay flap include a powerful, minimally invasive lift, good cosmesis, ease of titration or reversal, and a low incidence of complications.

This use of a lateral tarsoconjunctival flap secured to the lower eyelid margin was first described for paralytic lower eyelid malposition indications. An additional observation in this population was that in patients with a strong Bell (supraduction on eyelid closure) reflex, movement of the superior fornix upon supraduction resulted in some favorable movement of pre-operatively flaccid eyelids. This was due to transmission of superior fornix movement through the connected flap to the lower eyelid [6].

The flap was later described to be effective in other vectors of lower eyelid retraction. It may have a role in complications from lower eyelid blepharoplasty, such as in revision surgery for post-operative lower eyelid retraction or from cicatricial changes from other periocular surgeries. These patients who are often still seeking an optimal aesthetic outcome often will not accept the risks of visible scars or other stigmata of surgery associated with procedures such as skin grafts.

Tanenbaum et al. previously described a mechanistically similar tarsal pillar technique. Some key differences were a mid-posterior lamella recipient site (i.e., rather than margin) for the transconjunctival flap that may induce slight margin ectropion. Importantly their technique results in visible tissue bands at the medial and lateral limbus [5]. A far lateral positioning

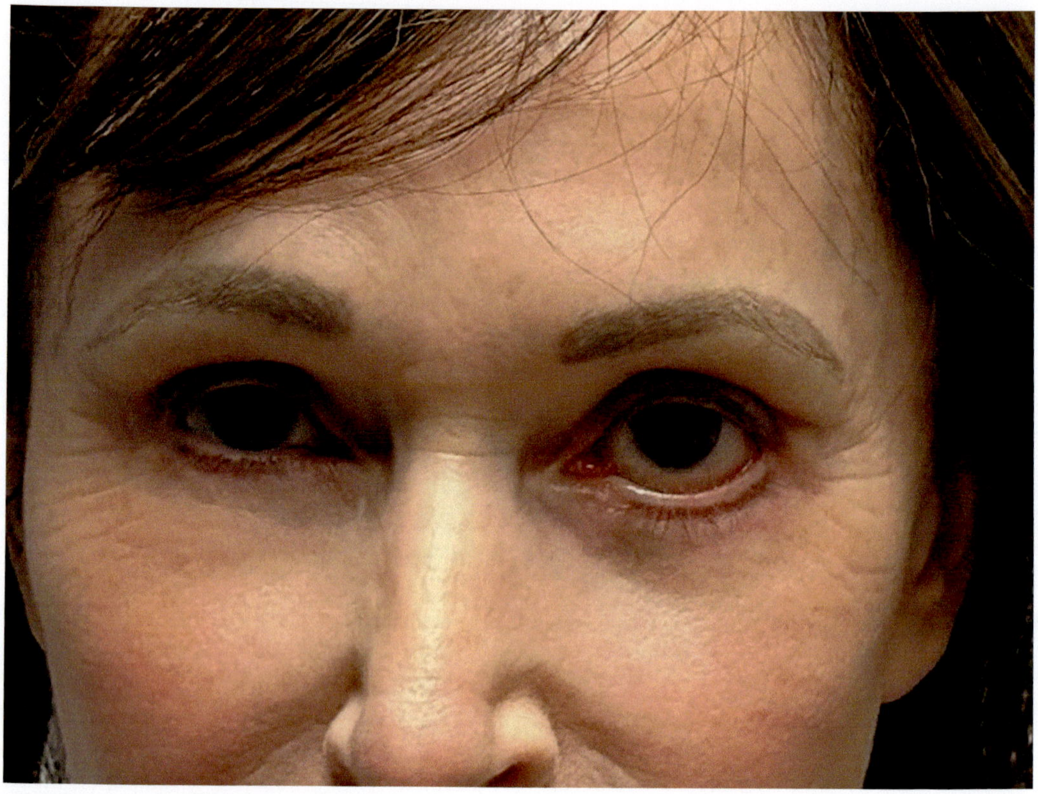

Fig. 5 Preoperative photograph of a patient with left lower eyelid retraction after blepharoplasty and who failed attempts at canthoplasty as well as a spacer graft

of the tarsoconjunctival flap, may achieve a more satisfactory cosmetic outcome because it is well hidden under the lateral upper eyelid and allows the lower eyelid to maintain its natural contour. The dominant, overriding lateral upper eyelid and superior lateral canthal tilt induced with flap placement conforms to facial beauty ideals [8]. Hence, the lateral tarsonjunctival onlay flap may have broader indications.

In a large series, patients treated with a lateral tarsoconjunctival onlay flap reported improvement in ocular surface disease related symptoms and cosmesis [6, 8]. Complications included flap dehiscence (2.6%), pyogenic granulomas (4.5%), need for additional medial tarsorrhaphy (6.4%), temporal peripheral vision restriction (6.4%) [6]. A single case required additional midface lift and lateral canthopexy for continued symptomatic eyelid retraction. Another case required partial flap resection because of a visible tarsoconjunctival flap [8].

Lastly, the degree of eyelid closure achieved by the tarsoconjunctival flap can be tailored to each patient and titrated postoperatively. The flap may be augmented, decreased, or even fully reversed as an in-office procedure with local anesthesia only. (Video 2) In cases of inadequate closure, augmentation can be achieved by adding an additional tarsoconjunctival flap adjacent to the prior or medial repositioning of the tarsoconjunctival flap. A partial or complete takedown is performed with sharp dissection of the flap off the lower eyelid margin. At the flap origin site, adhesions are released with scissors to forestall upper eyelid retraction and to allow the flap to reseat to its native position.

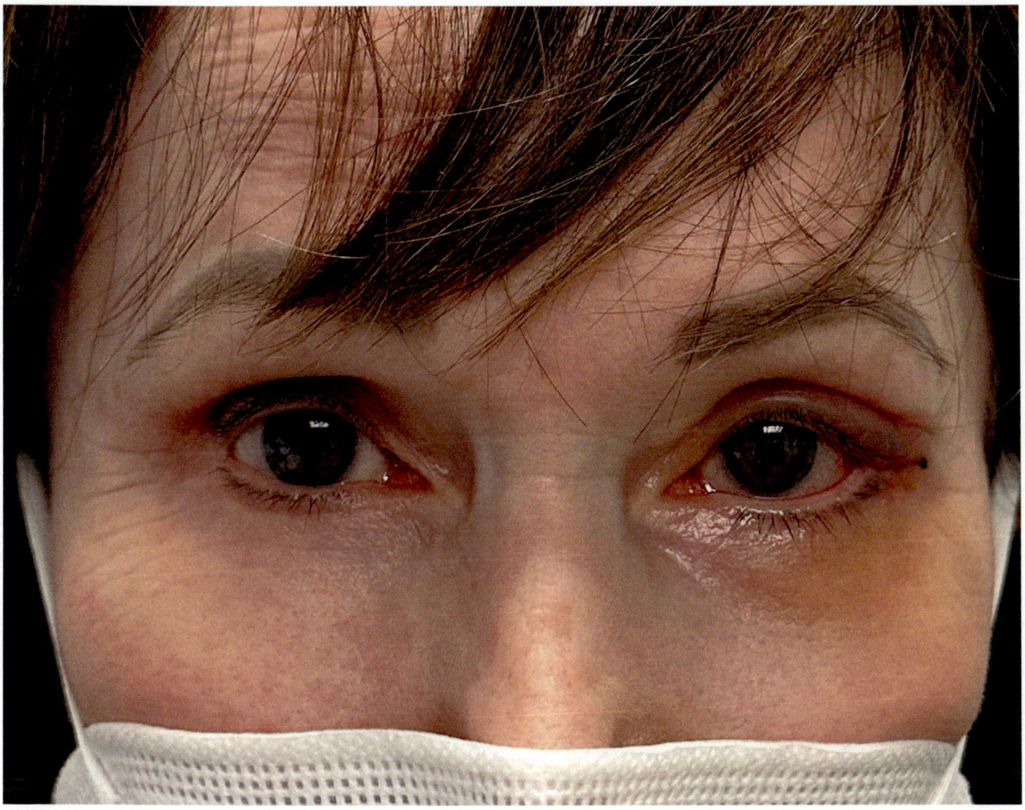

Fig. 6 Patient in Fig. 5 one week postoperative after a left tarsoconjunctival onlay flap and lateral tarsal strip

Serious complications are rare. Pyogenic granulomas are perhaps the most common side effect and can be treated with a topical antibiotic-steroid ointment, or surgical excision [9].

5 Conclusion

The lateral tarsoconjunctival onlay flap is a powerful, versatile, well-tolerated and cosmetically satisfactory solution to effectively manage lower eyelid retraction. It may be effective as a standalone procedure or as an adjunct to other surgeries in a variety of types of lower eyelid retraction.

References

1. Hahn S, Desai SC. Lower lid malposition: causes and correction. Facial Plast Surg Clin North Am. 2016;24(2):163–71.
2. Mojallal A, Cotofana S. Anatomy of lower eyelid and eyelid-cheek junction. Ann Chir Plast Esthet. 2017;62(5):365–74.
3. Boboridis KG, Bunce C. Interventions for involutional lower lid entropion. Cochrane Database Syst Rev. 2011;(12):CD002221.
4. Rathore DS, Chickadasarahilli S, Crossman R, Mehta P, Ahluwalia HS. Full thickness skin grafts in periocular reconstructions: long-term outcomes. Ophthalmic Plast Reconstr Surg. 2014;30(6):517–20.
5. Tanenbaum M, Gossman MD, Bergin DJ, Friedman HI, Lett D, Haines P, et al. The tarsal pillar technique for narrowing and maintenance of the interpalpebral fissure. Ophthalmic Surg. 1992;23:418–25.

6. Tao JP, Vemuri S, Patel AD, Compton C, Nunery WR. Lateral tarsoconjunctival onlay flap lower eyelid suspension in facial nerve paresis. Ophthalmic Plast Reconstr Surg. 2014;30(4):342–5.
7. Chien KH, Patel A, Lu DW, Tao J. Lateral tarsoconjunctival onlay flap in multi-vector lower eyelid retraction. J Med Si. 2016;36:171–4.
8. Conger JR, Grob SR, Limongi RM, Tao JP. Lateral tarsoconjunctival flap suspension treatment of post blepharoplasty lower eyelid retraction. Ophthalmic Plast Reconstr Surg. 2020;36(6):613–6.
9. Wollina U, Langner D, França K, Gianfaldoni S, Lotti T, Tchernev G. Pyogenic granuloma—a common benign vascular tumor with variable clinical presentation: new findings and treatment options. Open Access Maced J Med Sci. 2017;5(4):423–6.

Reverse Ptosis

Naomi E. Gutkind, Ying Chen and Chris R. Alabiad

Abstract

Reverse ptosis is defined as an abnormally elevated lower eyelid with a decrease in the margin to corneal light reflex distance 2 (MRD2). Patients may present with functional or aesthetic concerns due to asymmetry, obscuration of the visual axis on downgaze, or decreased visual acuity due to astigmatism. Causes of reverse ptosis can be mechanical or neurologic. Treatment is typically surgical. Surgical approaches may include addressing globe position, or in the case of isolated lower eyelid dysfunction, advancement of the lower eyelid retractors or inferior tarsal muscle-conjunctivectomy. This chapter details etiology and treatments for reverse ptosis of the lower eyelid.

Keywords

Reverse ptosis · Upside-down ptosis · Lower eyelid retractor

Illustrations by Michael Han

N. E. Gutkind · Y. Chen · C. R. Alabiad (✉)
Bascom Palmer Eye Institute, University of Miami, Miami, FL, USA
e-mail: CAlabiad@med.miami.edu

1 Introduction

Reverse ptosis, also known as upside-down ptosis, refers to lower eyelid malposition in which the margin of the lower eyelid is above the level of the inferior corneoscleral limbus. Clinically, this can be measured as a decrease in the margin to reflex distance 2 (MRD2) due to decrease in the distance from the corneal light reflex to the central portion of the lower eyelid (Figs. 1, and 2).

This condition can be caused by several conditions including globe dystopia, hypoglobus, involutional changes, orbital trauma, post-surgical, or neurological conditions. Patients may present with cosmetic or functional concerns leading to dry eye and potential decrease in visual acuity.

Techniques to restore lower eyelid function and anatomy include addressing abnormal globe position relative to the lower eyelid, performing an external/internal advancement of the lower eyelid retractors, or performing an inferior tarsal muscle-conjunctivectomy.

2 Presenting Symptoms

Patients with reverse ptosis may present with functional or cosmetic complaints. One of the most bothersome presenting symptoms of reverse ptosis is visual changes. The pupillary axis can be obscured by the lower eyelid

J. P. Tao (ed.), *Plastic Surgery of the Lower Eyelids*,
https://doi.org/10.1007/978-3-031-36175-3_23

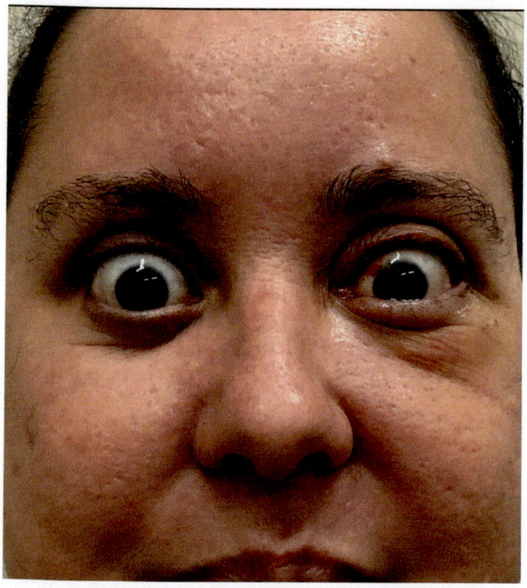

Fig. 1 Left reverse ptosis in a patient status post orbital floor decompression for thyroid eye disease (photo courtesy of Maria Belen Camacho)

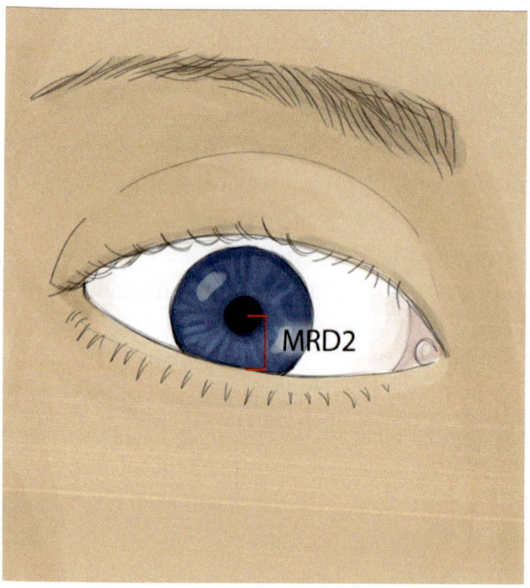

Fig. 2 Illustration of a patient with reverse ptosis. Note the lower lid resting above the inferior limbus

resulting in inferior visual field defects. When the normal retraction of the lower eyelid on downgaze is impaired, patients may present with reading difficulty due to the obscuration of visual axis in downgaze [1]. Furthermore, reverse ptosis has been previously reported to cause corneal steepening and with-the-rule astigmatism, leading to decreased visual acuity [2].

Many patients presenting with reverse ptosis may present with aesthetic concerns. Due to the asymmetry of one eyelid being abnormally elevated, patients can present complaining of an enophthalmic appearance of one eye. Exophthalmometry or MRD2 measurements may reveal the abnormally elevated lower eyelid position in the affected eye, with or without asymmetry in globe position.

3 Causes

There are multiple causes of reverse ptosis. Broadly, the causes can be divided into two categories: mechanical and neurologic.

3.1 Mechanical Causes

Mechanical causes of reverse ptosis include weakening/disinsertion of lower eyelid retractors, globe malposition, trauma, and iatrogenic or post-surgical. Although involutional change is more likely to cause lower eyelid laxity leading to ectropion and an increased MRD2, some patients have predominant weakening of the lower eyelid retractors without significant horizontal laxity. This combination ultimately results in reverse-ptosis, with a decreased MRD2 and a high-riding lower eyelid. In one series of eight patients with reverse ptosis, three were found to have reverse-ptosis due to involutional changes [1]. When lower eyelid retractor laxity is compounded with an upward force, as is the case in sticky eyelid syndrome, temporary adhesion between the upper eyelid and the abnormally lax lower eyelid results in a decrease in MRD2. This results in reverse-ptosis that can completely occlude the visual axis [3, 4].

Globe malposition, as in the setting of post-traumatic or anatomic globe dystopia, hypoglobus or enophthalmos, may also lead to a mechanical reverse-ptosis. In these cases, the depressed position of the globe itself thus makes the otherwise normal lower eyelid sit higher on the eye surface and leading to a decrease in MRD2 (Fig. 1).

Additionally, patients may experience reverse ptosis after eyelid, orbital, or ocular surgery. In a series of 32 patients undergoing orbital floor wall fracture repair, seven had reverse ptosis at their postoperative month three visit, as defined by a decrease in MRD2 by greater than 1 mm [5]. In a separate series of eight patients with reverse ptosis, five (62.5%) had previous ocular, orbital, or eyelid surgery [1]. This may be due to weakening of the lower eyelid retractors from direct trauma, intraoperative speculum use, or residual eyelid malposition.

3.2 Neurologic Causes

The muscles which contribute to lower eyelid retraction form the capsulopalpebral fascia. The inner division of the capsulopalpebral fascia is composed of smooth muscle fibers analogous to Müller muscle, and it is similarly innervated by sympathetic nerve fibers. The outer division is composed of fibers arising from the inferior rectus muscle innervated by the oculomotor nerve (CNIII) [6]. Thus, lesions along either of the innervation pathways, sympathetic or CNIII, can lead to reverse ptosis.

The sympathetic pathway begins at the hypothalamus. The first order neurons travel ipsilaterally in the brainstem and synapse in the spinal cord. These second order neurons then travel in the sympathetic chain and synapse in the superior cervical ganglion. The third order neurons then travel along the carotid artery into the cavernous sinus, where they enter the orbit via the superior orbital fissure to supply the superior and inferior tarsal muscles. Lesions along any point in this pathway can cause Horner syndrome, leading to reverse ptosis by denervation of the smooth muscle fibers of the lower eyelid retractors. In one study of 73 pediatric patients with Horner syndrome, 42% were congenital, 42% occurred after surgical procedure to the neck, thorax, or central nervous system, and 15% were acquired from trauma, tumors, or vascular malformation [7]. In a study of adults with Horner syndrome, post-procedural cases were most common (21%), followed by carotid dissection (9%) and trauma (8%) [8]. Horner syndrome can be intermittent, and thus patients with reverse ptosis should be carefully evaluated [9].

The motor division of CNIII supplies innervation to the medial rectus, superior rectus, inferior rectus, inferior oblique, and the levator palpebrae superioris. The motor nerve fibers arise in the oculomotor nucleus and join the autonomic motor component passing through the tegmentum of the midbrain to exit anteriorly between the cerebral peduncles. Then, they pass through the cranial cavity to enter the cavernous sinus. From there the nerve enters the orbit through the superior orbital fissure where it divides to supply the muscles of the orbit. A lesion along this pathway can cause upper eyelid ptosis, reverse ptosis, ocular motility deficit, and an efferent pupillary defect [10].

4 Treatment

Treatment of reverse ptosis is typically surgical repair. The type of surgical intervention will depend on the cause of reverse ptosis. The goal is to restore normal lower eyelid positioning relative to the globe for both cosmetic and functional purposes.

In the case of hypoglobus, globe dystopia, or enophthalmos, it is essential to address globe position and orbital volume by addressing the underlying cause. In these cases, restoration of globe position relative to the lower eyelid may restore adequate symmetry and function, and it should be performed prior to addressing the eyelid itself.

In the setting of appropriate globe position, two techniques have been described in the literature to address the lower eyelid position: advancement of lower eyelid retractors, and inferior tarsal muscle conjunctivectomy.

The authors' preferred method for repair is advancement of the lower eyelid retractors. Though this can be done from an anterior or

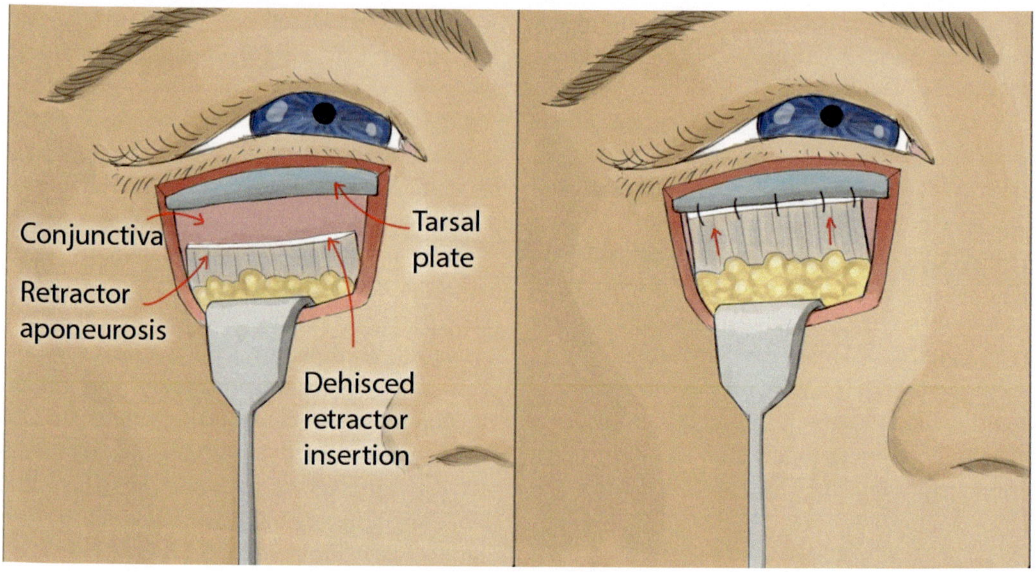

Fig. 3 Illustration of view of dehisced lower lid retractor after dissection of skin and orbicularis oculi muscle (Panel A) and post advancement of the lower lid retractor to the tarsal plate (Panel B) as described by Bartley et al. [1]

posterior eyelid approach, we describe the anterior approach in this chapter (Fig. 3). Bartley and colleagues described this technique of transcutaneous advancement of the lower eyelid retractors in eight patients with reverse ptosis from various causes [1]. Analogous to external levator advancement in upper eyelid ptosis repair, the procedure starts with local anesthesia (which can be supplemented with intravenous sedation) to achieve proper patient comfort. A Frost suture is placed along the lower eyelid to serve as traction. A subciliary incision is created, followed by a skin-muscle flap in the post orbicular fascial plane to expose the underlying orbital septum. The orbital septum is incised to expose the lower eyelid fat pads, which sit posterior to the orbital septum and anterior to the lower eyelid retractors. The disinserted lower eyelid retractors are then advanced and secured to epitarsal tissue with either slow-absorbing or permanent sutures. Some surgeons in the series preferred to bring the patient to the sitting position to inspect the eyelid position and assess motility in downgaze. The skin incision is closed with absorbable or permanent sutures. With this technique the mean MRD2 improved from 1.7 to 3.3 mm [1]. Symptoms improved in all patients, and there were no post-operative complications in the follow up period (average of 9 months) [1].

Adopting a technique similar to a conjunctivomullerectomy procedure, which is commonly used to address upper eyelid ptosis, Medel et al. described the use of a muscle-conjunctivectomy for the correction of reverse ptosis [11] (Fig. 4; see also Chap. "Repair of Tarsal Ectropion Using a Putterman Ptosis Clamp"). In this the lower eyelid is everted, and a caliper was used to mark the conjunctiva 3 mm below the inferior tarsal border. These marks were grasped, lifting conjunctiva and the adherent tarsal muscle, and a Putterman clamp was used to incarcerate 6 mm of muscle and conjunctiva. A 6-0 polypropylene suture is placed in a running mattress fashion, and the incarcerated tissue was excised. At post operative week one, the suture was removed. At post operative month one the authors reported a 1 mm increase in MRD2 with restoration of eyelid symmetry. Care must be taken to ensure adequate inferior fornix depth prior to this procedure to avoid inferior fornix foreshortening.

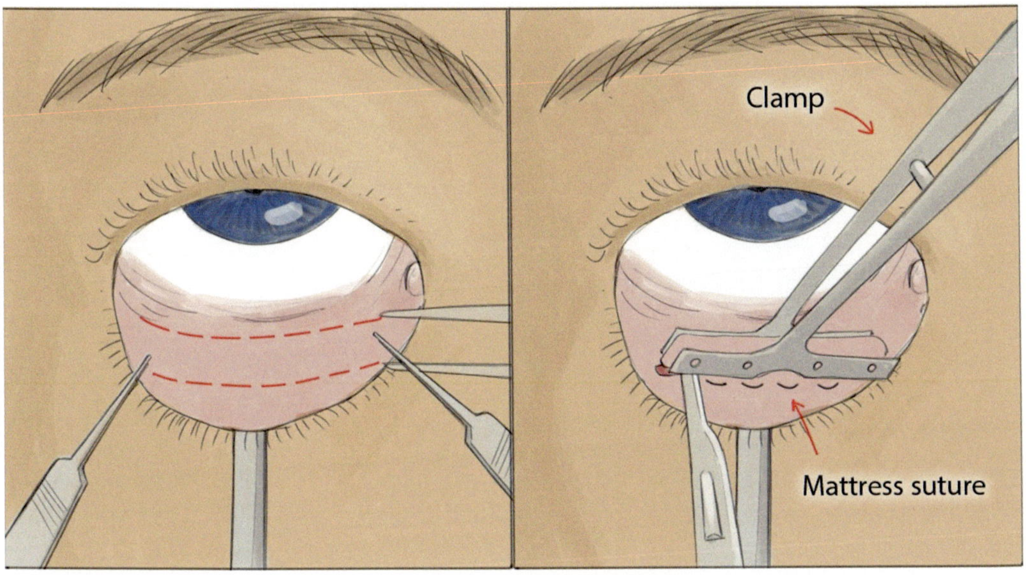

Fig. 4 The red hash lines demonstrate the area within the inferior fornix to perform a muscle conjunctivectomy (Panel A). These are clamped using a Putterman clamp (Panel B) and the edges approximated using a mattress suture as described by Medel et al. [11]

5 Conclusion

Reverse ptosis is defined as a decreased MRD2. Careful evaluation of the etiology is necessary, as the condition may be caused by globe malposition, mechanical dysfunction, or neurological insult to the lower eyelid. Surgical approaches include addressing the underlying cause and, when appropriate, advancement of lower eyelid retractors or inferior tarsal muscle-conjunctivectomy.

References

1. Bartley GB, Frueh BR, Holds JB, Linberg JV, Patel BC, Hawes MJ. Lower eyelid reverse ptosis repair. Ophthalmic Plast Reconstr Surg. 2002;18(1):79–83.
2. Ben Simon GJ, Goldberg RA, McCann JD. Reverse ptosis-induced corneal steepening and decreased vision after LASIK surgery. Cornea. 2004;23(8):831–2.
3. Chang M, Lee H, Park MS, Baek S. The clinical characteristics and new classification of sticky eyelid syndrome in East Asian patients. Acta Ophthalmol. 2014;92(8):e667–70.
4. Kortvelesy JS, Buerger GF Jr. Sticky eyelid syndrome. Am J Ophthalmol. 2004;138(5):882–4.
5. Park J, Kim S, Baek S. The Characteristics of lower eyelid reverse ptosis after reconstruction of orbital floor wall fracture using transconjunctival approach. J Craniofac Surg. 2019;30(7):e649–53.
6. Dutton JJ, Yanoff M, Duker JS. Ophthalmology. Elsevier Health Sciences; 2018.
7. Jeffery AR, Ellis FJ, Repka MX, Buncic JR. Pediatric horner syndrome. J Am Assoc Pediatr Ophthalmol Strabismus. 1998;2(3):159–67.
8. Sabbagh MA, De Lott LB, Trobe JD. Causes of Horner syndrome: a study of 318 patients. J Neuro-Ophthalmol: The Official J North Am Neuro-Ophthalmol Soc. 2020;40(3):362.
9. Cohen LM, Elliott A, Freitag SK. Acquired intermittent pediatric Horner syndrome due to neuroblastoma. Ophthalmic Plast Reconstr Surg. 2018;34(2):e38–41.
10. Champney TH. Essential clinical neuroanatomy. John Wiley & Sons; 2015.
11. Medel R, Balaguer Solé Ò, Vasquez LM. Inferior tarsal muscle-conjunctivectomy for reverse ptosis repair: a novel technique. Orbit. 2017;36(3):125–7.

Transconjunctival Blepharoplasty

Michael A. Rafaelof and Jeffrey M. Joseph

Abstract

Lower eyelid fat herniation may be treated with transconjunctival blepharoplasty. Fat may be resected or preserved and repositioned to fill the tear trough and other depressions at the eyelid cheek junction. Transconjunctival blepharoplasty is associated with a high safety profile and excellent aesthetic results but is limited in that it does not treat dermatochalasis. This chapter describes clinical and anatomical basics as well as a technique of transconjunctival blepharoplasty.

Keywords

Lower blepharoplasty · Eyelid bags · Under eye surgery · Fat transposition · Tear trough · Under eye hollows

1 Introduction

Transcutaneous lower eyelid blepharoplasty is frequently undertaken, and has a relatively high incidence of aesthetic and functional complications [1]. Surgery to rejuvenate the lower eyelids is a challenging procedure requiring careful planning and consideration.

One of the primary considerations is the surgical approach to the lower eyelid orbital fat pads, that are often targets of lower eyelid cosmetic surgery. The fat pads can be accessed through an anterior transcutaneous or posterior transconjunctival approach.

Transcutaneous blepharoplasty is the more traditional method and affords the opportunity to treat excess skin. However, a key disadvantage is a greater risk for eyelid malposition especially in inexperienced hands. This approach is appropriate for select patients and is discussed at length in Chap. "External Lower Eyelid Blepharoplasty".

Transconjunctival surgery, has gained prevalence in the modern landscape of periocular rejuvenation. The transconjunctival method directly approaches the orbital fat utilizing an incision through the lower eyelid conjunctiva. The orbicularis muscle and orbital septum are not disturbed which has been shown to produce less distortion of the periorbital anatomy postoperatively, leading to less eyelid retraction, ectropion, and cosmetic lower eyelid distortion;

Supplementary Information The online version contains supplementary material available at https://doi.org/10.1007/978-3-031-36175-3_24.

M. A. Rafaelof · J. M. Joseph (✉)
Gavin Herbert Eye Institute, University of California, Irvine, CA, USA
e-mail: joseph11881@gmail.com

J. P. Tao (ed.), *Plastic Surgery of the Lower Eyelids*,
https://doi.org/10.1007/978-3-031-36175-3_24

problems which have plagued the transcutaneous approach [2–5]. While the external approach is highly safe in experienced hands, the transconjunctival approach has gained popularity owing to lower complications and possibly quicker recovery.

The transconjunctival approach, however, is limited since it does not address the excess tissue (skin/muscle) or eyelid laxity that may be present in a patient. Adjunctive procedures, including skin excision, muscle plication, eyelid tightening, and skin resurfacing can be performed concomitantly to address some of these variables [2]. Volume preservation and volume augmentation principals corroborate the aesthetic benefits of transconjunctival surgery. In this chapter, the authors detail the transconjunctival approach to eyelid rejuvenation.

2 Lower Eyelid Anatomy

The lower eyelid can be broken down into three layers, or lamellae. The outer (anterior) lamella is composed of skin and orbicularis, the middle lamella contains the orbital septum, and the inner (posterior) lamella contains conjunctiva, the tarsus, and the eyelid retractors [2].

The orbicularis oculi muscle has two parts; the outer orbital and inner palpebral segments. The medial components join at the lacrimal crest to contribute to the medial canthal tendon, and similarly the lateral components insert onto the lateral orbital tubercle to contribute to the lateral canthal tendon [6]. Deep to the orbicularis oculi muscle lies the orbital septum that cover the three orbital fat pads of the lower eyelid. Figure 1 this fibrous septal tissue originates from the periosteum at the orbital rim (arcus marginalis) and fuses with the capsulopalpebral fascia, a collective term for the lower eyelid retractors, below the inferior tarsal border. The protrusion of the orbital fat contributes to poor cosmesis, and as such, these fat pads are often a key target of facial rejuvenation surgery. The medial and central fat pads are separated by the inferior oblique muscle while the central and lateral fat pads are separated by the arcuate extension of the oblique muscle [7]. When dissecting and contouring the fat pads during lower blepharoplasty, special attention should be paid to the inferior oblique to avoid damage. The tarsus

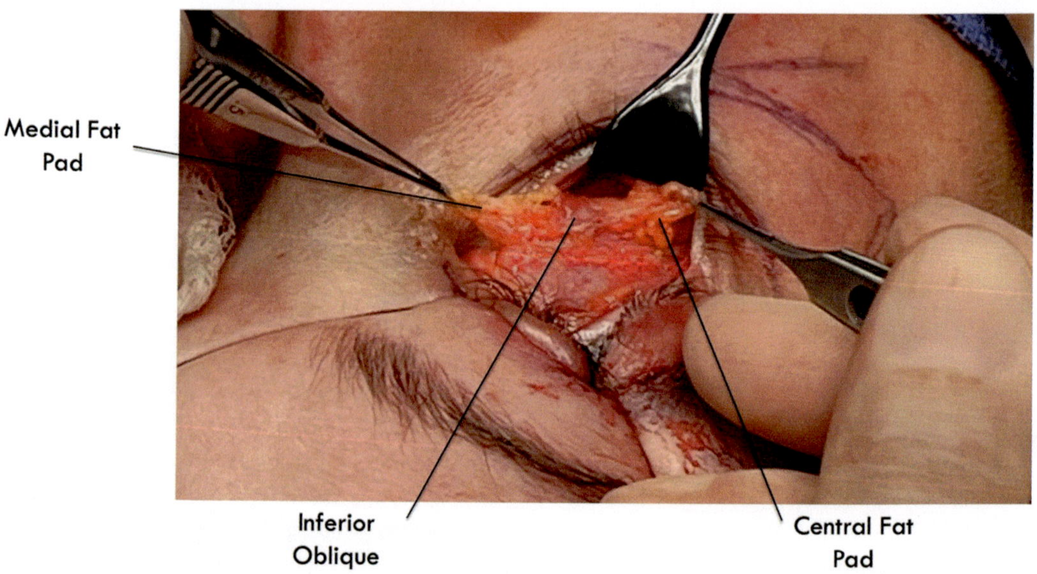

Fig. 1 Intra-operative photo of the medial and central fat pads in relation to the inferior oblique muscle

itself, is the scaffolding of the eyelid margin, providing support and structure. Below the tarsus, the conjunctiva then continues further to the inferior fornix. Here, the lower eyelid retractors are closely connected and adherent to the conjunctiva. These retractors arise from fibers of the inferior rectus and inferior oblique muscles and eventually fuse with the septum roughly 5 mm below he inferior border of the tarsal plate [7].

Midface anatomy:

The midface and its aging process indirectly contributes to the aging of the lower eyelid. The midface and lower eyelid should be evaluated and treated as a complex rather than individual aesthetic units. The orbicularis retaining ligament (ORL) is osseo-cutaneous structure that maintains the position of the eyelid and cheek soft tissues [8]. The ORL originates from the periosteum near the orbital septum and fuses with the orbital rim. When surrounding soft tissue descends or changes in volume, the ORL becomes more evident, manifesting as grooves of the eyelid-cheek interface [8–10]. In preparation for surgical intervention, the fat pats of the midface must also be considered. The sub-orbicularis oculi fat (SOOF), lies on the bone below the lateral half of the infraorbital rim [11]. The SOOF can be visualized from the sub-orbicularis space during blepharoplasty [11, 12]. The SOOF should be distinguished from orbital fat (Fig. 2). The SOOF is analogous with the retro-orbicularis oculi fat (ROOF), an area of superior fat tissue deep and superior to the upper eyelid at the level of the brow and located between the muscles (orbicularis/frontalis) and the orbital septum [13]. The infraorbital neurovascular bundle must also be considered during surgical planning. The infraorbital neurovascular bundle exits through the infraorbital foramen approximately 0.7–1.0 from the orbital rim and provides sensation to the lower eyelid skin, lateral nose, cheek, and upper lip [11]. The nerve and vessels in this area can be easily damaged in midface dissection if not appropriately identified and protected.

3 Preoperative Considerations

Evaluation for lower eyelid blepharoplasty requires detailed evaluation of anatomic changes that should be correlated to complaints. In addition, there are both anatomic and physiologic factors that may influence the surgeon's

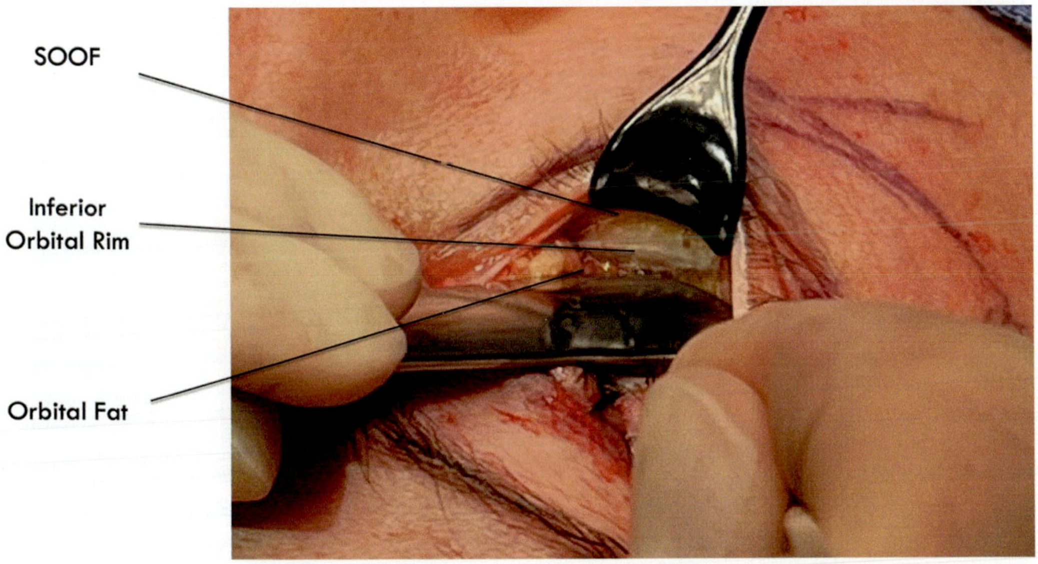

Fig. 2 Intra-operative photo of the dissection landmarks during fat reposition lower blepharoplasty. Appreciate the sub-orbicularis oculi fat (SOOF) in relation to the inferior orbital rim and surrounding orbital fat pads

approach and if may lead to complications if not appreciated.

Patients often complain of puffy eyelids or herniation of the lower eyelid orbital fat. One can appreciate the fat in primary gaze when there is true herniation. Having the patient look up during the exam, highlights the fat. A patient's cosmetic concerns can include excess skin, eyelid laxity, and periocular volume deficits (Fig. 3).

Importantly, aesthetic concerns are often correlated to involutional tissue changes that diminish lower eyelid support and increase risk of post-operative eyelid retraction. Involutional changes of the tarsal plate and the canthal tendons can lead to eyelid instability. Loss of soft tissue and skeletal support in the midface over time can also predispose patients to inferior migration of the lower eyelid position. Gravitational change and changes in muscle tone must also be considered.

Surgical planning must be individualized. For example, if a patient only has fat prominence, then tranconjunctival blepharoplasty with fat excision alone may be sufficient. However, if excess skin is present, an additional skin excision or resurfacing may be necesariy to achieve desired results [14, 15]. If eyelid laxity is present or muscle tone is reduced, an eyelid tightening or muscle plication should be added [16]. Moreover, if there are volume deficits, fat grafting, fat preservation, or post-operative filler treatment could be considered.

4 Surgical Technique (Video 1)

The eyelid is pre-operatively injected with local anesthetic containing epinephrine. If fat repositioning is planned, the infraorbital hollow at the orbital rim is also marked and injected with the same anesthetic.

To expose the conjunctival surface for incision, the lower eyelid is everted and reflected inferiorly and using manual pressure on the globe, the orbital fat prolapses forward and causes the conjunctival surface to bow forward. Next, using sharp dissection, an incision is

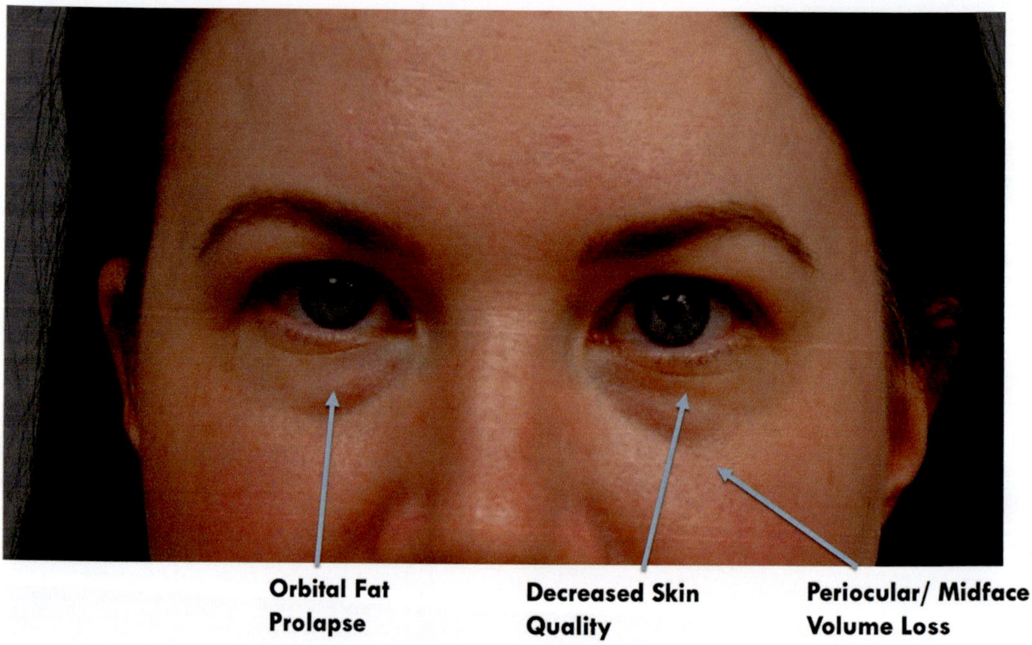

Fig. 3 Pre-operative considerations in transconjunctival blepharoplasty. This photo highlights orbital fat prolapse, decreased skin quality, and periocular and midface volume loss

made approximately 4–5 mm below the tarsal plate across the horizontal extent of the eyelid. This incision enters the post-septal space and provide direct access to the fat pads. A 4-0 silk traction suture is then placed through the inferior cut edge of the conjunctiva and retractors. This suture is placed on superior stretch further exposing the surgical field and protecting the globe. A retractor can then be used to reflect and protect the tarsus, orbicularis muscle and skin.

Inferior traction with the retractor coupled with the superior traction suture creates wide exposure of the orbital fat. Blunt and sharp dissection is used to expose all three fat pads. If the surgical plan involves fat excision, the fat pads are then evaluated and partially excised until they are flush with the orbital rim. When there is volume deficit in the infraorbital hollow, fat preservation and transposition of fat to these areas is an excellent choice. It is imperative to fully dissect the fat from the surrounding soft tissue structures and connective tissue. Medially it is particularly important to free the medial and central fat pad from the inferior oblique muscle so traction is not placed on the muscle when the fat is transposed. The fat may need to be trimmed and tailored for each patient to avoid overfilling and prominence post-operatively.

Dissection is carried inferiorly to prepare for fat transposition. Using the retractor, firm inferior pressure is placed on the eyelid, draping the soft tissues over the orbital rim and exposing the arcus marginalis. Further blunt dissection can be used to push the anterior soft tissues (orbicularis muscle and SOOF) away from the orbital rim inferiorly in a sub- or pre-periosteal dissection plane.

Sub- or pre-periosteal pockets are then formed by using sharp or blunt dissection. After achieving hemostasis, the fat pads are further dissected maintaining posterior (vascular) attachments and then they are transposed into the sub- or pre-periosteal pockets. Sutures can be used to secure that fat transposition. They can be externalized by using a 4-0 permanent monofilament suture passed through the skin ath the level of the inferior tear trough. Alternatively, internal dissolvable (5-0 chromic or similar) sutures can be at the inferior aspect of the dissection, securing fat to periosteum inferior to the rim on the malar face. Several interrupted sutures can be placed as needed to individualize the contour as needed.

After this fat repositioning, the volumizing effects of the fat should be visible externally on the face.

The traction suture is released and the conjunctiva is reapproximated.

Adjunctive procedures can now be added if necessary to achieve the desired result or help prevent post-operative complications. Figures 4, 5, 6 and 7 for instance, if there is excess skin, a subcilliary excision can be performed, the remaining skin undermined, and a primary closure completed. Other possible procedures include canthal suspension to treat eyelid laxity, facial fat grafting to address further midface volume deficiency, and skin resurfacing via laser, radiofrequency or chemical peel to address finer rhytids.

5 Complications

Complications are usually minor and self-limiting. These include dry eye, bruising, swelling, chemosis and subconjunctival hemorrhage [17, 1]. These patients need reassurance but can also be treated with a short course of topical and/or oral steroid. Chemosis, if not resolving with ocular lubrication, may require patching, suture tarsorrhaphy, or further surgery.

Cosmetic complications are most often related to under or over reduction of the lower eyelid fat. leading to persistent prominence or new hollowness. Under correction can be treated with further fat excision, but over excision of fat may require placement of additional volume in

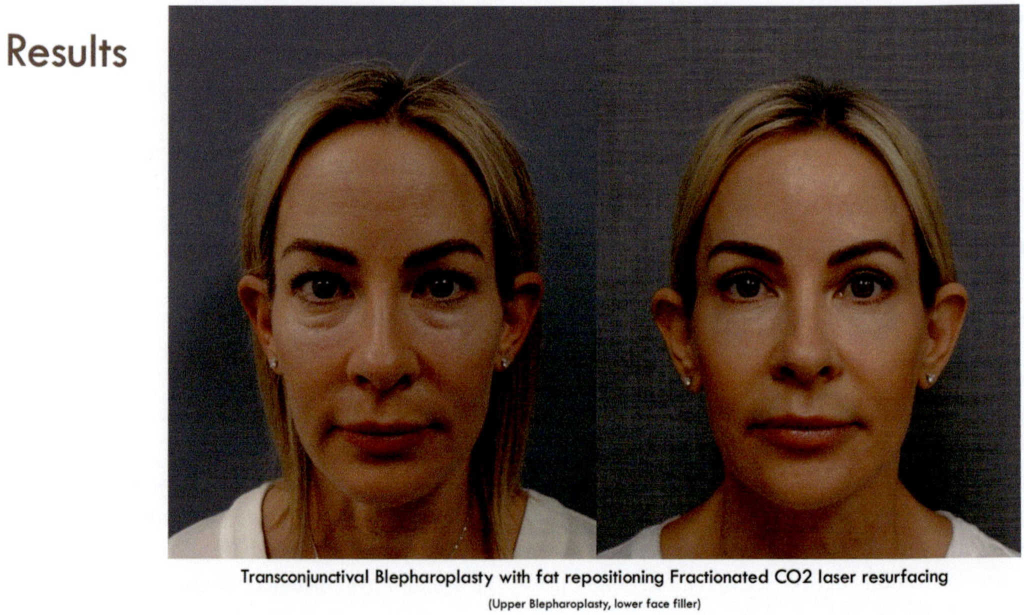

Fig. 4 Pre-operative (left) and post-operative photos of transconjunctival lower blepharoplasty with CO_2 laser

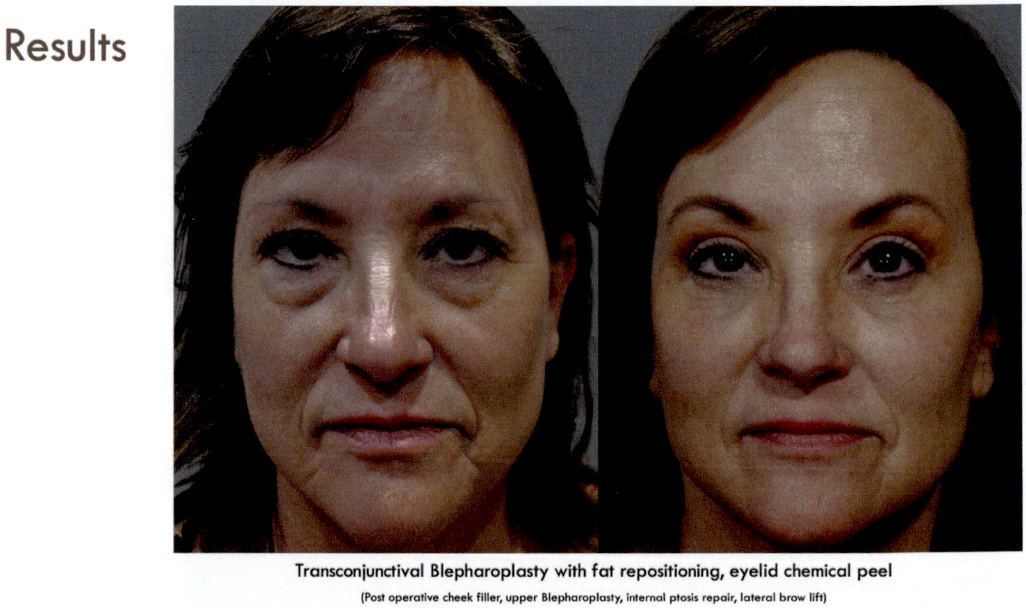

Fig. 5 Pre-operative (left) and post-operative photos of transconjunctival lower blepharoplasty with chemical peel (patient also underwent upper eyelid blepharoplasty and ptosis repair and brow lift)

Results

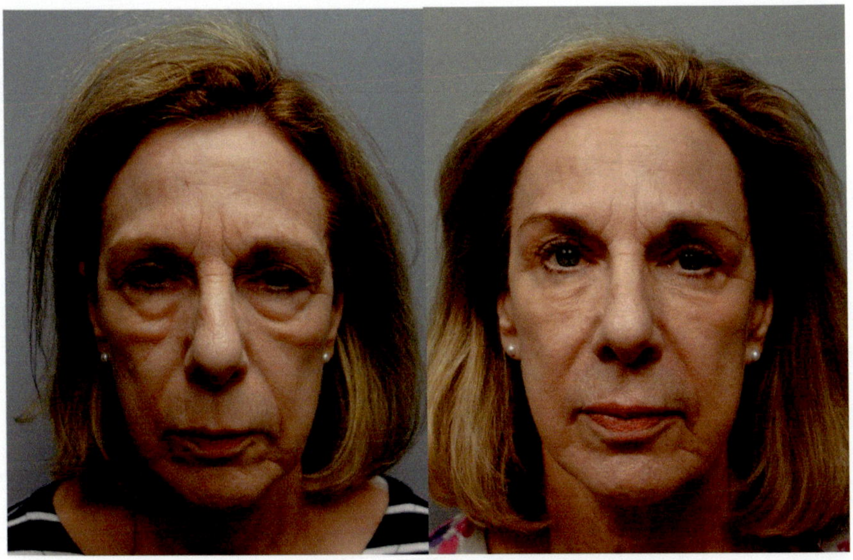

Fig. 6 Pre-operative (left) and post-operative photos of transconjunctival lower blepharoplasty with CO_2 laser resurfacing (patient also underwent upper eyelid blepharoplasty and ptosis repair and brow lift)

the form of hyaluronic acid gel filler or autologous fat grafts.

More serious complications involve eyelid malposition in the form of eyelid retraction, entropion or ectropion and trichiasis [18 19]. While these complications are well known and more frequently associated with transcutaneous surgery, they can occur with a transconjunctival approach as well.

Fat repositioning has its own unique complications including diplopia (rarely), fat granulomas, prolonged edema, and tear trough irregularities [20]. Transient diplopia may be secondary to anesthesia versus muscle injury. This can be treated with steroids, or expectantly. While most cases of diplopia resolve over time strabismus surgeon evaluation may be indicated for persistent diplopia especially after 6–12 months (see Chap. "Extraocular Muscle Considerations in Lower Eyelid Surgery"). Fat granulomas are rare but can be treated with injections of steroid or 5-fluorouracil.

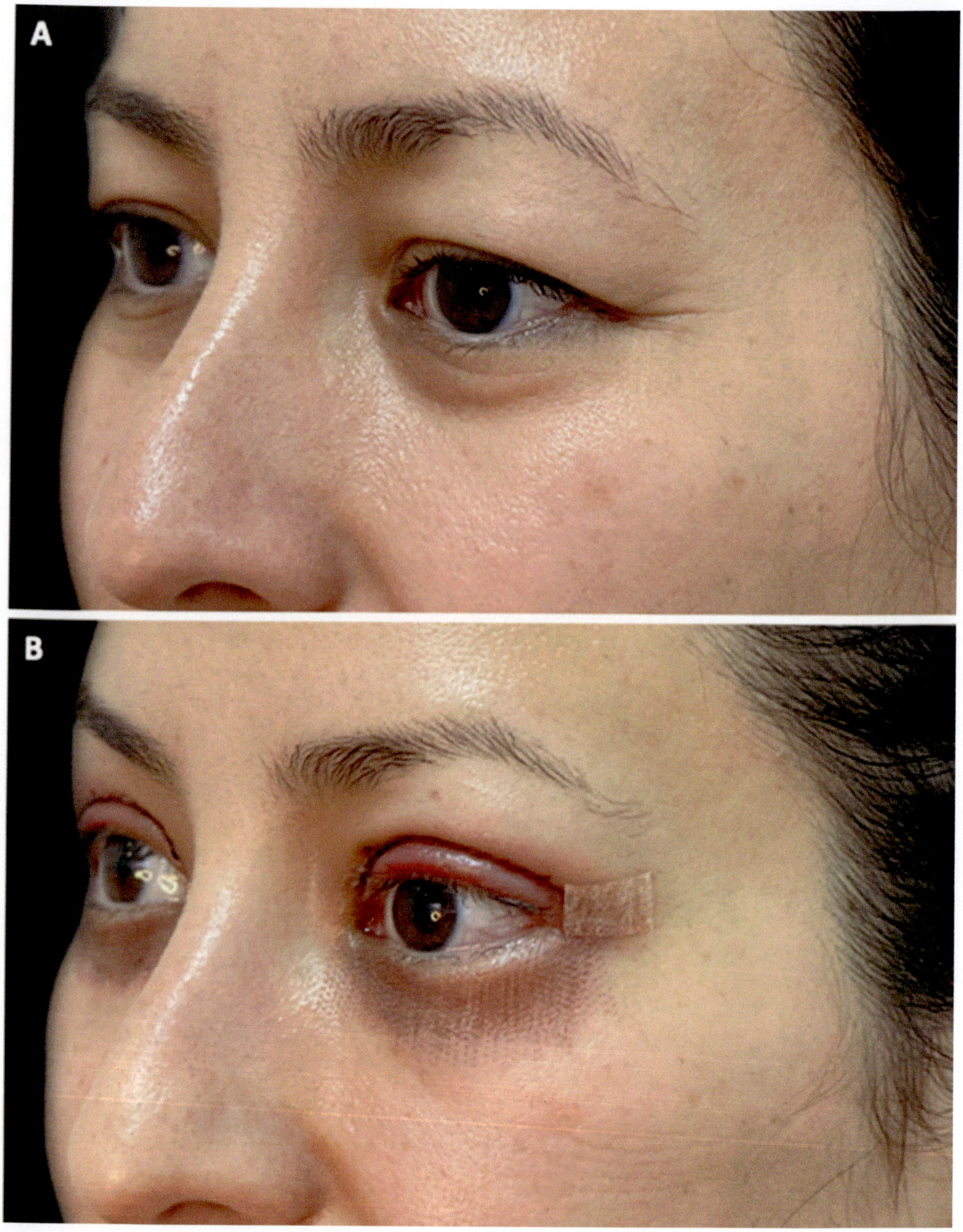

Fig. 7 A. Preoperative photograph of a patient with mild lower eyelid skin laxity mild under eye hollows; B. Postoperative photograph days post transconjunctival lower blepharoplasty with CO_2 laser skin resurfacing (patient also underwent upper eyelid blepharoplasty) (*photos courtesy of Andre Borba*)

6 Conclusion

Transconjunctival blepharoplasty is increasingly popular and offers highly safe and effective aesthetic outcomes. Owing to less distortion of the eyelid anatomy, these procedures may be associated with a lower incidence of complications than external blepharoplasty approaches but are limited because they do not treat the skin or midface soft tissues.

References

1. Lelli GJ, Lisman RD. Blepharoplasty complications. Plast Reconstr Surg. 2010;125(3):1007–17. https://doi.org/10.1097/PRS.0B013E3181CE17E8.
2. Massry GG, Murphy MR, Azizzadeh B. Master techniques in blepharoplasty and periorbital rejuvenation; 2011.
3. Davison SP, Irio M. Transconjunctival lower blpeharoplasty with and without fat repositioning 2015;42:51–6.
4. Goldberg RA, Lessner AM, Shorr N, Baylis HI. The transconjunctival approach to the orbital floor and orbital fat. A prospective study. Ophthal Plast Reconstr Surg. 1990;6(4):241–6. https://doi.org/10.1097/00002341-199012000-00003.
5. Jacono AA, Moskowitz B. Transconjunctival versus transcutaneous approach in upper and lower blepharoplasty. Facial Plast Surg. 2001;17(1):21–7. https://doi.org/10.1055/S-2001-16366/ID/21.
6. Jacono AA, Malone MH. Transcutaneous lower blepharoplasty. Master Tech Facial Rejuvenation 2018:142–51.e1. https://doi.org/10.1016/B978-0-323-35876-7.00013-3.
7. Sykes JM, Suárez GA, Trevidic P, Cotofana S, Moon HJ. Applied facial anatomy. Master Tech Facial Rejuvenation 2018:6–14. https://doi.org/10.1016/B978-0-323-35876-7.00002-9.
8. Kwon H-J, Choi Y-J, Cho T-H, Yang H-M. Three-dimensional structure of the orbicularis retaining ligament: an anatomical study using micro-computed tomography OPEN. https://doi.org/10.1038/s41598-018-35425-0.
9. Muzaffar AR, Mendelson BC, Adams WP. Surgical anatomy of the ligamentous attachments of the lower eyelid and lateral canthus. Plast Reconstr Surg. 2002;110(3):873–84. https://doi.org/10.1097/00006534-200209010-00025.
10. Schiller JD. Lysis of the orbicularis retaining ligament and orbicularis oculi insertion: a powerful modality for lower eyelid and cheek rejuvenation. Plast Reconstr Surg. 2012;129(4). https://doi.org/10.1097/PRS.0B013E31824423C7.
11. Hwang K. Surgical anatomy of the lower eyelid relating to lower blepharoplasty. Anat Cell Biol. 2010;43(1):15. https://doi.org/10.5115/ACB.2010.43.1.15.
12. Aiache A. The suborbicularis oculi fat pad: An anatomic and clinical study. Plast Reconstr Surg. 2001;107(6):1602–4. https://doi.org/10.1097/00006534-200105000-00050.
13. Wang X, Wang H. Anatomical study and clinical observation of retro-orbicularis oculi fat (ROOF). Aesthetic Plast Surg. 2020;44(1):89–92. https://doi.org/10.1007/S00266-019-01530-2.
14. Nassif PS. Lower blepharoplasty: transconjunctival fat repositioning. Facial Plast Surg Clin North Am. 2005;13(4):553–9. https://doi.org/10.1016/J.FSC.2005.06.006.
15. Seckel BR, Kovanda CJ, Cetrulo CL, Passmore AK, Meneses PG, White T. Laser blepharoplasty with transconjunctival orbicularis muscle/septum tightening and periocular skin resurfacing: a safe and advantageous technique. Plast Reconstr Surg. 2000;106(5):1127–41. https://doi.org/10.1097/00006534-200010000-00024.
16. Kim EM, Bucky LP. Power of the pinch: pinch lower lid blepharoplasty. Ann Plast Surg. 2008;60(5):532–7. https://doi.org/10.1097/SAP.0B013E318172F60E.
17. Prischmann J, Sufyan A, Ting JY, Ruffin C, Perkins SW. Dry eye symptoms and chemosis following blepharoplasty: a 10-year retrospective review of 892 cases in a single-surgeon series. JAMA Facial Plast Surg. 2013;15(1):39–46. https://doi.org/10.1001/2013.JAMAFACIAL.1.
18. Baylis HI, Nelson ER, Goldberg RA. Lower eyelid retraction following blepharoplasty. Ophthal Plast Reconstr Surg. 1992;8(3):170–5. https://doi.org/10.1097/00002341-199209000-00002.
19. Griffin G, Azizzadeh B, Massry GG. New insights into physical findings associated with postblepharoplasty lower eyelid retraction. Aesthetic Surg J. 2014;34(7):995–1004. https://doi.org/10.1177/1090820X14544306.
20. Klapper SR, Patrinely JR. Management of cosmetic eyelid surgery complications. Semin Plast Surg. 2007;21(1):80. https://doi.org/10.1055/S-2007-967753.

External Lower Eyelid Blepharoplasty

André Borba

Abstract

External lower eyelid blepharoplasty aims to improve contour irregularities, fat herniation, and excess skin. Good anatomic understanding and good surgical technique are essential since the lower eyelids are very prone to eyelid malposition complications that can both worsen appearance and cause ocular surface exposure. In this chapter, principles and techniques of external lower eyelid blepharoplasty are described.

Keywords

Lower eyelid blepharoplasty · Under eye bags · Dark circles · Lower eyelid lift

1 Introduction

The lower eyelids are highly visible and are a common target for aesthetic improvement. Commonly, patients seek lower eyelid surgery to correct a tired, aged, or sad appearance or for eyelid bags [1–3].

Understanding facial aging at different layers and facial levels is important in rejuvenation of the periorbital region. In youth, there is a smooth transition between the lower eyelid and the malar region in a single convexity and there exist no or few static rhytids [3]. Aging vertically elongates the lower eyelid through ptosis of the malar region and cheek complex and sagging of the lower eyelid skin. In addition, orbital fat may prolapse or herniate through a weakened orbital septum [4]. Together, these processes can lead to a double convexity and a deepened nasojugal fold. These changes can be attributed to specific changes in the supporting ligaments and tissues of the face and eyes [3, 5].

Anatomical concepts guide surgical rejuvenation of the lower eyelid. Historically, an aged appearance was believed to be due to tissue redundancy. Hence, subtractive procedures that excised the skin, orbicular oculi muscle, and fat pads prevailed. The initial descriptions of lower blepharoplasty were of the transcutaneous approach. Transconjunctival approaches were described later and are increasing in popularity since they may be less prone to eyelid malposition. The external approach remains highly relevant for specific aims.

Whether from a transconjunctival or transcutaneous approach, most modern blepharoplasty concepts advocate for preservation of tissues.

A. Borba (✉)
Division of Oculoplastic Surgery, Department of Ophthalmology, University of São Paulo, Sao Paulo, Brazil
e-mail: prof.dr.andreborba@gmail.com

J. P. Tao (ed.), *Plastic Surgery of the Lower Eyelids*,
https://doi.org/10.1007/978-3-031-36175-3_25

Resection versus transposition of tissue is individualized to the patient.

Retraction or ectropion of the lower eyelid margin is a key risk with lower blepharoplasty. Lateral canthal reinforcement is often necessary during lower blepharoplasty to prevent eyelid malposition.

This chapter will address the anatomy and aging of the lower eyelid complex, and describe the external blepharoplasty approach. The included techniques include those for correction of eyelid laxity to avoid complications such as retraction and ectropion.

2 The Anatomy of the Aging Lower Eyelid

The first layer of this complex lower eyelid region is the skin, which unlike other areas of the body, is extremely thin and elastic, which allows the eyes to close [6]. The skin of the eyelids is the thinnest in the body, often less than 1 mm thick [3, 7]. A thin layer of fat can be observed laterally but not medially. The skin covering the malar region is thicker and has a more abundant subcutaneous tissue; this difference between the two types of skin accentuates the cheek junction deformity. During aging, subcutaneous fat atrophies at the lateral lower eyelid, which can increase the deformity of the palpebromalar sulcus, leading to a skeletonized appearance [8, 9].

Immediately posterior to the skin is the orbicularis oculi muscle, composed of a palpebral portion with pre- and post-tarsal components and an orbital part [3, 10]. The orbicularis muscles fuse with the orbital retaining ligament, the attachment to the zygomatic bone [11, 12]. Medially, a tear trough or nasojugal groove is formed due to the attachment of the orbicularis just below the orbital ridge [3]. Deeper to the orbicularis muscle is the orbital septum, which the eyelid into separates the anterior and posterior lamella. The posterior lamella consists of the inferior tarsus and the palpebral conjunctiva. Inferior to the tarsus, the lower eyelid retractors, also known as the capsulopalpebral fascia, also contribute to the posterior lamella. The lateral canthal tendon provides lateral anchorage for the eyelids and vertical anchorage for the eyeball and lower eyelid. It has a bony attachment to the lateral orbital tubercle, located near the lateral orbital ridge on the orbit wall [1].

Posterior to the orbital septum exist three orbital fat pads: nasal, central, and temporal. The medial and central fat pads are divided by the inferior oblique muscle, an important anatomical landmark during inferior eyelid or orbital surgery. The central pad is separated from the temporal by the arcuate expansion of the Lockwood ligament, which forms an inferior suspension band for the globe [9, 13].

The signs of aging in this region stem from the changes in these anatomical structures. Starting with the skin, rhytids and crow feet laterally may be evident [1]. These results from ultraviolet exposure and age-related collagen remodeling. In addition, the laxity of the lateral canthal tendon imposes a more rounded shape on the lateral canthal angle [14, 15].

The appearance of the inferior palpebral bags arises from a complex aging process and not from increase in adipose volume. Progressive laxity of the eyeball support apparatus (Lockwood suspensory ligament and lateral canthal tendon), causes the eyeball to descend posteriorly, displacing the post-septal fat anteriorly, causing the appearance of a bulge or pseudo-herniation across the orbital septum [1, 3]. This effect contributes to dark circles and shadowing under the eyes. Most of the infraorbital bulge is caused by anteriorly post-septal fat projecting, with its inferior margin being contained by the orbicularis retaining ligament [10, 16, 17].

In the malar region, the fat compartment anterior to the SMAS corresponds to the malar compartment and the posterior to the suborbicular oculi fat (SOOF). The malar compartment contributes significantly to the volume of the middle third of the face; its atrophy and descent result in depression, highlighting the lower orbital fat pockets [5, 18].

3 Fundamental Aspects of Patient Selection

3.1 Clinical Indications

The most common indications for inferior blepharoplasty are aging changes such as excess skin, inferior palpebral laxity, orbicular muscle laxity or hypertrophy, orbital fat pad protrusion, and malar festoon, or nasojugal folds [16]. Zoumalan et al. [19] proposed an algorithm to determine whether a patient was a candidate for lower blepharoplasty, considering seven criteria, which include the presence and extent of orbital fat herniation, amount of excess skin, volumetric loss of the middle third of the face, cheek vector, and others [19].

Patients should be carefully examined, and the goals of blepharoplasty should be clear. In many patients, less invasive approaches, such as ablative resurfacing with lasers, plasma jets, and fillers such as hyaluronic acid, may be useful alternatives if surgery is not indicated nor desired.

3.2 Preoperative Assessment

The medical history includes a history of previous ocular or facial surgery, comorbidities, use of anticoagulant medication, immunosuppression, smoking, and history of hypertrophic/keloid scarring. Dry eye symptoms and history of ocular changes such as blepharitis, epiphora, and conjunctivochalasis should be identified.

One should assess the degree and location of fat pad prolapse, quantity, and quality of excess skin. Ridges and depressions, scleral show, eyelid malposition, negative vector, midface ptosis, festoons, malar bags, and facial asymmetry should be recorded.

In cases where a negative vector is observed preoperatively, a midface or SOOF lift may be indicated concomitant to lower blepharoplasty. The ideal patients for transcutaneous lower blepharoplasty are those with orbital fat prolapse and significant redundancy of skin.

4 Transcutaneous Lower Blepharoplasty

4.1 Surgical Technique (Fig. 1)

The procedure can be performed with local anesthesia with or without sedation or general anesthesia, depending on the individual needs of a patient. Before anesthesia, and with the patient seated, assessment with the patient looking upwards can be useful. In eye elevation, the prolapse of the orbital fat is accentuated, and the fat pockets can be better demarcated.

With a corneal protector in place, the infraciliary incision is created 1–2 mm below the ciliary line with a number 15 blade. The skin is then dissected from the orbicular oculi muscle to the inferior border of the tarsus to preserve the pre-tarsal portion of the orbicular oculi muscle. The orbicular oculi muscle is incised in its pre-septal portion and a myocutaneous flap is dissected by blunt dissection. Small openings are created in the septum to access the orbital fat pockets, which must be dissected with gentle traction. Gentle pressure on the globe can help expose the fat herniation, especially the lateral pad.

Hemostasis during the procedure is important. When resecting fat pedicles many advise clamping with a hemostat before excision, with cauterization of the stump prior to hemostat release. Alternatively direct coagulation of bleeding vesels within the fat can be performed with monopolar cautery, bipolar cautery, or laser.

Next, the amount of skin to be resected is assessed. The skin is resected chiefly laterally, with progressively less medially. The skin resection should be conservative to reduce the risk of postoperative eyelid retraction. The patient can be asked to open his or her mouth to assess for the amount of skin removal.

Once the skin is excised, orbicularis muscle suspension is performed. The muscle is fixed to the periosteum of the lateral orbital ridge with two simple sutures using 5-0 absorbable thread. Finally, the skin incision is closed with a continuous 6-0 polypropylene or nylon suture.

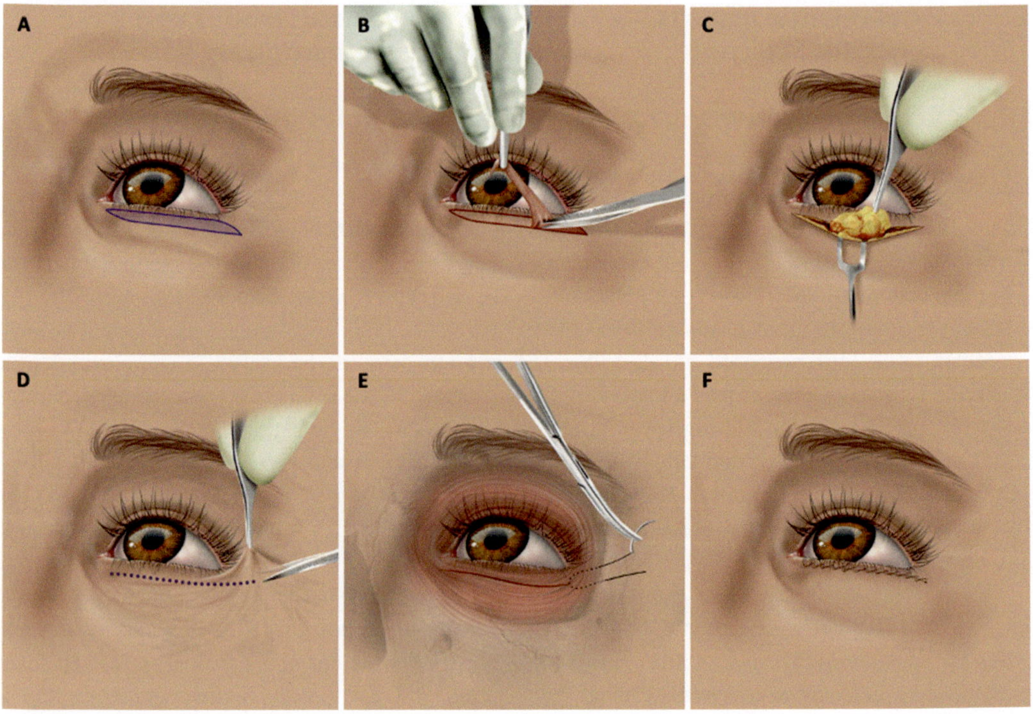

Fig. 1 Step by step of the external lower blepharoplasty technique. a Demarcation of the 3 mm strip of skin and muscle resection; b Resection of skin and orbicularis oculi muscle; c Resection or transfer of the fat pad; d Skin trimming if necessary; e Orbicualiris oculi muscle myopexy to periosteum; f. Skin closure

Concomitant procedures may be performed with the aforementioned technique. In particular, midface lift, also known as a suborbicularis oculi fat (SOOF) lift, or an extended blepharoplasty may be performed. These are described in detail in other chapters but in brief, cheek attachments at the inferior orbital rim are released to augment or extend the tightening effects of blepharoplasty.

Skin resurfacing techniques may be performed concomitantly as well. In particular, and as described in other chapters, the CO_2 laser imposes a slight retraction in the skin, with subsequent intense collagen stimulation [16, 20]. Fine rhytids are removed with an overall tightening effect to that improves skin quality (Figs. 2, 3, 4, 5).

4.2 Fat Repositioning Variation

In some patients, fat repositioning helps fill inferior orbital hollows. In this technique, the orbicularis retaining ligament must be released using a blunt dissection. An absorbsable suture is passed through the fat pedicle and into the periosteum below the inferior orbital rim or the sutures can be passed externally through skin. The repositioning of the fat results in a volume increase in the inferior orbital sulcus along the orbital rim.

Depending on the patient's degree of eyelid laxity, additional lateral canthal procedures (canthopexy or canthoplasty) may be indicated. These techniques are useful in preventing post-blepharoplasty retraction and are described in detail in other chapters.

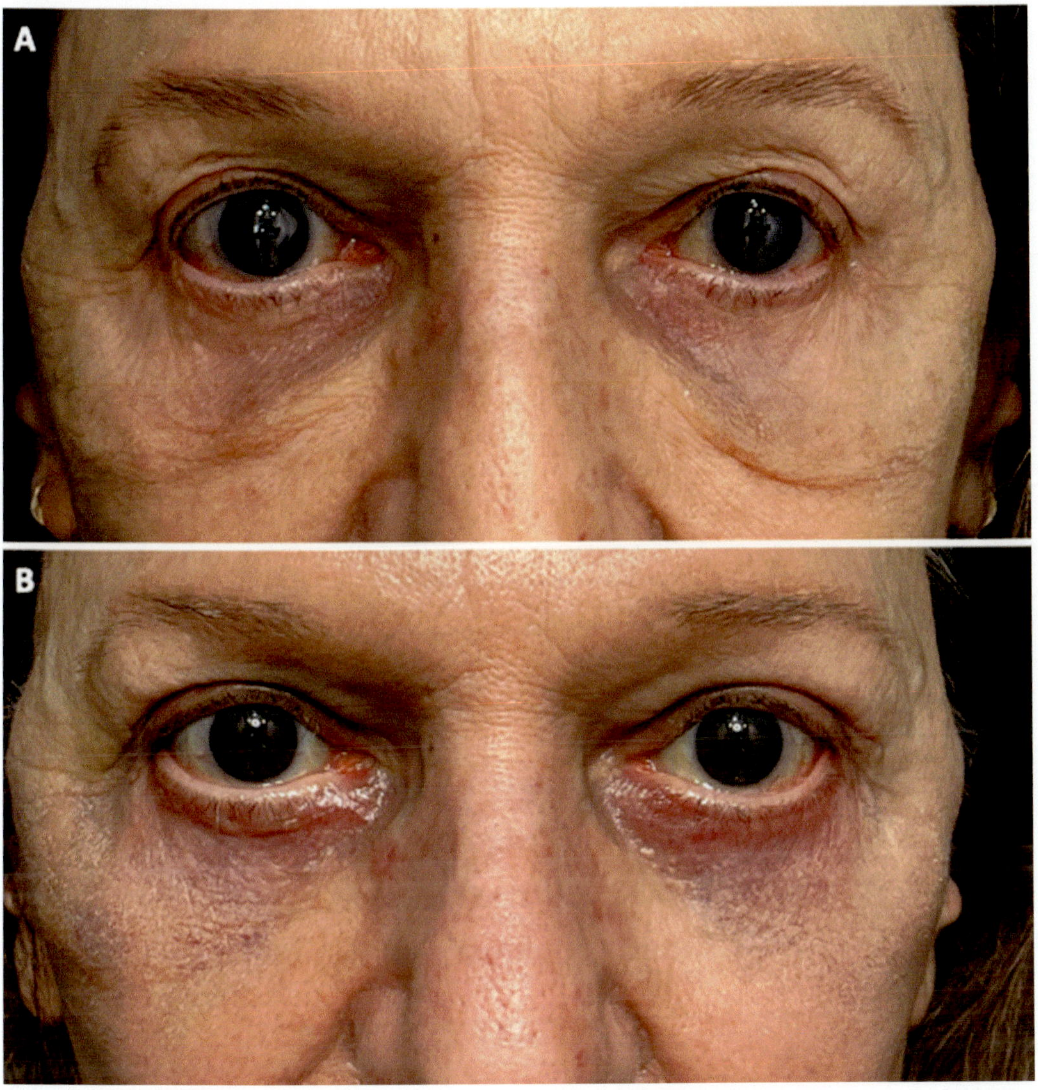

Fig. 2 **a** Preoperative photograph of a patient who presented with malar edema and lower eyelid laxity; **b** Postoperative day 15 photograph demonstrating improvement in palpebral laxity and malar edema after external lower blepharoplasty

5 Complications

Orbital fat prolapse through the lower eyelids can be over- or under-corrected. Undercorrection is typically seen in the lateral fat pocket and can be corrected with additional resection. Excessive fat removal can lead to hollowing. If it occurs, it can be treated with injectable fillers or fat grafting.

Eyelid retraction and ectropion are often present in the first postoperatrive weeks. Patients should be advised to aggressively lubricate the eyes as the edema and inflammation subsides. If eyelid malposition persists after several months, surgical intervention may be indicated. A variety of approaches are described in other chapters.

Diplopia is rare, but can result after eyelid surgery. It may be transient due to edema

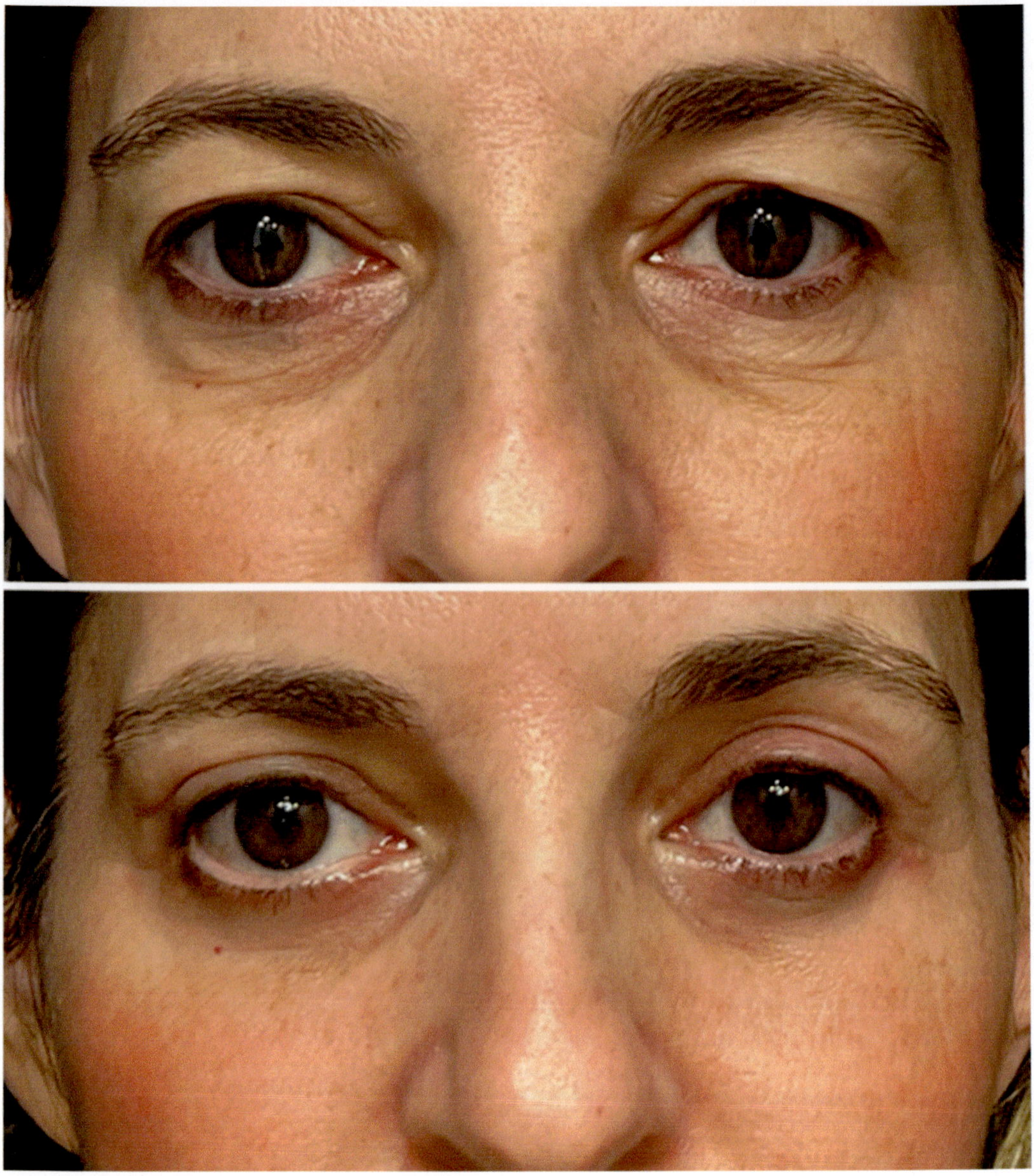

Fig. 3 **a** Preoperative photograph lower palpebral laxity and rhytids; **b** Postoperative photograph after external lower blepharoplasty demonstrating improvement in skin rhytids and laxity

or hematoma. Importantly, injury to the inferior oblique muscle is possible. Avoidance is key, with careful dissection of the fat pads and care to visualize and avoid the inferior oblique muscle located between the medial and central fat pads. Careful use of cautery in this region is advised. Referral to an adult strabismus specialist may be advised for inferior oblique injury that does not recover after many months.

Hematomas are often self limited, but large ones may require surgical drainage. This is rare but may occur in up to 1% of cases and usually within the first 24 h after surgery. To reduce the risk of this complication, the suspension of anticoagulants before surgery should be evaluated and discussed with the patient's clinician/cardiologist, and systemic arterial hypertension should be controlled. During surgery,

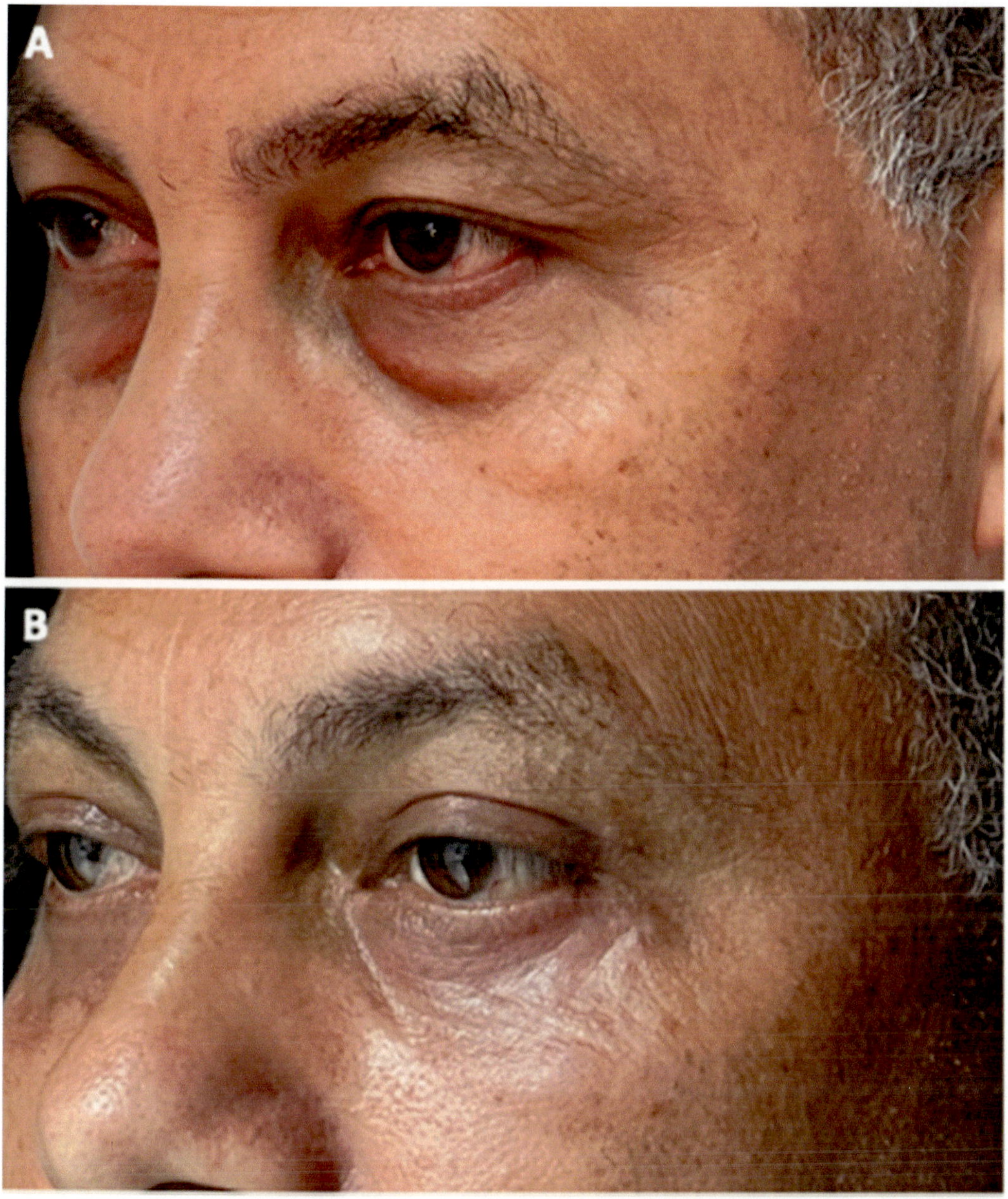

Fig. 4 **a** Preoperative photograph of a patient with fat herniation and a tear trough deformity; **b** Postoperative photograph 30 days post external lower eyelid blepharoplasty with fat transposition to the hollows

meticulous hemostasis should be performed, particularly during the removal of orbital fat. Postoperatively, cold compresses and restrictions of physical activity are recommended.

Chemosis complicates a small percentage of lower eyelid blepharoplasty patients. Predisposing factors include inflammation, venous congestion, and disruption of lymphatic drainage. It can also occur due to inflammation due to allergy, trauma, or infection. Recognition and correction of pre-existing ocular surface changes, conjunctivochalasis, palpebral malocclusion, and lower eyelid laxity should be considered during the preoperative evaluation to

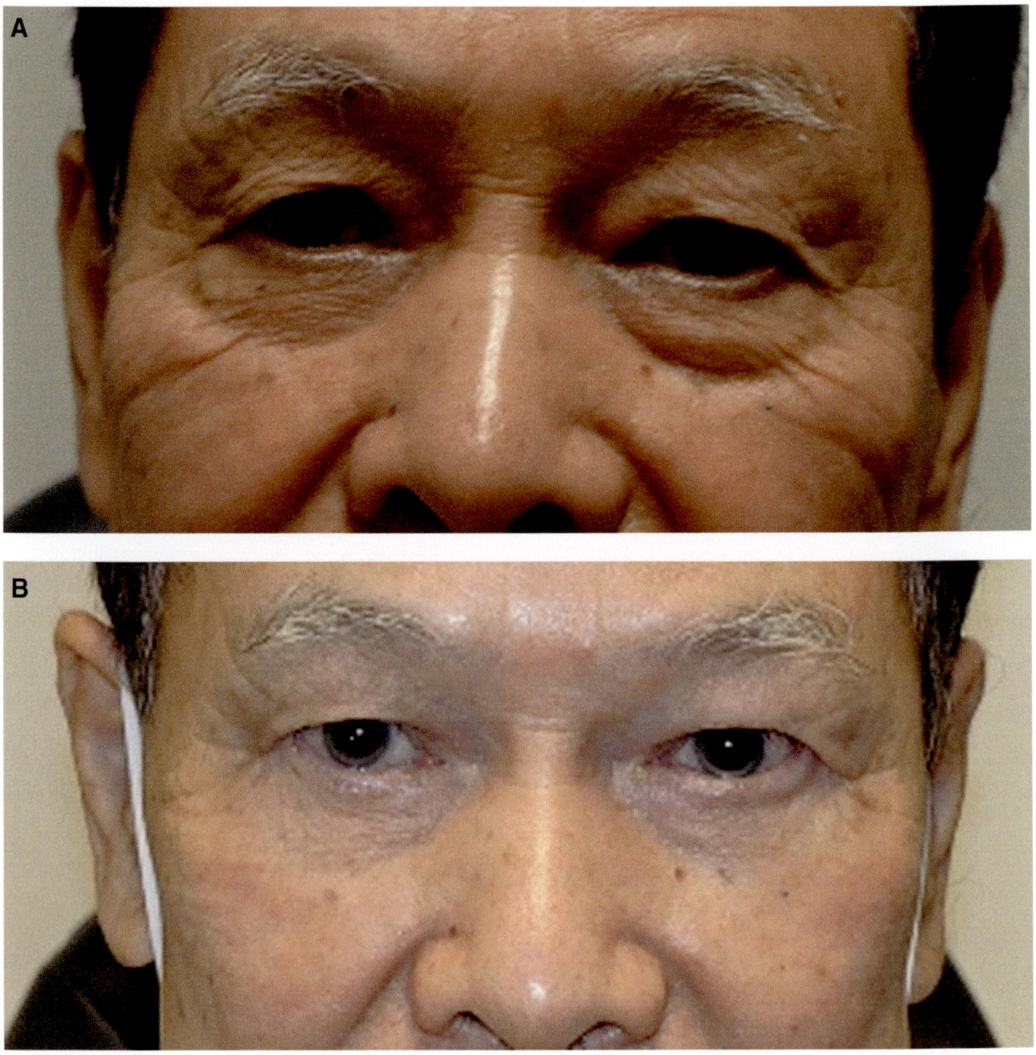

Fig. 5 **a** Preoperative photograph of a patient with lower eyelid rhytids and mild fat herniation. **b** Patient in (**a**) 4 months after bilateral lower eyelid external blepharoplasty

avoid or minimize this complication postoperatively. Prophylactic treatment with anti-inflammatory drugs such as topical steroid eye drops, and systemic steroids can reduce inflammation and possibly reduce or prevent postoperative chemosis. Aggressive lubrication is advised. Rarely a suture tarsorrhaphy is indicated and most chemosis subsides over time.

6 Conclusion

External lower blepharoplasty can achieve excellent results for under eye rhytids and contour abnromalities. There exists a risk for eyelid malposition and dry eye with these proceudres. Attention to other variables such as eyelid laxity or other vectors predisposing to eyelid malposition are key. With a good understanding of anatomy and with good technique, favorable results may be achieved with external blepharoplasty for patients desiring aesthetic improvements to their lower eyelids.

References

1. Pack S, Quereshy FA, Altay MA, Baur DA. Transconjunctival lower blepharoplasty. Atlas Oral Maxillofac Surg Clin [Internet]. 2016;24:147–51. Available from https://linkinghub.elsevier.com/retrieve/pii/S106133151630018X
2. Smith CB, Waite PD. Lower transcutaneous blepharoplasty. Atlas Oral Maxillofac Surg Clin. 2016;24:135–45. Available from https://linkinghub.elsevier.com/retrieve/pii/S1061331516300142
3. Branham GH. Lower eyelid blepharoplasty. Facial Plast Surg Clin North Am. 2016;24:129–38. Available from https://linkinghub.elsevier.com/retrieve/pii/S1064740615001418
4. Reilly MJ, Tomsic JA, Fernandez SJ, Davison SP. Effect of facial rejuvenation surgery on perceived attractiveness, femininity, and personality. JAMA Facial Plast Surg. 2015;17:202–07. Available from https://www.liebertpub.com/doi/10.1001/jamafacial.2015.0158
5. Cotofana S, Fratila A, Schenck T, Redka-Swoboda W, Zilinsky I, Pavicic T. The anatomy of the aging face: A review. Facial Plast Surg. 2016;32:253–60. Available from http://www.thieme-connect.de/DOI/DOI?10.1055/s-0036-1582234
6. Most SP, Mobley SR, Larrabee WF. Anatomy of the eyelids. Facial Plast Surg Clin North Am. 2005;13:487–92. Available from https://linkinghub.elsevier.com/retrieve/pii/S1064740605000490
7. Hwang K. Surgical anatomy of the lower eyelid relating to lower blepharoplasty. Anat Cell Biol. 2010;43:15. Available from https://synapse.koreamed.org/DOIx.php?id=10.5115/acb.2010.43.1.15
8. Shams P, Ortiz-Pérez S, Joshi N. Clinical anatomy of the periocular region. Facial Plast Surg. 2013;29:255–63. Available from http://www.thieme-connect.de/DOI/DOI?10.1055/s-0033-1349365
9. Mojallal A, Cotofana S. Anatomy of lower eyelid and eyelid–cheek junction. Ann Chir Plast Esthétique. 2017;62:365–74. Available from https://linkinghub.elsevier.com/retrieve/pii/S0294126017301516
10. Rohrich RJ, Arbique GM, Wong C, Brown S, Pessa JE. The anatomy of suborbicularis fat: Implications for periorbital rejuvenation. Plast Reconstr Surg. 2009;124:946–51. Available from http://journals.lww.com/00006534-200909000-00031
11. Palermo EC. Anatomy of the periorbital region. Surg Cosmet Dermatol. 2013;5:245–56.
12. Codner MA, Mccord CD. Eyelid and periorbital surgery. 2nd ed. St. Louis: Taylor & Francis; 2017.
13. Kruglikov I, Trujillo O, Kristen Q, Isac K, Zorko J, Fam M, et al. The facial adipose tissue: A revision. Facial Plast Surg. 2016;32:671–82. Available from http://www.thieme-connect.de/DOI/DOI?10.1055/s-0036-1596046
14. Fezza JP, Massry G. Lower eyelid length. Plast Reconstr Surg. 2015;136:152e–159e. Available from http://journals.lww.com/00006534-201508000-00007
15. Raschke GF, Rieger UM, Bader R-D, Schaefer O, Guentsch A, Schultze-Mosgau S. Transconjunctival versus subciliary approach for orbital fracture repair—an anthropometric evaluation of 221 cases. Clin Oral Investig. 2013;17:933–42. Available from http://link.springer.com/10.1007/s00784-012-0776-3
16. Murri M, Hamill E, Hauck M, Marx D. An update on lower lid blepharoplasty. Semin Plast Surg. 2017;31:046–50. Available from http://www.thieme-connect.de/DOI/DOI?10.1055/s-0037-1598632
17. Rohrich RJ, Pessa JE, Ristow B. The youthful cheek and the deep medial fat compartment. Plast Reconstr Surg. 2008;121:2107–12. Available from https://journals.lww.com/00006534-200806000-00034
18. Cotofana S, Lachman N. Anatomy of the facial fat compartments and their relevance in aesthetic surgery. JDDG J der Dtsch Dermatologischen Gesellschaft. 2019;17:399–413. Available from https://onlinelibrary.wiley.com/doi/abs/10.1111/ddg.13737
19. Zoumalan CI, Roostaeian J. Simplifying blepharoplasty. Plast Reconstr Surg. 2016;137:196e-213e. Available from http://journals.lww.com/00006534-201601000-00064
20. Omi T, Numano K. The role of the CO_2 laser and fractional CO_2 laser in dermatology. LASER Ther. 2014;23:49–60. Available from https://www.jstage.jst.go.jp/article/islsm/23/1/23_14-RE-01/_article

Midface Lift

Meleha Ahmad, Amanda Miller, Michael Han,
Jeremiah P. Tao and Seanna Grob

Abstract

The midface is comprised of the lower eyelid subunit and cheek extending to the nasolabial fold. Several aging changes occur to the midface, including skin descent, orbicularis attenuation, reduced malar prominence, and skeletonizing of the inferior orbital rim. Midface lifting may be performed for cosmetic indications to address these changes or for functional indications such as lower eyelid malposition due to trauma, prior surgery, or facial nerve dysfunction. In both, vertical malposition is improved through suspensory mechanisms. This chapter describes approaches to midface lifting.

Illustrations by Michael Han

Supplementary Information The online version contains supplementary material available at https://doi.org/10.1007/978-3-031-36175-3_26.

M. Ahmad · A. Miller · S. Grob
Department of Ophthalmology, University of California San Francisco, San Francisco, CA, USA
e-mail: Meleha.Ahmad@ucsf.edu

A. Miller
David Geffen School of Medicine, University of California Los Angeles, Los Angeles, CA, USA

M. Han · J. P. Tao (✉)
Department of Ophthalmology, University of California, Irvine, CA, USA

Keywords

Cheek lift · Midface · Extended blepharoplasty · Malar suspension · Midface lift

1 Introduction

The midface is the region between the lateral canthus, oral commissure, and the nasolabial fold. Midface lifting aims to address ptosis of the midface (Fig. 1), with goals of aesthetic enhancement or functional malposition correction or both. A midface lift can be used to rejuvenate eyelid and cheek contour. Midface lifting can correct midface atrophy and descent, improve the tear trough deformity, and reposition the malar fat pad [1]. While more extensive than most lower blepharoplasty techniques, midface lifting may add support to the lower eyelid that in turn reduces lower eyelid retraction complications.

2 Anatomy and Pathophysiology

Key anatomical landmarks in midface lifting include the lower eyelid skin, orbicularis oculi muscle, orbital septum, sub-orbicularis oculi fat, malar fat pads, lateral canthal tendon, and the zygomatic and orbicularis retaining ligament

J. P. Tao (ed.), *Plastic Surgery of the Lower Eyelids*,
https://doi.org/10.1007/978-3-031-36175-3_26

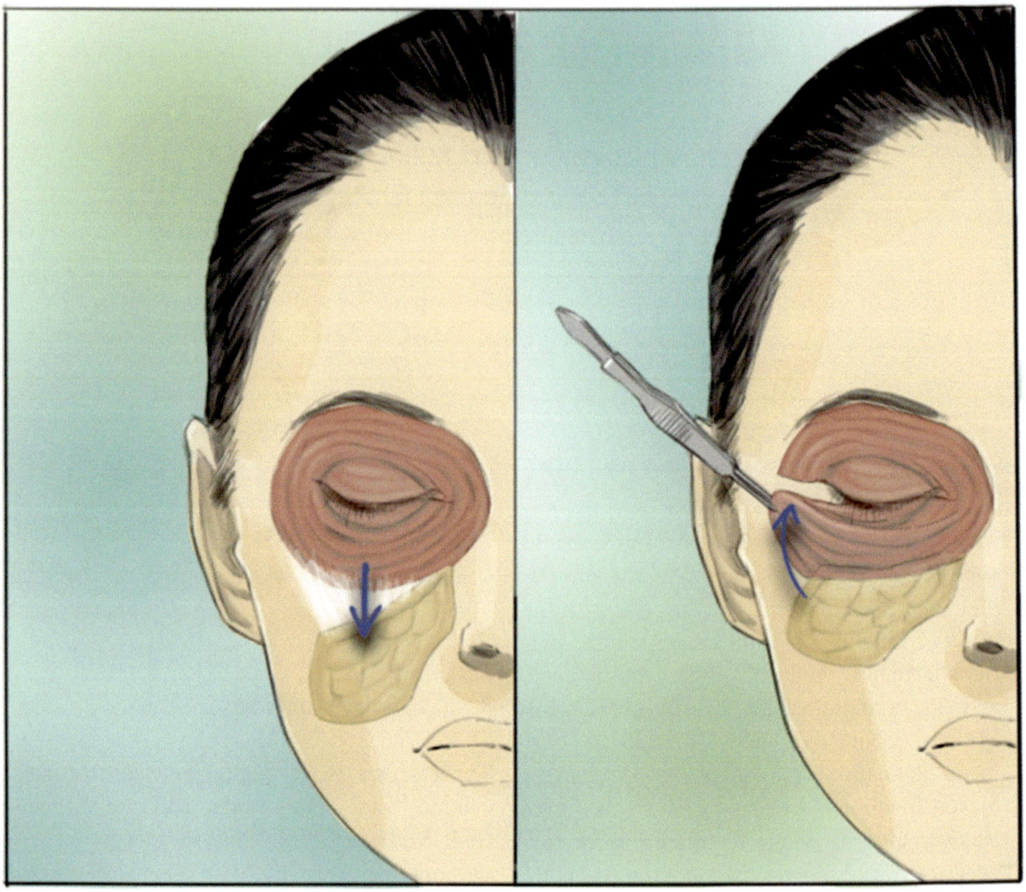

Fig. 1 Diagram showing effects of aging with midface descent (Left) and improvement in midface positioning with midface lift surgery (Right). With aging, grooves can be seen over the ligamentous attachments in the face that accentuate the outpouching or bulging of the lower eyelid fat pads and also malar mounds or festoons

(ORL). The orbicularis oculi muscle is an eyelid protractor that is just deep to skin and spans just over 1 cm superior and inferior to the orbital rims, and over 2 cm lateral to the lateral rims [2]. It has a close association with the thin eyelid skin due to the absence of subcutaneous fat. The ORL, also known as the orbitomalar ligament [3], is a collagen-elastin osseocutaneous structure that originates 4–6 mm below the inferior orbital rim and extends anteriorly to insert at the level of the dermis between the eyelid and the cheek [4] (Fig. 1). It spans the orbital rim just lateral to the medial limbus, up to the lateral canthus where it merges with the lateral orbital thickening, a triangular condensation of the superficial and deep fascia. The ORL is strongest at its lateral extent, and weakest centrally. Inferior and lateral to the ORL is the prezygomatic space which contains the zygomaticofacial foramen and nerve, and is bordered inferiorly by the zygomatic ligament [5] (Fig. 1).

The fat of the face is divided into discrete fat compartments. The four relevant fat pads involved in midface lifting include: supraperiosteal, nasolabial, buccal, and orbital [6]. The supraperiosteal fat pad, a component of which is the suborbicularis oculi fat (SOOF), contributes to the malar crescent and is bound both to periosteum and bone (Fig. 2). The nasolabial, also known as malar, fat pad is held to the malar eminence by true ligaments, and can be subdivided into three separate compartments: medial, middle and lateral [7]. The buccal fat pad is held by false ligaments. The lower eyelid has three

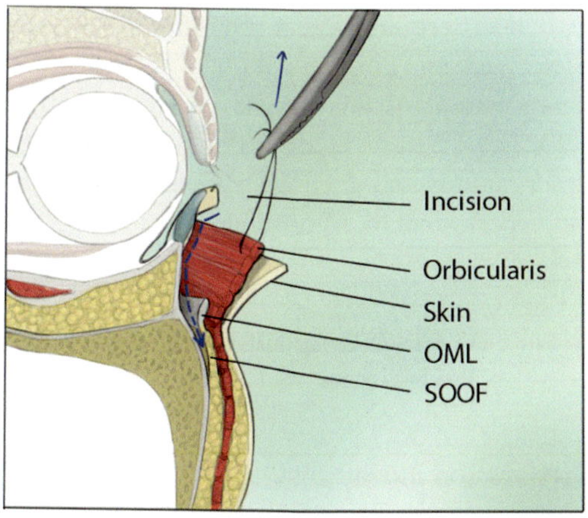

Fig. 2 Diagram showing the dissection plane starting at the subciliary incision, extending down to the orbital rim in the preseptal, postorbicularis oculi plane and release of the orbital retaining ligament (ORL). Once a muscle flap is created, the orbicularis flap is elevated superolaterally and secured to the lateral orbital rim

postseptal fat compartments—nasal, central, and lateral. With age, the septum weakens causing the orbital fat to bulge anteriorly over the orbital rim creating lower eyelid bags. The SOOF, which lies deep to the orbicularis muscle of the lower eyelid and caudal to the orbitomalar ligament, consists of a medial and a lateral component separated by the lateral canthus [8] (Fig. 2).

2.1 Aging Changes

Change occurs within each of the layers of the midface, with differences noted as early as the third decade of life [9]. Gravitational descent of the skin and subcutaneous fat is perhaps the first to occur and the most obvious change in most patients (Fig. 1). Other external findings include grooves correlating to underlying ligamentous attachments that serve as tethers and bulges that overly spaces between these attachments. The nasojugal groove medially and the palpebromalar groove laterally create the classic lower eyelid bulge, highlighted due to attenuation of the ORL and descent of the postseptal orbital fat pads. The mid-cheek groove is a continuation of the nasojugal groove downward and outward and corresponds to the zygomatic-cutanaeous ligaments and give rise to the malar mound (also known as festoons) inferior to the lower eyelid bulge [5, 10]. Ligamentous laxity of the medial and lateral canthi and lower eyelid retractors may also contribute to the aging changes of the lower eyelid and midface.

Other aging phenomena include skin and orbicularis attenuation and differential adipose volume loss [11]. In addition, the concept of pseudoptosis, described by Rohrich, involves the selective loss of volume of the deep fat compartments compared to the more superficial ones and can also lead to deepening of the nasolabial fold and decreased midface projection [12]. There is also possible contribution of facial skeleton changes to the aging appearance of the midface [13]. Certain areas of the midface skeleton including the pyriform region of the maxilla, the superomedial and inferolateral orbital rim, and the prejowl mandible are more predisposed to bone resorption over time. Failing to note and address these bony changes may present the upper limit to aesthetic results by manipulation of skin and soft tissues during midface lifts.

3 Preoperative History and Evaluation

Specific features of the patient history, including patient complaints, aesthetic and functional goals should be identified. Ophthalmic and periocular surgical history is crucial to understanding the patient's anatomy, possible areas of scarring, and placement and orientation of the lower eyelid. A complete eye exam should be performed, noting any corneal pathology or functional abnormalities of eyelid position, including ectropion, lower eyelid retraction, laxity or floppy eyelid syndrome, or facial nerve palsy as midface lifting can provide a chance for surgical correction. In these instances, adjunctive procedures such as tarsal strip, lateral canthoplasty, or lower eyelid spacer graft may be indicated to address these issues at the time of cosmetic midface surgery [14].

Additionally, cosmetic concerns such as prominence of the orbital rim, nasolabial or nasojugal folds, lower eyelid fat prolapse, dermatochalasis, or festoons should be identified. Pressure on the globe with observation for further herniation can be used to differentiate between herniated orbital fat and fat in other parts of the midface [15]. The presence of a negative inferior eyelid vector or midface volume loss is extremely important to note as midface lifting without volume augmentation (with hyaluronic acid fillers, lipofilling or implants) have been associated with lower long-term patient satisfaction and need for additional procedures [16]. In the setting of a negative vector, care must be taken in lower eyelid or midface surgery to prevent further lower eyelid retraction or eyelid malposition.

4 Surgical Technique

4.1 Overview

A variety of surgical and non-surgical approaches have been used to correct abnormalities in the midface, dictated primarily by preoperative findings. Non-surgical approaches include hyaluronic acid fillers or autologous fat transfer for volume augmentation, laser resurfacing or chemical peels, or threads. The majority of surgical approaches consist of some combination of skin removal, fat grafting or repositioning, lateral canthopexy or lateral tarsal strip, lower eyelid blepharoplasty (fat removal or repositioning) and ORL release [11, 17]. Variations in surgical approach include eyelid-based approaches such as temporal (often performed in conjunction with lateral tarsal strip), transconjunctival or transcutaneous approaches (depending on the amount of excess skin), endoscopic approaches from the temporal region, or preauricular or temporal incisions that are often avoided due to risk of facial nerve injury [18, 19]. A skin-muscle flap may be utilized to provide cheek suspension. ORL release may allow better effacement of the tear trough [4, 11, 17, 20] and is required if fat repositioning is being performed concurrently with midface lifting. The lateral extent of this release can be performed selectively based on the extent of tear trough deformity formation [17]. Dissection planes may be preperiosteal [4, 4] or subperiosteal [11].

4.2 Transcutaneous Preperiosteal Technique

Preparation for Surgery

This procedure is performed under local anesthesia with intravenous sedation or general anesthesia if needed. Local anesthesia is injected subcutaneously and diffusely across the eyelids, lateral canthal area, and midface. The patient's entire face is prepared with povidone-iodine and then the patient is draped. Corneal protectors are placed.

Surgical Procedure (Video 1)

Methylene blue or a surgical marking pen is used to mark a lateral canthal line that begins at the lateral canthus and extends approximately 1.5 cm horizontal and slightly superolateral. The skin is incised with a #15 Bard-Parker blade along this mark. A subciliary incision is then made along the lower eyelid which connects to the lateral canthal incision. Sharp dissection is carried in the preseptal plane (Fig. 2). Then using curved tenotomy scissors, blunt dissection is continued in the preseptal plane across the lower eyelid and the orbicularis oculi is separated from the underlying septum across the subciliary incision. The skin and muscle are retracted to expose the septum and lower eyelid fat pads that emerge from the deeper orbit (Fig. 3A). Using both blunt dissection and sharp dissection with electrocautery, the orbital rim is identified and preperisoteal dissection is performed across the midface, with special attention to release of the ORL. Care is taken to avoid the infraorbital nerve. The orbital fat pads are then exposed and repositioned or draped over the orbital rim to create a smooth eyelid cheek junction. If excess orbital fat is present, the fat pads are also sculpted and resected accordingly. The inferior oblique, that is often found between the medial and central fat pads, is avoided and preserved. In the majority of patients, especially those over 50 years old, but also many younger horizontal eyelid tightening is advised to forestall eyelid malposition. A canthotomy incision is made using a #15 blade and straight iris scissors which is then followed by cantholysis of the inferior canthal tendon. The free tarsal edge is secured to the inner rim periosteum with a 4-0 braided polyester or polyglactin suture with or without creating a small tarsal strip. The orbicularis muscle is sharply dissected away from the skin laterally on the skin-muscle flap just lateral to the lateral canthus (Fig. 3A). The muscle flap is then advanced superotemporally, some excess muscle is resected, and the cut edge is secured to the outer rim periosteum and temporalis fascia with a 4-0 or 5-0 polyglactin suture (Fig. 3B). Excess superior skin past the lateral canthus is draped with a slight vertical vector and excess is marked with methylene blue or a surgical marking pen and is then excised (Fig. 3C). Most of the skin removal is lateral to the lateral canthus with minimal skin (often 2 mm or less) removed along the subciliary lower eyelid to prevent lower eyelid retraction or ectropion. The skin wounds should be under no or minimal tension. The subciliary incision is closed with a running 6-0 plain gut suture and the skin is closed laterally with deep 6-0 polyglactin sutures and 6-0 nylon or prolene sutures to the skin (often in a running vertical mattress technique with good eversion of this thicker, visible skin).

Pre- and post-operative photographs are shown in Fig. 4. Outcomes on 80 cosmetic patients of 2 surgeons demonstrated good to excellent aesthetic outcomes [21]. There were few complications, with only one case of ectropion requiring subsequent tarsal strip, and 5% of cases developing lateral "mounding" that required elliptical excision and repair. This complication is likely mitigated with modifications to the technique above, with a small increased risk of lateral hollowing when orbicularis is resected [22].

Variations in Technique

Several variations in the authors' technique have been described [23, 24]. The primary variation is the use of a subperiosteal dissection plane [18, 25]. The periosteum is extensively elevated off the facial skeleton from the gingivobuccal sulcus inferiorly to the malar eminence laterally and the nasomaxillary junction medially with care to preserve the infraorbital nerve and zygomaticofacial nerves. Dissection along the zygomatic arch is generally avoided to evade frontal nerve injury. A 3-0 polydioxanone suture is used to fixate the elevated soft tissues to the cuff of periosteum at the inferior orbital rim (stronger than lateral orbital rim periosteum), sometimes with 3-5 sutures [26]. A similar technique with extensive dissection to nasolabial fold in the preperiosteal plane has also been described [27].

Adjunctive therapies can be performed at the same time as midface lifting such as soft tissue volume augmentation via autologous fat transfer [11] at the level of the prezygomatic space and the medial midfacial fat compartment in the suborbicuarlis oculi plan. Festoons can be addressed using nonsurgical options such as radiofrequency ablation, carbon dioxide laser, chemical peel, dermal filler, and injections, or surgical options such as direct excision or skin-muscle flap [15].

A further modification to the midface lift technique is the use of endoscopic guidance. Through a temporal incision, the orbicularis oculi and malar fat pad are elevated through direct visualization with selective disruption of the midfacial ligaments. This technique can be performed in the preperiosteal or subperiosteal planes, [28, 29] and may be performed in conjunction with endoscopic forehead lift. Fixation is typically performed with a single suture suspending the malar fat pad to the deep temporalis fascia, however endotines or multiple suture suspension may also be employed.

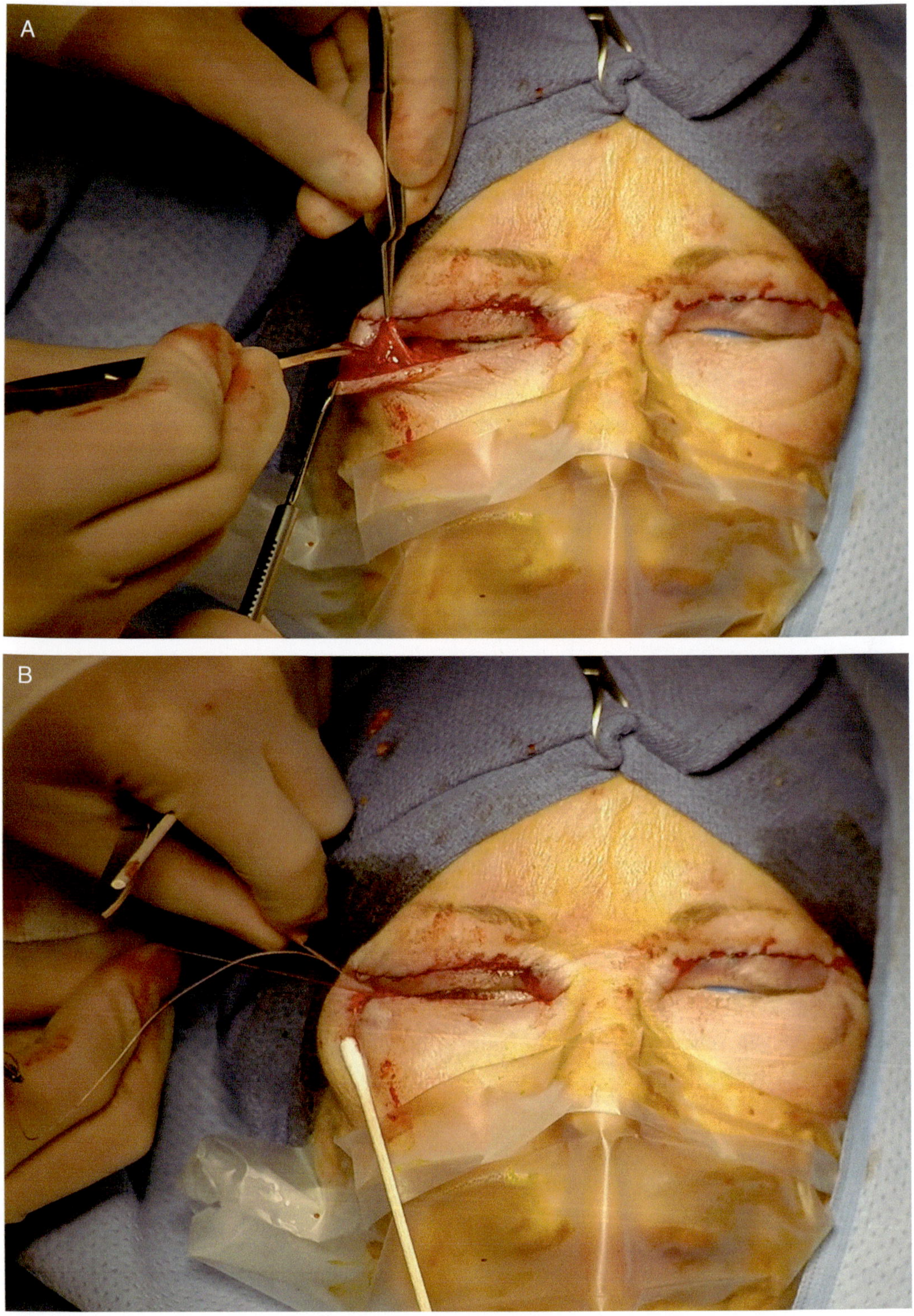
A
B

Fig. 3 A: Development of orbicularis oculi muscle flap for midface lift. The orbicularis is sharply dissected away from the skin lateral to the lateral canthus. A two-pronged skin hook is used to retract the skin while the surgeon elevates the muscle flap. Care should be taken to avoid a button-hole while dissecting muscle off the skin. It is helpful to have the assistant lift the skin more vertically, rather than folding it back over inferiorly over the cheek. B: Fixation of orbicularis oculi muscle flap to periosteum. A 5-0 polyglactin suture is used to engage the muscle flap lateral to the lateral canthus. The muscle flap is then secured to the periosteum at the lateral orbital rim superiorly to achieve a tightening and lifting of the lower eyelid and midface. C: Resection of excess skin is mostly lateral to the lateral canthus with minimal skin removed along the inferior eyelid. The excess skin is marked and then excised with straight iris scissors. Usually 2 mm or less of skin is excised along the subciliary incision to prevent lower eyelid malposition

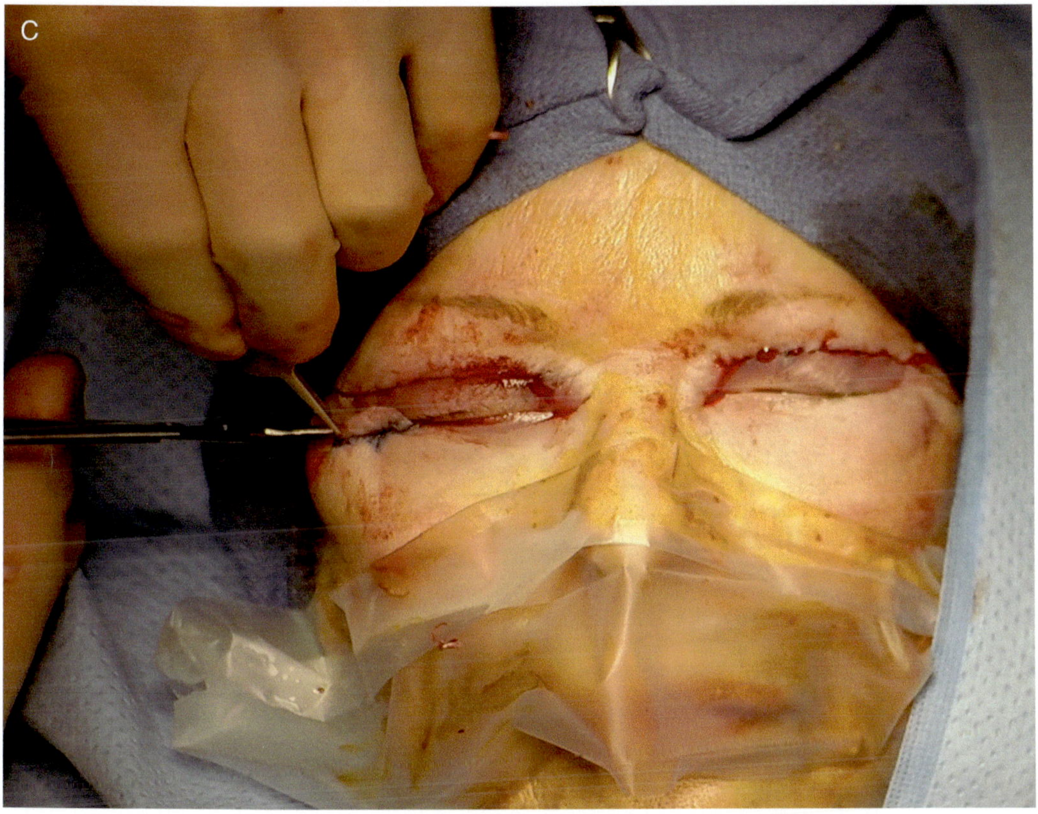

Fig. 3 (continued)

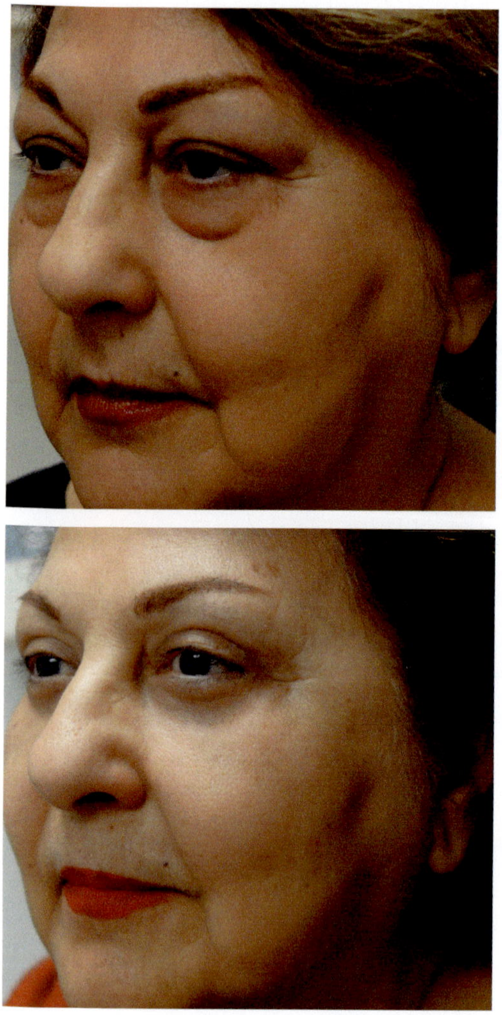

Fig. 4 Pre-operative (top) and post-operative (bottom) photos of authors' transcutaneous preperiosteal midface lift technique

5 Postoperative Considerations and Complications

Several complications can arise during midface lifting, both functional and aesthetic (Table 1), with some groups demonstrating a revision rate of up to 20% [18]. The most prevalent functional complication associated with midface lifting is lower eyelid malposition, including lower eyelid retraction and ectropion, which has been shown to occur in 5–11% of cases [21, 30]. Causes for lower eyelid malposition after midface lift are often multifactorial but most often occur due to aggressive skin removal or unidentified lower eyelid laxity or negative vector. Care to ensure canthal stabilization and support, especially in patients with pre-existing eyelid laxity, can minimize this risk. Also, excision of excess skin should be focused lateral to the lateral canthus after the skin-muscle flap is elevated with minimal (often 2 mm or less) skin removed from the subciliary location. Subperiosteal dissection may be associated with a higher rate of ectropion [31], as can trimming rather than plication of the orbicularis muscle [11]. Other functional complications include orbital hemorrhage, infraorbital nerve injury, postoperative swelling and chemosis. These complications can be minimized by careful preoperative patient selection and care during dissection intraoperatively. Aesthetic complications such as asymmetry, canthal rounding or webbing, lower eyelid contour abnormalities, and cutaneous scarring, are also possible and can be mitigated as described in Table 1.

6 Closed Techniques

There are several options for nonsurgical correction of midface ptosis. Some of these are described in more detail in other chapters. These include placement of polydioxanone (PDS) threads, applying bipolar fractionated radiofrequency, and the use of fillers or autologous fat transfer [16, 32–35].

7 Conclusions

Midface lifting is a safe and effective treatment for the lower eyelids and cheeks. When performed correctly in the appropriate patient, it is an excellent adjunct to lower eyelid blepharoplasty and may improve irregular contours due to underlying ligamentous attachments and forestall eyelid retraction. Midface lifting techniques may also have utility for functional or reconstructive eyelid malposition indications.

Table 1 Complications of midface lifting

Complication	Cause	Ways to mitigate
Functional		
Cicatricial ectropion	Aggressive skin removal	Conservative skin excision, especially in the subciliary location
Dry Eye	Orbicularis paralysis due to orbicularis resection or superior buccal branch injury	• Transconjunctival approach • Subperiosteal dissection
Lower eyelid retraction	• Aggressive skin or fat removal (transcutaneous) • Aggressive conjunctival closure (transconjunctival)	• Conservative skin excision, especially in the subciliary location, as well as conservative fat excision • Transconjunctival approach • Closure of conjunctiva with single or several sutures • Identification of negative vector preoperatively • Postoperative Frost suture [9]
Involutional ectropion/ Laxity	• Inadequate lateral canthal support • Possible orbicularis disruption during ORL release	• Lateral canthoplasty or canthopexy • ORL release [30] • Consider subperiosteal dissection [31]
Postoperative swelling/ Chemosis	Multifactorial	ORL release [30]
V2 anesthesia	Infraorbital nerve injury	Care to avoid infraorbital nerve during dissection
Orbital Hemorrhage	• Aggressive fat removal • Failure to stop blood thinners • Inadequate hemostasis • Post-operative Valsalva maneuvers	• Careful removal of fat • Intraoperative hemostasis • Stopping anticoagulants • Avoidance of post-operative Valsalva maneuvers
Aesthetic		
Lower eyelid or cheek contour abnormality	Orbicularis redundancy	Appropriate redraping or resection of orbicularis oculi
Asymmetry	• Too much or too little fat excision on one side compared to other • Asymmetry skin excision • Development of eyelid malposition	• Care during procedure to match fat and skin-muscle excision on either side, unless preoperative asymmetry needs to be addressed
Lateral canthal mounding	• Orbicularis redundancy • Skin redundancy after closure	• Careful redraping of skin muscle flap • Resection of excess lateral orbicularis oculi muscle flap • Careful closure of lateral canthal incision
Lateral canthal dystopia rounding or webbing	Unaddressed lower eyelid laxity	Lateral canthoplasty without canthotomy when appropriate
Cutaneous scarring	Cutaneous incision	• Transconjunctival incision when skin is not removed • 5FU or triamcinolone injection postoperatively

References

1. Paul MD, Calvert JW, Evans GRD. The evolution of the midface lift in aesthetic plastic surgery. Plast Reconstr Surg. 2006;117:1809–27.
2. Costin BR, Sakolsatayadorn N, McNutt SA, Rubinstein TJ, Trichonas G, Rocha KM, McClintic JI, Huang L, McBride JM, Perry JD. Dimensions and anatomic variations of the orbicularis oculi muscle in nonpreserved, fresh-frozen human cadavers. Ophthal Plast Reconstr Surg. 2014;30:198–200.
3. Kikkawa DO, Lemke BN, Dortzbach RK. Relations of the superficial musculoaponeurotic system to the orbit and characterization of the orbitomalar ligament. Ophthal Plast Reconstr Surg. 1996;12:77–88.
4. Schiller JD. Lysis of the orbicularis retaining ligament and orbicularis oculi insertion: a powerful modality for lower eyelid and cheek rejuvenation. Plast Reconstr Surg. 2012;129:692e–700e.
5. Mendelson BC, Muzaffar AR, Adams WP. Surgical anatomy of the midcheek and malar mounds. Plast Reconstr Surg. 2002;110:885–96; discussion 897–911.
6. Keller G, Quatela VC, Antunes MB, Sykes JM, Magill CK, Seth R. Midface lift: panel discussion. Facial Plast Surg Clin N Am. 2014;22:119–37.
7. Rohrich RJ, Pessa JE. The fat compartments of the face: anatomy and clinical implications for cosmetic surgery. Plast Reconstr Surg. 2007;119:2219–27.
8. Rohrich RJ, Arbique GM, Wong C, Brown S, Pessa JE. The anatomy of suborbicularis fat: implications for periorbital rejuvenation. Plast Reconstr Surg. 2009;124:946–51.
9. Sclafani AP, Dibelius G. Transpalpebral midface lift. Facial Plast Surg Clin N Am. 2015;23:209–19.
10. Muzaffar AR, Mendelson BC, Adams WP. Surgical anatomy of the ligamentous attachments of the lower lid and lateral canthus. Plast Reconstr Surg. 2002;110:873–884; discussion 897–911.
11. Nakra T. Biplanar contour-oriented approach to lower eyelid and midface rejuvenation. JAMA Facial Plast Surg. 2015;17:374–81.
12. Rohrich RJ, Pessa JE, Ristow B. The youthful cheek and the deep medial fat compartment. Plast Reconstr Surg. 2008;121:2107–12.
13. Mendelson B, Wong C-H. Changes in the facial skeleton with aging: implications and clinical applications in facial rejuvenation. Aesthetic Plast Surg. 2012;36:753–60.
14. Kahana A, Lucarelli MJ. Adjunctive transcanthotomy lateral suborbicularis fat lift and orbitomalar ligament resuspension in lower eyelid ectropion repair. Ophthal Plast Reconstr Surg. 2009;25:1–6.
15. Krakauer M, Aakalu VK, Putterman AM. Treatment of malar festoon using modified subperiosteal midface lift. Ophthal Plast Reconstr Surg. 2012;28:459–62.
16. Barone M, Cogliandro A, Salzillo R, Ciarrocchi S, Abu Hanna A, Russo V, Tenna S, Persichetti P. Midface lift plus lipofilling preferential in patients with negative lower eyelid vectors: a randomized controlled trial. Aesthetic Plast Surg. 2021;45:1012–9.
17. Rohrich RJ, Ghavami A, Mojallal A. The five-step lower blepharoplasty: blending the eyelid-cheek junction. Plast Reconstr Surg. 2011;128:775–83.
18. Hester TR, Codner MA, McCord CD. The "centrofacial" approach for correction of facial aging using the transblepharoplasty subperiosteal cheek lift. Aesthet Surg J. 1996;16:51–8.
19. Weng C, Quatela V. Achieving a youthful midface: examination of midface anatomy improvement following lower blepharoplasty with fat transposition and transtemporal midface lift with lower lid skin pinch. Aesthet Surg J. 2019;39:NP416–NP428.
20. Sullivan PK, Drolet BC. Extended lower lid blepharoplasty for eyelid and midface rejuvenation. Plast Reconstr Surg. 2013;132:1093–101.
21. Tao JP, Limongi RM. Short-incision midface-lift in lower blepharoplasty. JAMA Facial Plast Surg. 2016;18:313–4.
22. Hirabayashi KE, Tao JP. Midface-lift with lateral orbicularis oculi flap excision or imbrication. Dermatol Surg Off Publ Am Soc Dermatol Surg Al. 2014;40:743–7.
23. Massry GG, Hartstein ME. The lift and fill lower blepharoplasty. Ophthal Plast Reconstr Surg. 2012;28:213–8.
24. Perry CB, Allen RC. The subperiosteal, drill hole, midface lift. Orbit. 2016;35:250–3.
25. Gunter JP, Hackney FL. A Simplified transblepharoplasty subperiosteal cheek lift. Plast Reconstr Surg. 1999;103:2029–35.
26. Ben Simon GJ, Lee S, Schwarcz RM, McCann JD, Goldberg RA. Subperiosteal midface lift with or without a hard palate mucosal graft for correction of lower eyelid retraction. Ophthalmology. 2006;113:1869–73.
27. Marshak H, Morrow DM, Dresner SC. Small incision preperiosteal midface lift for correction of lower eyelid retraction. Ophthal Plast Reconstr Surg. 2010;26:176–81.
28. Engle RD, Pollei TR, Williams EF. Endoscopic midfacial rejuvenation. Facial Plast Surg Clin N Am. 2015;23:201–8.
29. Shtraks JP, Fundakowski C, Yu D, Hartstein ME, Sarcu D, Lu X, Wulc AE. Investigation of the longevity of the endoscopic midface lift. JAMA Facial Plast Surg. 2019;21:535–541.
30. Chan NJ, Nazemzadeh M, Hartstein ME, Holds JB, Massry GG, Wulc AE. Orbicularis retaining ligament release in lower blepharoplasty: assessing efficacy and complications. Ophthal Plast Reconstr Surg. 2018;34:155–61.
31. Moelleken BRW. Midfacial rejuvenation. Facial Plast Surg FPS. 2003;19:209–222.
32. Martin JC, Dokic Y, Munavalli G, Malone CH. Bipolar fractionated radiofrequency midface

lift: a retrospective review. J Cosmet Dermatol. 2022;21:268–70.
33. Myung Y, Jung C. Mini-midface lift using polydioxanone cog threads. Plast Reconstr Surg Glob Open. 2020;8: e2920.
34. Stein R, Holds JB, Wulc AE, Swift A, Hartstein ME. Phi, fat, and the mathematics of a beautiful midface. Ophthal Plast Reconstr Surg. 2018;34:491–6.
35. Trevidic P, Kaufman-Janette J, Weinkle S, Wu R, Dhillon B, Antunes S, Macé E, Maffert P. Injection guidelines for treating midface volume deficiency with hyaluronic acid fillers: the ATP approach (anatomy, techniques, products). Aesthet Surg J sjac007. 2022.

Autologous Fat Grafting to the Malar Region

Jenny N. Wang, Maria Belen Camacho and D. J. John Park

Abstract

Autologous fat grafting is a powerful method to treat malar depressions in facial rejuvenation surgery. It is an excellent adjunct to lower blepharoplasty. Autologous grafting of the adipose fraction of lipoaspirate from the abdomen of lower body treat the contour depressions below the tear trough. Autologous fat grafting has both advantages and disadvantages compared to hyaluronic fillers. This chapter describes technique for fat extraction, purification, and injection to the malar region.

Keywords

Fat graft · Adipose tissue · Autologous transfer · Volumetric augmentation · Midface hollowing · Rejuvenation

J. N. Wang · M. B. Camacho
Gavin Herbert Eye Institute, University of California, Irvine, CA, USA

D. J. J. Park (✉)
Plastic Surgery, Newport Beach, CA, USA
e-mail: Johnparkmd@gmail.com

1 Introduction

Fat grafting is the autologous transfer of the adipose fraction of lipoaspirate from one area of the body to a different area to augment the area to which the fat is transferred. The general process by which fat grafting is completed is to first extract the fat (using liposuction), purify the fat, and injecting the purified fat into the area of interest.

The first instance of fat grafting was documented in 1893 when plastic surgeon Gustav Neuber extracted fat from the arm and reinjected it into the orbital region to enhance the appearance of scars [1]. Since then, fat grafting was used but the technique was not widely adopted until the 1990s when Sydney Coleman popularized his surgical technique of 'lipostructure' [2]. Coleman harvests fat with a 3 mm blunt cannula and 10 mL syringe with low negative pressure, centrifuges the fat to separate the adipocytes from oil and water, and injects the fat using an 18-gauge cannula into several adjacent sites in the tissue via needle puncture port sites.

Autologous fat grafting to the malar area is useful in revitalizing the midface by softening the harsh shadows that can be cast by the contour depressions in the malar area which cannot be adequately addressed with lower blepharoplasty alone.

J. P. Tao (ed.), *Plastic Surgery of the Lower Eyelids*,
https://doi.org/10.1007/978-3-031-36175-3_27

2 Anatomy

Knowledge of the anatomy of the lower eyelids and the malar area is a critical first step in consideration for malar autologous fat grafting. Topographically, there are two convergent lines, or more accurately convergent shadows, that worsen with age; one at the lower eyelid/cheek junction (nasojugal groove medially and palpebromalar groove laterally) and the other between the medial and lateral malar fat pads (mid cheek furrow) [3]. Where the lines converge at the infero central arcus marginalis, there is a triangular zone of volume loss that the authors refer to as the intra malar triangle. The mid cheek furrow and the intra malar triangle is the primary target for fat grafting. (Fig. 1) At the lower eyelid/cheek junction, which corresponds to the arcus marginalis, pseudo herniation of the lower eyelid fat pads creates a prominence, the lower portion of which casts a shadow. In addition, loss of volume at the subjacent uppermost portion of the malar fat pads creates a contour depression, which will exaggerate the shadow from the pseudo herniation. However, in some instances the reverse can occur in those who have an abundance of facial fat, where the lateral malar fat pad is more prominent than that of the eyelid. This feature is commonly seen laterally, where there is often less eyelid fat pseudo herniation and limited volume loss.

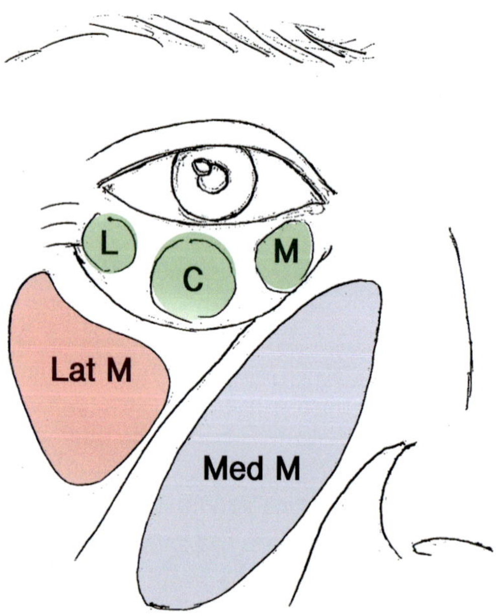

Fig. 1 Three discrete orbital fat pads: medial (M), central (C), and lateral (L) lower eyelid fat pads that become more evident with age. The mid cheek furrow can be a subtle depression or a more obvious groove between the lateral malar fat pad and the medial malar fat pad. Where there mid cheek furrow converges with the nasojugal groove at the eyelid cheek junction, there is a triangular area of soft tissue deflation that should be augmented with fat grafting

The relevant anatomy for the lower eyelid fat pads includes orbital fat pads that are separated into three compartments—the medial, central, and lateral fat compartments. The inferior oblique muscle separates the medial and central fat compartments, and the central and lateral fat compartments are separated by the Lockwood ligament's arcuate expansion [4, 5] (Fig. 1). The orbital septum separates the orbital space from the pre-septal facial anatomic planes. It is bound circumferentially at the arcus marginalis in line with the orbital rim periosteum and the orbicularis retaining ligament inferiorly [6]. As with other cutaneous ligaments of the face, such as the McGregor patch at the malar eminence, pre-auricular Furnas ligament, and the mental ligament, the orbicularis retaining ligament attaches the skin to the underlying periosteum and restrains movement of the skin. Medially, the orbicularis retaining ligament coincides with the muscular origin of the lower orbicularis muscle.

3 Fat Graft vs. Filler

Both fat grafts and hyaluronic acid fillers can be used in the midface. Compared to fillers, one of the advantages of fat grafting is its durability. However, as autologous fat grafting involves the transfer of fat globules into a recipient area with graft survival in mind, its efficacy depends on adequate circulation around the grafts. Even under ideal circumstances, approximately half of the fat volume will be lost. Because the fat transfer is autologous, there is maximal biocompatibility and minimal immunogenicity possible in injecting fat compared to filler [7]. In addition, fat grafting is not likely to induce the Tyndall effect, the blueish hue sometimes left after filler injection. Lastly, fat grafting may prove more economical for the patient, as fillers usually need to be repeated.

Fat grafting presents several challenges. As noted above, not all of the graft volume remains owing to atrophy. As such, the final volume retention is uncertain. Also, unlike hyaluronic fillers which comes out of the needle or cannula tips predictably and consistently as a single cohesive stream, fat grafts remain globular, and are more difficult as a thin consistent stream. Unlike hyaluronic acid fillers which by nature is temporary and can be dissolved with hyaluronidase, reversing fat grafting is difficult. Because of the less predictable and more permanent nature of fat grafting, it is important to prevent problems with good technique and to be abundantly conservative in the amount, as it is always easier to graft more fat than to take away overly done fat grafts.

4 Purification of Fat Grafts

Fat grafts must be purified, as there is aqueous solution, cellular fragments, and fibrous tissue that require removal. Harvested adipocytes are fragile, which makes the purification and processing technique a crucial step in the fat grafting procedure. There are several ways to process harvested fat. Here we will review the most common current methods of fat processing, and the next section will detail the technique.

Fat grafting processing methods include centrifugation, cotton gauze rolling, gravity separation (also known as sedimentation or decantation), filtration and washing [8, 9]. Centrifugation was introduced by Sydney Coleman to spin down the fat graft at high speeds form 3–5 minutes to separate out the denser blood and aqueous solution from the adipocytes. Cotton gauze rolling involves placing the fat onto cotton non-adherent gauze (Telfa®), surgical towels, or gauze pads and rolling the fat back and forth to remove the aqueous and free oil fractions of the lipoaspirate. With gravity separation, the lipoaspirate is allowed to settle into layers by density with the aqueous solution at the bottom, fat cells in the middle, and free oil from lysed cells on top. Commercial products for gravity separation include AquaVage (MD Resource, Livermore, CA) and Red Head (Miami Fat Supply, Groveland, FL) which allow separation to occur in a closed sterile device. This technique is used for large volume fat grafting and not appropriate for facial fat grafting. Washing involves rinsing the harvest with saline or sodium lactate multiple times. Filtration involves using membranes or metal sieves to separate out the adipocytes from the other materials. Washing is usually done in conjunction with filtration. Commercial products that complete both washing and filtration include Revolve (LifeCell, Branchburg, NJ) and Puregraft (Cytori Therpeutics, Plano, TX) which process fat in a closed system. Tissu-Trans Filtron (Tulip Medical Products, San Diego, CA) and LipiVage (Genesis Biosystems, Lewisville, TX) are commercial products that perform filtration only. One technique of fat purification has not been conclusively shown to be more effective than others [8].

5 Surgical Technique and Clinical Pearls

Autologous facial fat grafting requires: (1) harvesting of the lipoaspirate, (2) processing and purification of the lipoaspirate, followed by (3) microaliquot fat grafting.

Harvesting of the lipoaspirate first requires infiltration of a diluted local anesthetic and vasoconstrictive solution followed by liposuction via syringe. Commonly, Klein solution (0.1% lidocaine with 1:1,000,000 epinephrine) made up in a liter IV bag is used for larger volume liposuction. The author advocates the simple dilution of 1% lidocaine with 1:100,000 epinephrine by mixing 1-part local anesthetic and 4 parts injectable saline bringing the final concentration to 0.2% lidocaine with 1:500,000 epinephrine. With the lower volumes of infiltration (typically ~60–80cc per site), there is essentially no risk of toxicity. Optionally, tranexamic acid can be added to 1 mg/cc concentration to reduce bruising at the donor site.

The ideal donor site should have ample fat redundancy from which to harvest, elastic skin with moderate thickness to camouflage any secondary contour irregularities, and be readily accessible with the patient in supine position. Common donor sites for fat harvesting are the anterior abdomen (either supraumbilical or more likely infraumbilical), flanks, or lateral thighs. The senior author's preference is for anterior abdominal fat, as the 5 mm puncture incision can be hidden in the umbilicus and the fat is easily accessible in a supine patient.

Undiluted 1% lidocaine with 1:100,000 epinephrine is injected under the planned port site. This step can be skipped if the patient is under general anesthesia. A #11 blade is used to make the puncture incision. A multiport infusion cannula (Fig. 2 A, B) is used on a 20cc syringe to infiltrate approximately 40–60cc of the above diluted anesthetic solution. If done under local anesthesia, about twice as much infiltration will be needed with the area of infiltration going beyond the planned limit of the liposuction area.

After a period of 10 minutes, a Coleman harvesting cannula (Fig. 2C) on a 20cc syringe is used to perform the liposuction. For efficient liposuction, even firm compression with the non-dominant hand is critical. The fat should preferentially be harvested from the deeper aspect of the fatty deposit so as not to create secondary contour irregularity at the skin level. The cannula should be fairly tangential to the deep facial plane to prevent inadvertent violation of the abdominal wall. While applying firm pressure overlying the liposuction site, the cannula is rapidly passed in a fan-shaped manner in the deeper fat tissue planes. In instances where the vacuums seal is broken, the air should be expressed, and liposuction resumed under syringe suction. Excess suction pressure applied to the syringe can cause more cell lysis [10].

When available, centrifugation of the lipoaspirate is performed. (Fig. 3A) The harvested fat is transferred to a 10-cc syringe and the Luer-lock capped. The plunger is removed prior to placing the syringe in the sterilizable

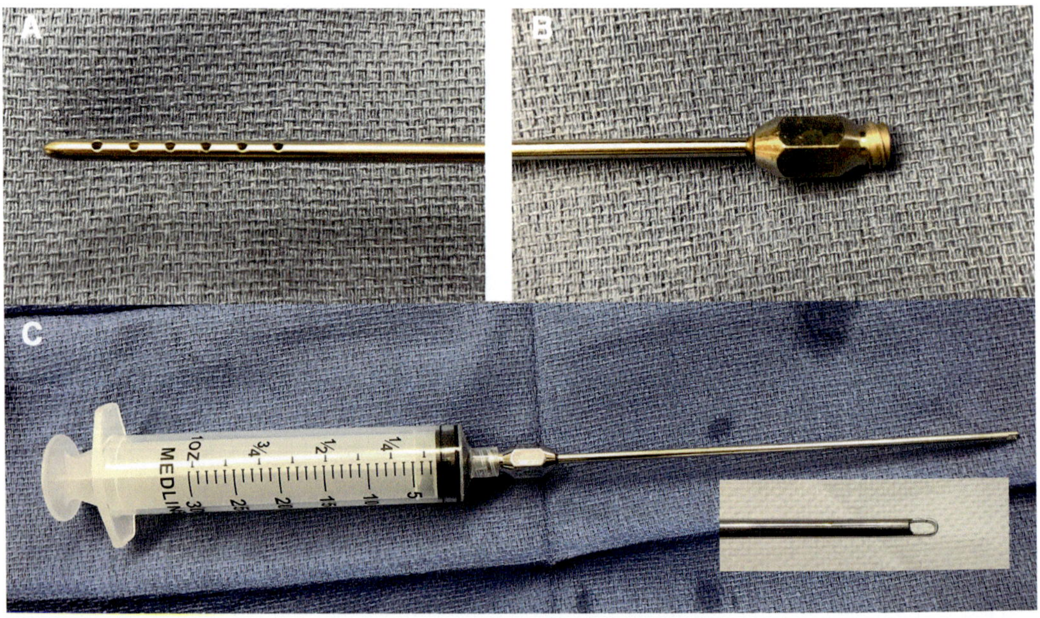

Fig. 2 (A) multiport infiltration cannula tip. (B) Lure lock for both infiltration and harvesting cannula to interface with syringe. (C) Coleman harvesting cannula with bucket handle style tip

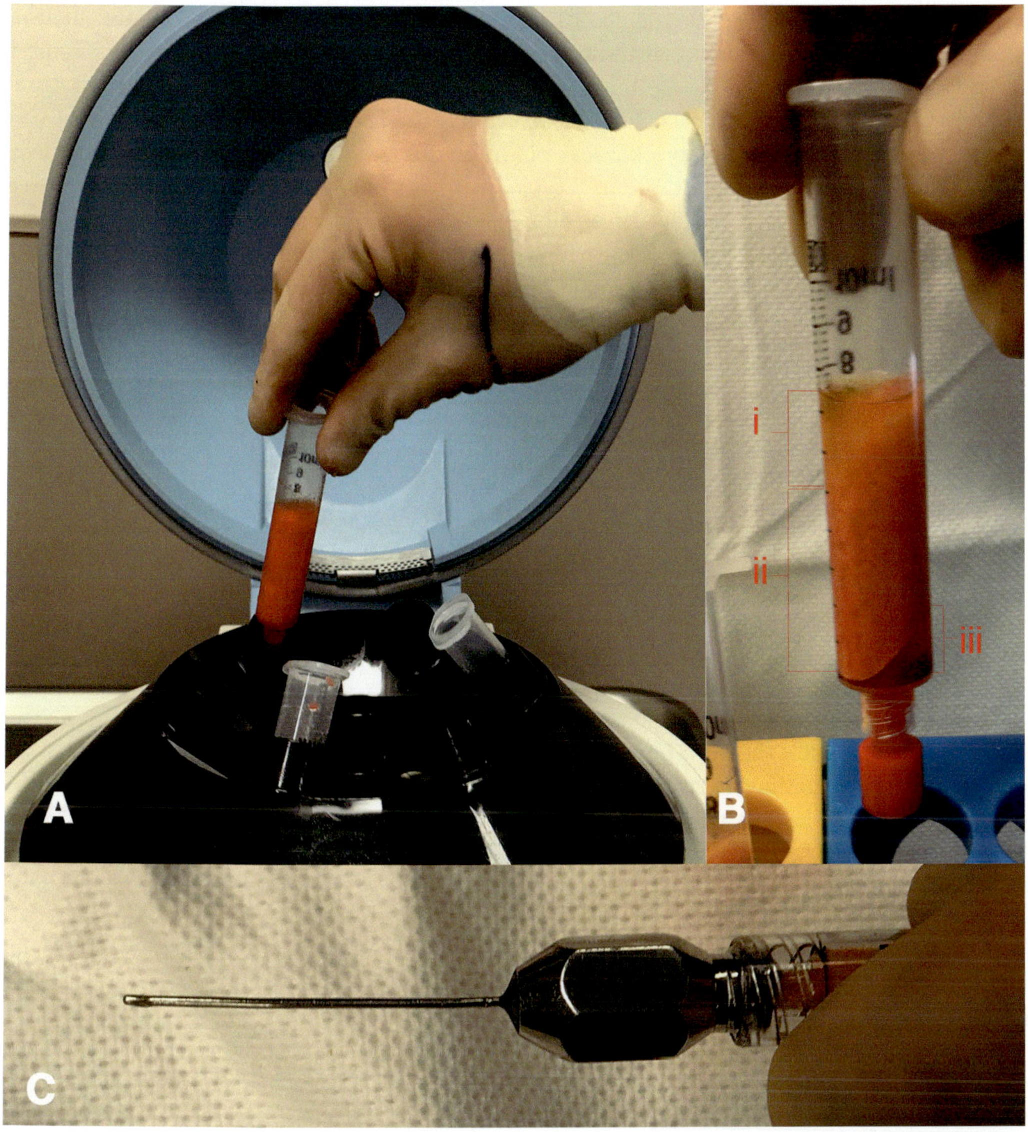

Fig. 3 (A) Lipoaspirate in a 10cc syringe without the plunger placed into a centrifuge to separate the viable from the nonviable components. (B) The component fractions separate and layer by density. [i] Uppermost layer with free oil from ruptured cells. Less healthy fat cells or more traumatic harvesting/processing will have more free oil. [ii] The middle fraction is the cellular layer. The bottom most portion of this cellular layer is rich in adipose derived stem cells and shows as a thin white line. [iii] The bottom aqueous layer is the densest and is primarily composed of the infiltration fluid and some blood as well. (C) Injection cannula and syringe with blunt tip and side port

rotor inserts of the centrifuge. The lipoaspirate is then centrifuged at 3000 rpm (1200 g) for 3 minutes. Following centrifugation, three distinct fractions are formed: an aqueous layer that includes tumescent fluid at the bottom, fat in the middle layer, and a scant amount of oil on top (Fig. 3B). With excessive shear forces either with increased vacuum pressure, a narrow cannula, or with older patients, the free oil fraction may be more substantial. After aspirating the oil and decanting the aqueous fraction, the fat cell fraction is transferred to 1-cc syringes.

Care should be taken when reinserting the 10-cc syringe plunger to allow the fat cell fraction to fall onto plunger prior to setting the seal of the plunger. Otherwise, the air pocket will not be able to be evacuated without projectile loss of some of the valuable fat fraction.

When centrifuge is not available, the lipoaspirate may be filtered and washed with a small, sterilized kitchen sieve and sterile injectable saline. The lipoaspirate is expressed into the sieve and then washed with injectable saline with gentle agitation with the back end of a forceps until the blood fraction washes out. The remaining fat is then scooped into the back end of a 10-cc syringe with the plunger removed, then transferred to 1-cc syringes for grafting.

For the fat grafting, an 18-gauge needle is used to make a puncture incision approximately 1.5 cm lateral to the nasal ala between the nasolabial fold and the intramalar groove. In this manner, the cannula can conveniently reach the desired graft sites including the nasolabial folds, which should always be done with the malar fat grafting so as not to aggravate the nasolabial shadow with added volume in the medial malar fat pad. Also, the puncture incision should be at least 1 cm from the nearest planned graft site because of the difficulty of grafting fat immediately under the port site. The grafts should be applied with microaliquots with each pass to maximize vascularity of the grafts, thereby increasing survival of the grafts and reducing the chances of fat necrosis. The senior author uses an 18G, (Fig. 3C) single side port, injection cannula to apply the grafts. The grafts should be processed and grafted as soon as possible to limit ischemia time of the graft material. Because adequate vascularity is critical to retention and take of the grafts, care should be taken with planned serial grafting in instances of excessive scarring with compromised circulation or radiation. With compressed and scarred planes, there is a limited amount of fat that can be grafted without increasing the tissue pressure to the extent that graft perfusion is compromised. However, with successive and more conservative grafting, the scars will soften and the tissue planes will be thicker allowing for more volume to be grafted with subsequent sessions.

As a final note, because of the relative ease of performing additional fat grafting under local anesthesia, and the difficulty of removing overdone or poorly done fat grafting, as well as the unpredictable nature of the proportion of fat that will take hold, care should be taken to hedge on the side of underdoing the fat grafting until more experience can be gained. Also, extreme care should be taken when grafting directly into the tear trough at the eyelid/cheek junction where contour irregularities are more likely to show with the very thin eyelid skin overlying the grafts.

Post-operative oral antibiotics and a methylprednisolone taper dose pack is prescribed. The patient should also sleep with his/her head elevated and ice-cold compresses applied to reduce edema. (Figs. 4 and 5).

6 Complications

Problems related to malar fat grafting primarily fall into the category of undercorrection, overcorrection, or asymmetry. With a conservative approach as noted above, overcorrection should be very uncommon, with undercorrection being relatively more likely. Instances of minor overcorrection can be addressed with triamcinolone steroid injection to induce fat atrophy. More significant overcorrection requires surgical excision. Minor complications such as bruising and excessive edema are usually self-limiting. Prolonged edema can be seen in instances of fat necrosis which is very uncommon given the inherent vascularity of the recipient site and may require excision if not responsive to steroid injections. Infections are exceedingly rare with sterile technique. Major complications such as vascular embolization and sequelae of vision loss of neurologic compromise is even more rare with side port blunt cannula use and care to not graft under resistance or increased turgor or tissue pressure.

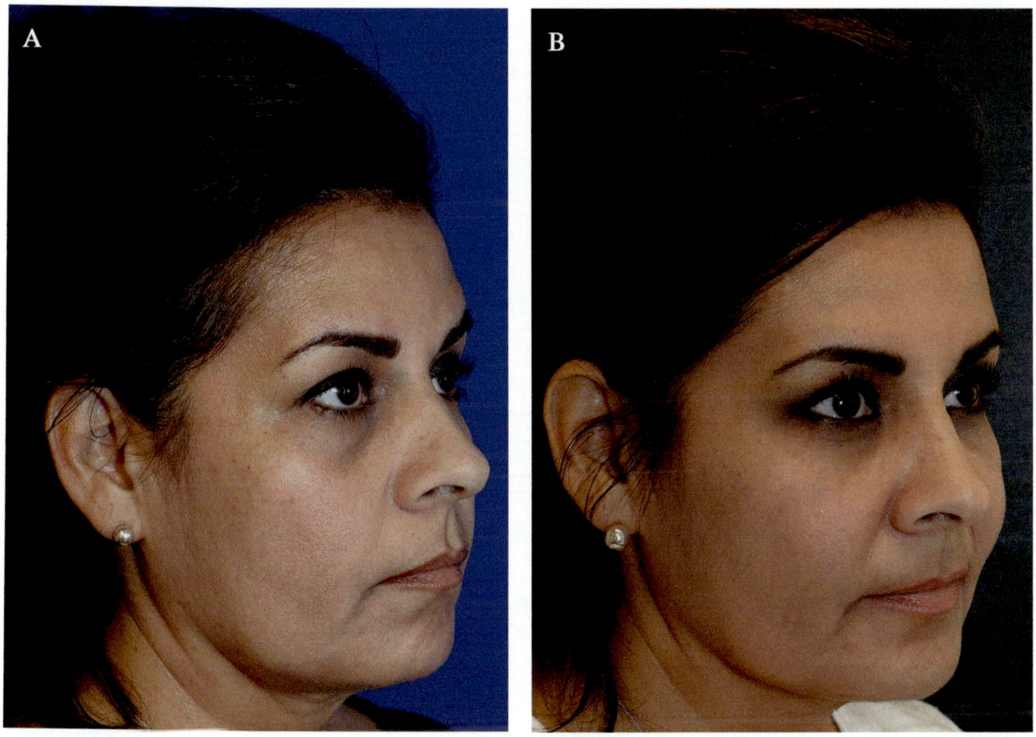

Fig. 4 A. Patient with malar deflation before intervention. B. Patient in Fig. 4A after autologous malar fat grafting

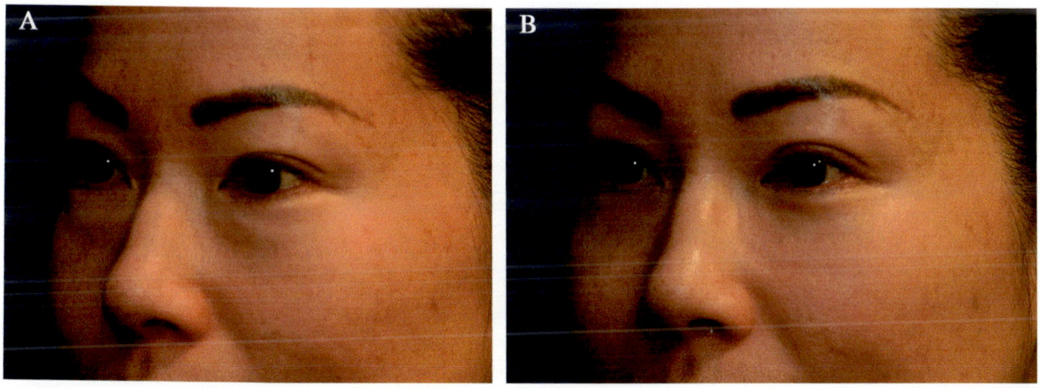

Fig. 5 A. Patient with prominent lower eyelid fat pads and malar deflation before intervention. B. Patient in Fig. 5A after transconjunctival lower blepharoplasty and autologous malar fat grafting. The shadow just below the eyelid cheek junction is effaced with volume augmentation at the medial malar area

7 Conclusion

Autologous malar fat grafting can achieve excellent improvements to the lower eyelid cheek region (Figs. 4 and 5). While there exist a small risk for complications, sound technique and a conservative approach achieves safe and effective adjuncts to lower blepharoplasty and a durable method to rejuvenate the lower eyelid and midface region.

References

1. Mazzola RF, Mazzola IC. The fascinating history of fat grafting. J Craniofac Surg. 2013;24(4):1069–71. https://doi.org/10.1097/SCS.0b013e318292c447.
2. Coleman SR, Katzel EB. Fat grafting for facial filling and regeneration. Clin Plast Surg. 2015;42(3):289–vii. https://doi.org/10.1016/j.cps.2015.04.001.
3. Mendelson BC, Jacobson SR. Surgical anatomy of the midcheek: facial layers, spaces, and the midcheek segments. Clin Plast Surg. 2008;35(3):395–393. https://doi.org/10.1016/j.cps.2008.02.003.
4. Kakizaki H, Malhotra R, Madge SN, Selva D. Lower eyelid anatomy: an update. Ann Plast Surg. 2009;63(3):344–51. https://doi.org/10.1097/SAP.0b013e31818c4b22.
5. Oh CS, Chung IH, Kim YS, Hwang K, Nam KI. Anatomic variations of the infraorbital fat compartment. J Plast Reconstr Aesthet Surg. 2006;59(4):376–9. https://doi.org/10.1016/j.bjps.2005.11.001.
6. Mojallal A, Cotofana S. Anatomy of lower eyelid and eyelid-cheek junction. Ann Chir Plast Esthet. 2017;62(5):365–74. https://doi.org/10.1016/j.anplas.2017.09.007.
7. Xie Y, Huang RL, Wang W, Cheng C, Li Q. Fat grafting for facial contouring (temporal region and midface). Clin Plast Surg. 2020;47(1):81–9. https://doi.org/10.1016/j.cps.2019.08.008.
8. Xue EY, Narvaez L, Chu CK, Hanson SE. Fat processing techniques. Semin Plast Surg. 2020;34(1):11–6. https://doi.org/10.1055/s-0039-3402052.
9. Lin Y, Yang Y, Mu D. Fat processing techniques: a narrative review. Aesthetic Plast Surg. 2021;45(2):730–9. https://doi.org/10.1007/s00266-020-02069-3.
10. Lipham WJ, Mellicher J. Cosmetic and clinical applications of Botox and dermal fillers, 3rd ed. SLACK;2015.

Midfacial Implants

Sathyadeepak Ramesh and Kenneth Morgenstern

Abstract

In midface hypoplasia or in a negative vector morphology, midfacial implants can be useful. They may be used in unique congenital or traumatic deformities but are also can be adjunct to cosmetic lower eyelid surgery. This chapter describes indications and technique for placement of implants to the cheeks or malar area.

Keywords

Midfacial implant · Cheek implant · Alloplastic implant · Autogenous implant · Fat grafting · Tear trough implant · Facial implant · Malar implant · Cheek implant

Supplementary Information The online version contains supplementary material available at https://doi.org/10.1007/978-3-031-36175-3_28.

S. Ramesh (✉) · K. Morgenstern
The Center for Eye and Facial Plastic Surgery, Somerset, NJ, USA
e-mail: info@deepakrameshmd.com

K. Morgenstern
The Morgenstern Center for Orbital & Facial Plastic Surgery, Wayne, PA, USA

1 Introduction

To surgically restore a youthful appearance, the underlying bony and structural anatomy may be appropriate surgical targets. Patients with midfacial hypoplasia can have a tear trough deformity, negative vector, inferior scleral show, or dark circles under the eye. Recognizing the hypoplastic maxilla and intervening appropriately [1] can improve the overall results of lower eyelid plastic surgery.

2 Patient Evaluation

Evaluation of the patient with midfacial hypoplasia must focus on three main areas—the bony maxilla/vector of the eye, deep facial fat, and lower eyelid tone. All interface with one another in overall lower eyelid appearance.

Patients with maxillary bone deficiency, shallow orbits with a prominent globe, or both can present with a negative vector morphology [2] wherein most of the globe lies anterior to the inferior orbital rim. This can be due to genetics, ethnicity [3], or trauma (accidental or surgical) (Fig. 1). The inferiorly and posteriorly displaced eyelid-cheek junction, gives the appearance of a long lower eyelid with a dark shadow at the eyelid-cheek junction itself. In severe cases, this can contribute to lagophthalmos (Fig. 2). To assess

J. P. Tao (ed.), *Plastic Surgery of the Lower Eyelids*,
https://doi.org/10.1007/978-3-031-36175-3_28

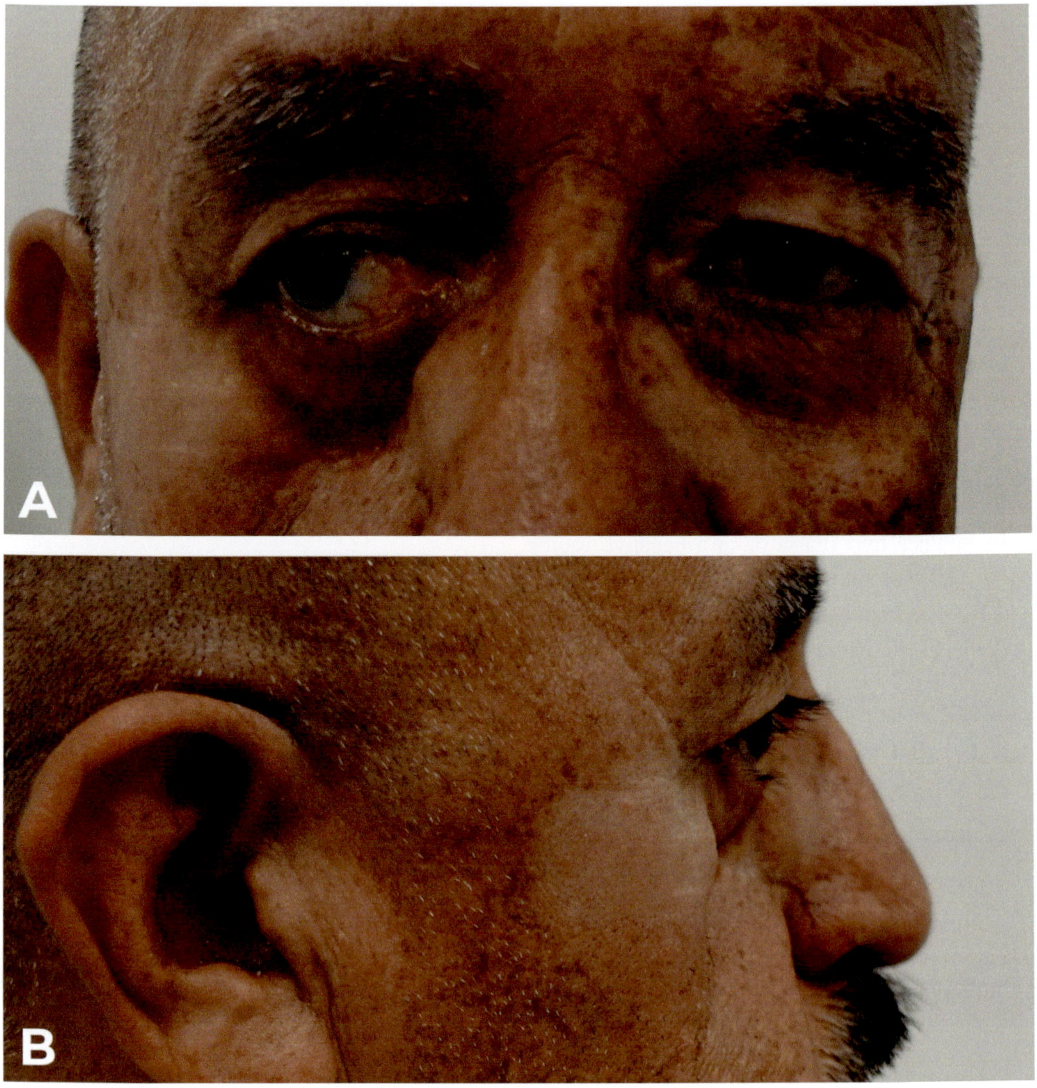

Fig. 1 Frontal (a) and profile (b) views of maxillary underprojection from facial trauma

maxillary hypoplasia versus axial globe position, the surgeon should examine the side profile and compare the anterior most point of the cornea to both the inferior and superior orbital rims. If the globe is in line with the superior orbital rim, then the eye is not relatively proptotic and addressing the maxilla alone can achieve a desirable result.

The volume and position of the deep facial fat must also be considered. Patients with an atrophic or descended malar fat pad will have volume deficiency at the eyelid-cheek junction, compounding underlying bony deficiencies [4]. This can be augmented with grafted fat to fill the deep medial fat compartment on top of any alloplastic implant placement. Finally, lower eyelid laxity at the lateral and medial canthal tendons due to aging can add ectropion to the negative vector. However, for patients with true negative vector morphology, simple eyelid tightening

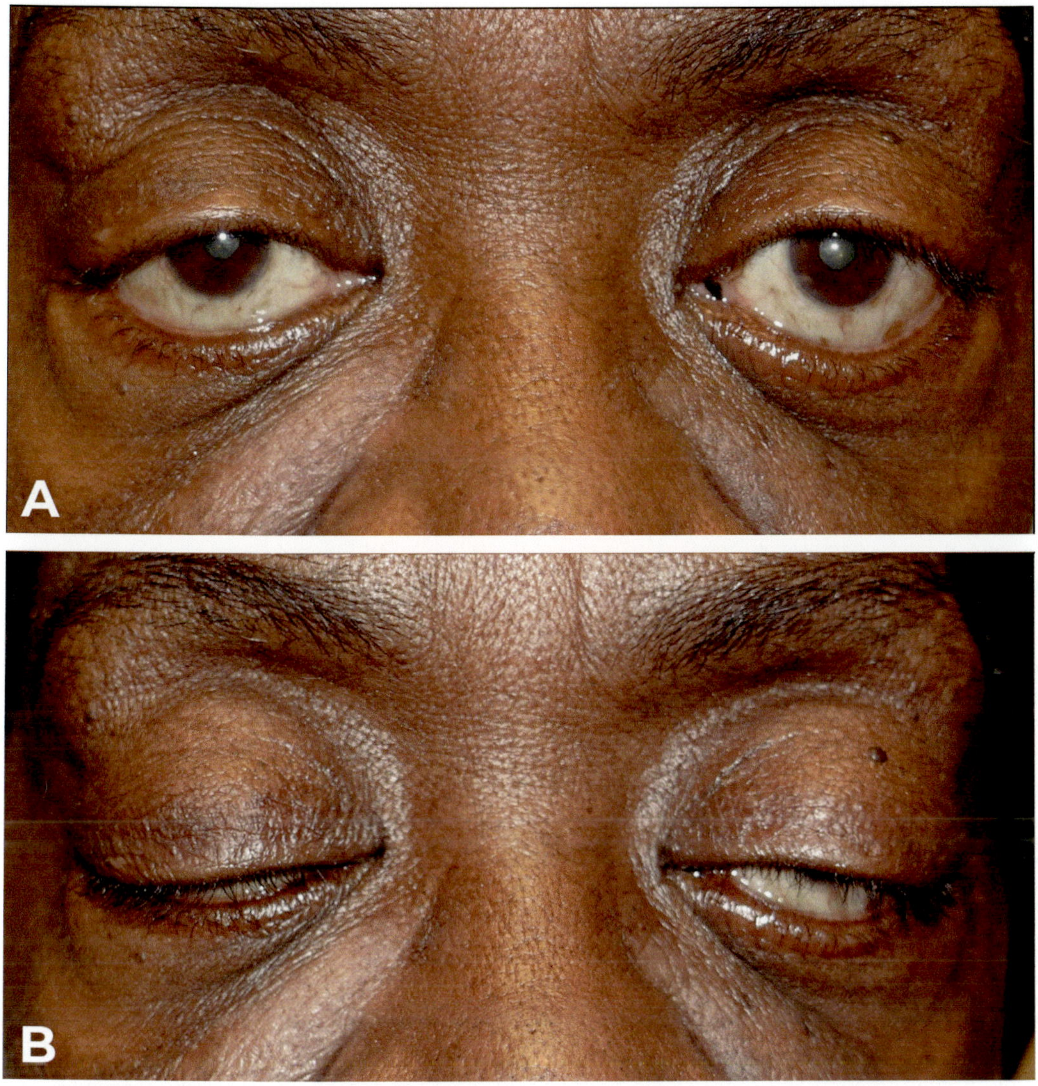

Fig. 2 Congenital maxillary hypoplasia causing significant lower eyelid retraction (a) and lagophthalmos (b)

may worsen appearance and eyelid positioning; a spacer graft placement to elevate the lower eyelid may be indicated [5]. This is particularly salient in patients with cicatricial changes from prior lower blepharoplasty. In these patients, elevation of the eyelid alone will again create a long lower eyelid that is unsupported at its base. Midfacial implant placement with alloplastic or autogenous tissue can provide a wide base of support, onto which the lower eyelid can rest and stay elevated.

3 Types of Implants

Midfacial implants include silicone (Implantech, Ventura, CA) (Fig. 3a), porous polyethylene (Su-Por, Newnan, GA), (Fig. 3b) and expanded polytetrafluoroethylene (ePTFE) (Surgiform, Lugoff, SC). These implants come in left- and a right-sided versions, with several sizes and shapes with varying coverage and anterior projection. Each type of implant has advantages and disadvantages.

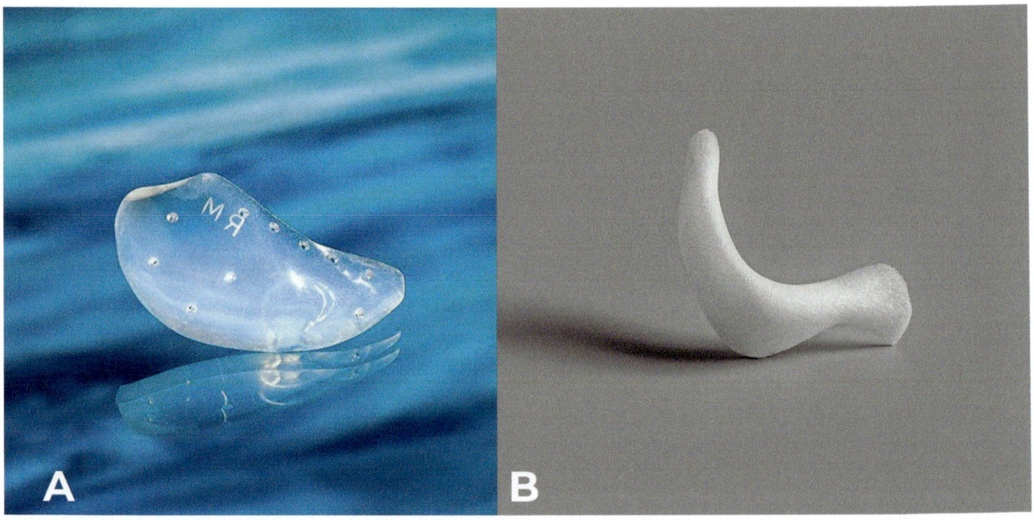

Fig. 3 Representative midfacial implants made from silicone (a) (Implantech, Ventura, CA), and porous polyethylene (Su-Por, Newnan, GA)

Silicone tends to be easy to insert as it is foldable and can placed through a small incision. Given its lack of porosity, it is also relatively straightforward to remove, if necessary. Silicone implants can be trimmed with scissors or a blade at their horizontal or vertical margins. Most silicone implants come with perforations through which a suture or screw can be passed; a common cutting needle can also pierce the silicone implant to fixate it to soft tissues or an osseous drill hole.

Porous polyethylene implants are rigid and must be implanted through a larger incision. The porosity of the implant is purported to allow tissue ingrowth and more stable fixation. Conversely, this makes the implant very difficult to remove once the ingrowth has occurred. Moreover, these devices may be more prone to infection or inflammation. These implants are typically fixated with titanium screws, and once attached to the bone, can be sculpted in all dimensions with a cutting burr or blade.

4 Surgical Technique

Preoperatively, the boundaries of the zygoma can be outlined with a skin marker. After the patient has been sufficiently anesthetized, tumescent anesthetic to the midface can help hydro dissect the soft tissue. A transconjunctival or transoral approach may be taken. In the transconjunctival approach, a Desmarres retractor is placed in the lower eyelid and a malleable retractor is placed to retract the inferior orbital tissues posteriorly (Fig. 4). A needle-tip monopolar cautery device is used to dissect through the conjunctiva and eyelid retractors until the inferior orbital rim is visible. A periosteal elevator is then used to gently dissect inferiorly on the preperiosteal plane, until the arcus marginalis is visualized. The cautery is then used to incise the periosteum inferior to the arcus marginalis and open the subperiosteal pocket. The elevator is then used to widely dissect the pocket that will receive the implant (Fig. 5), with care to not create too large of a compartment. In the transoral approach, the gingivobuccal sulcus is incised with cutting cautery until the same plane is visualized and the pocket dissected.

At this point, the implant sizers can be used to check the appropriate volume. Care is taken to make sure that the implant is right-side-up and the correct side is used (right versus left-Etchings on the implant undersurface aid in identifying correct orientation. The desired implant is then trimmed at its inferomedial

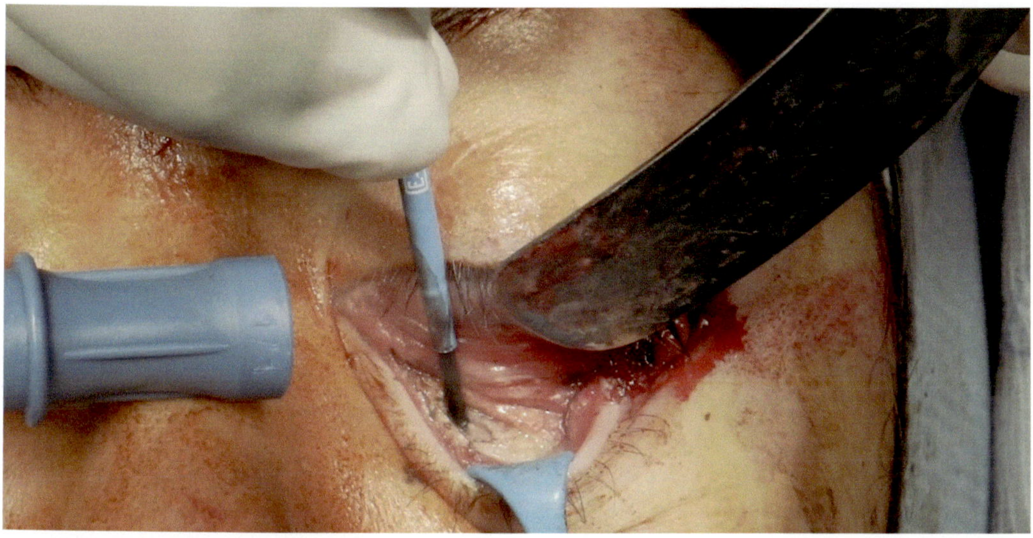

Fig. 4 Intraoperative view of transconjunctival approach to midface

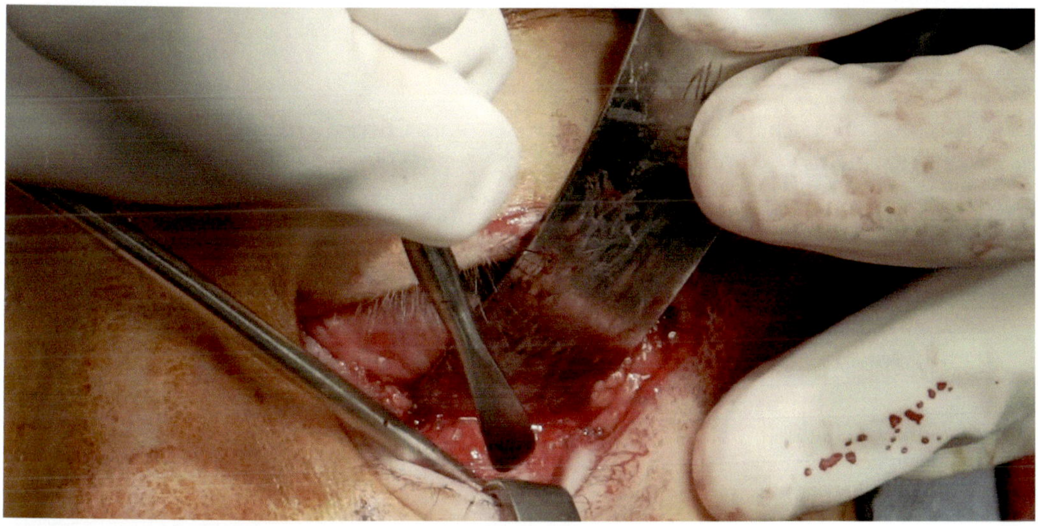

Fig. 5 Intraoperative view of periosteal elevator dissecting midface in the subperiosteal plane

border to forestall impingement of the infraorbital nerve. Many implants have a perforation or a cutout at this location that can be adjusted or enlarged as necessary.

The implant is then slipped into the subperiosteal pocket (Fig. 6). Care is taken to ensure appropriate position. Titanium screws (self-drilling, 3.5 × 5 mm) may be used to fixate the implant to the inferior orbital rim. The periosteum can then be closed with the desired sutures (the author prefers 5-0 poliglecaprone 25 (Monocryl, Ethicon, Inc., Raritan, NJ)). The conjunctiva or oral mucosa is then closed with plain gut suture, and a pressure dressing placed (Fig. 7).

Midfacial implants can be placed in isolation or in combination with adjunctive procedures such as lower blepharoplasty, orbital

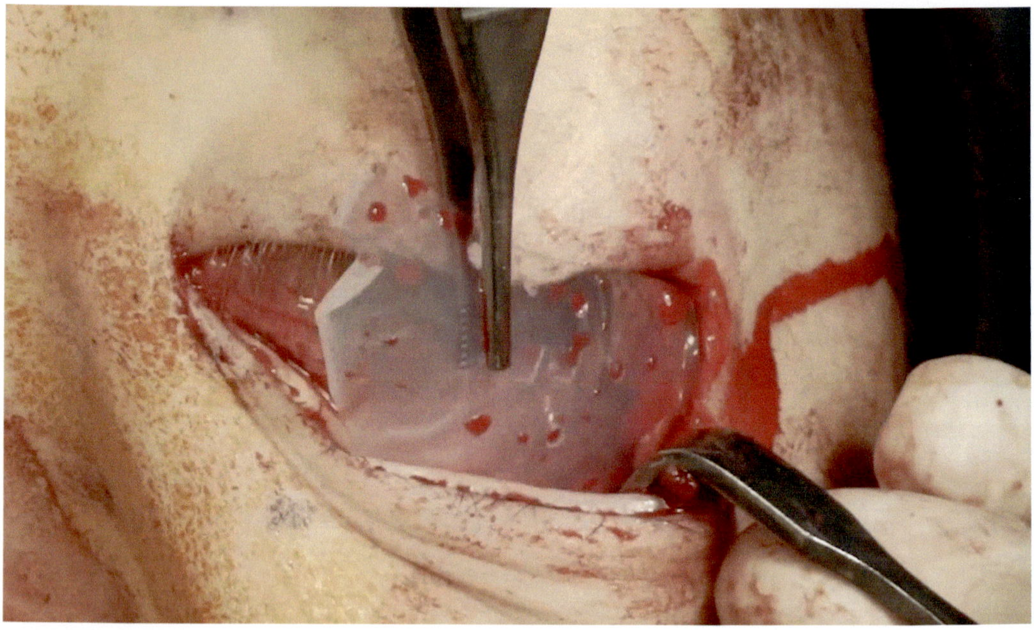

Fig. 6 Transconjunctival placement of silicone implant

decompression, or concomitant facial implant placement. Drains are typically not necessary if sufficient tumescent anesthetic is placed initially, and ice and pressure is used postoperatively.

5 Postoperative Care

Patients use cold compresses and gentle pressure for the first 4 days, and transition to warm compresses thereafter. If skin incisions are present, erythromycin ophthalmic ointment is preferred, whereas if the transconjunctival wound is the only incision, antibiotic eye drops are used. The patient is seen at 5–8 days after surgery to ensure appropriate implant placement and check for infection. Patients are advised edema and ecchymosis can last 6–12 weeks and the tissue will take time to feel flexible and compliant again.

6 Complications

Complications of midfacial implant placement can be divided into early and late complications. Early complications include implant malposition, infection, seroma, and pain or paresthesia from infraorbital nerve impingement. Late complications include implant migration, implant pocket infection, eyelid retraction, or bony resorption.

Infections are treated with systemic antibiotic treatment. If there is significant purulence, the implant pocket should be irrigated and implant removal should be considered. Silicone implants, given their nonporous nature, tend to be easier to clear of infection than porous implants. ePTFE implants can be impregnated with antibiotics to reduce infection risk. Seroma and hematoma should be drained appropriately. Late infections can cause compromise of the implant itself. Silicone implants can lose their

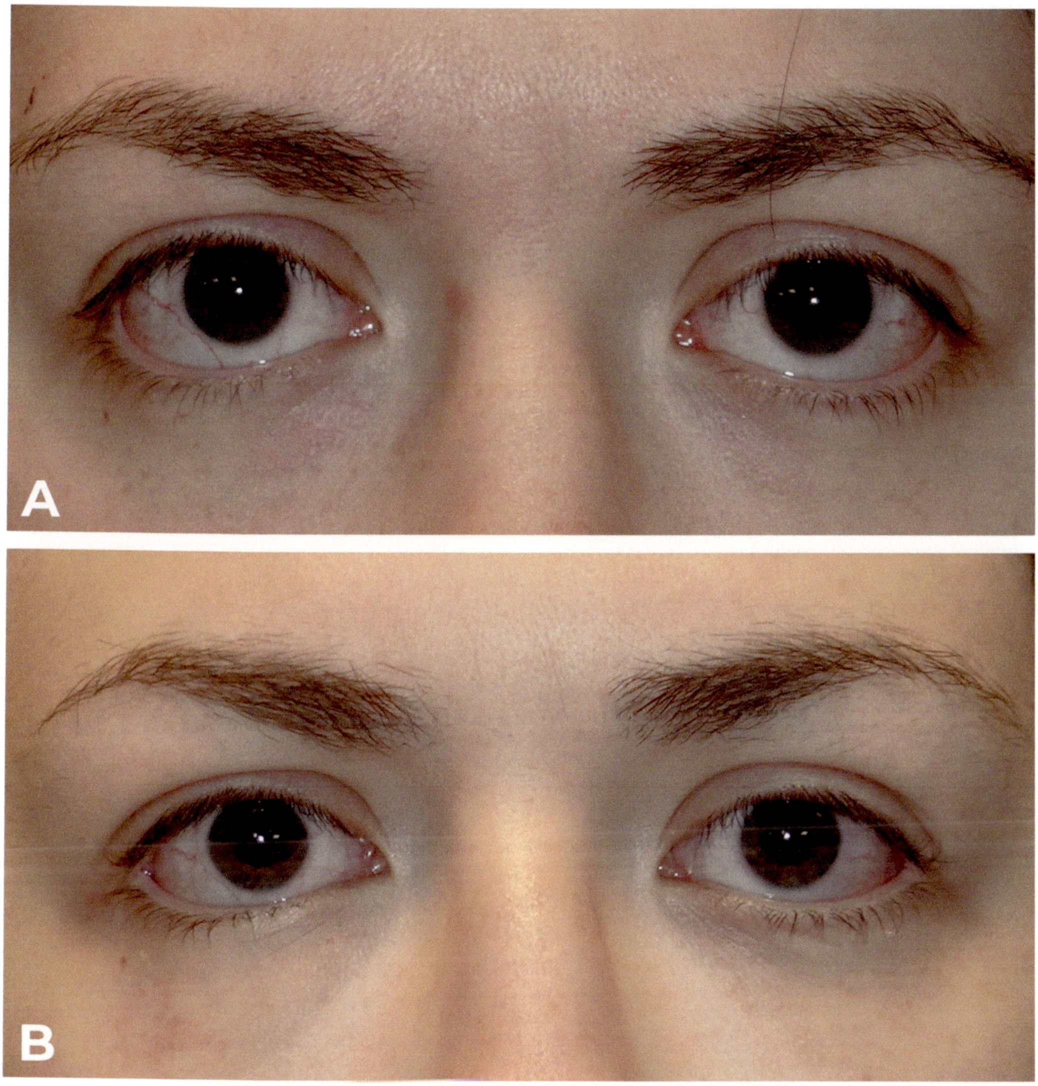

Fig. 7 Preoperative (a) and 6 month post-operative (b) view of patient after transconjunctival silicone cheek augmentation

rigidity and can even be suctioned out. Tissue ingrowth into porous implants makes late infection difficult to deal with, as implant removal requires extensive dissection. Antibiotic prophylaxis can be considered prior to treatments such as dental procedures.

Implant migration or malposition due to improper placement or facial movement requires surgical revision. Impingement on V2 also requires surgical intervention. Eyelid retraction can occur from aggressive tissue cautery, excessive skin resection, or inflammatory reaction to the implant. This may require injections or surgical revision. Bony resorption can also occur long-term at the site of implant placement, which may require further alloplastic or autologous augmentation.

7 Conclusion

Midfacial implants can provide durable and effective augmentation of bony deformities. Complications are rare, and patients can experience long-lasting improvement in the lower eyelid hollows, inferior scleral show, and negative vector morphology. Implant placement is a valuable adjunct to traditional lower blepharoplasty procedures and provides important aesthetic benefit in certain patients.

References

1. Flowers RS. Tear trough implants for correction of tear trough deformity. Clin Plast Surg. 1993;20:403–15.
2. Yaremchuk MJ. Improving periorbital appearance in the "morphologically prone." Plast Reconstr Surg. 2004;114:980–7. https://doi.org/10.1097/01.PRS.0000133202.32981.08.
3. Mcqueen CT, Diruggiero DC, Campbell JP, Shockley WW. Orbital osteology: a study of the surgical landmarks. Laryngoscope. 1995;105:783–8. https://doi.org/10.1288/00005537-199508000-00003.
4. Rohrich RJ, Pessa JE, Ristow B. The youthful cheek and the deep medial fat compartment. Plast Reconstr Surg. 2008;121:2107–12. https://doi.org/10.1097/PRS.0b013e31817123c6.
5. Patel MP, Shapiro MD, Spinelli HM. Combined hard palate spacer graft, midface suspension, and lateral canthoplasty for lower eyelid retraction: a tripartite approach. Plast Reconstr Surg. 2005;115:2105–7. https://doi.org/10.1097/01.PRS.0000164677.25488.49.
6. Pessa JE, Garza JR. The malar septum: the anatomic basis of malar mounds and malar edema. Aesthet Surg J;17:11–7. https://doi.org/10.1016/s1090-820x(97)70001-3.

Lower Eyelid Considerations in Lower Facelift

Donovan S. Reed and Tanuj Nakra

Abstract

Lower blepharoplasty and facelifting offer synergistic enhancements for patients seeking facial rejuvenation. However, risks can be heightened when both procedures are performed concurrently. Anatomy is the basis of safe procedure design and effective preoperative planning and surgery itself. There are various considerations when rejuvenating periorbital structures along with the lower face. This chapter details facelifting considerations in the context of the lower eyelids.

Keywords

Facelift · Rhytidectomy · Superiosteal facelift · Blepharoplasty · Blepharoplasty complications · Facial ligaments

Illustrations by Michael Han

D. S. Reed · T. Nakra (✉)
TOC Eye and Face, Austin, TX, USA
e-mail: tnakra@tocaustin.com

D. S. Reed · T. Nakra
Department of Ophthalmology, Dell Medical School, The University of Texas at Austin, Austin, TX, USA

1 Introduction

Rejuvenation of periorbital aging changes at the time of lower facelifting is often performed to rejuvenate the eyelid and facial continuum. Standard lower facelifting techniques yield a superolateral elevation of the midface, augmenting lower eyelid rejuvenation results and providing an improved overall cosmetic outcome. On the other hand, resection of lower facial tissues can contribute to greater risk for lower eyelid retraction, especially when performed concomitant to eyelid surgery.

Though the two procedures can be staged, concomitant periorbital rejuvenation maneuvers at the time of rhytidectomy can be effective and safe simultaneously, with an intimate understanding of the anatomical complexities and using good technique. This chapter describes anatomy, evaluation and surgical principals of lower eyelid rejuvenation at the time of lower facelifting to achieve good results while avoiding eyelid retraction, orbicularis muscle denervation, and ocular surface exposure keratopathy.

2 Anatomy

Cosmetic concerns of the lower eyelid commonly include steatoblepharon, the tear trough deformity, rhytids, infraorbital dark circles, and malar festoons. Myriad factors may ultimately

J. P. Tao (ed.), *Plastic Surgery of the Lower Eyelids*,
https://doi.org/10.1007/978-3-031-36175-3_29

contribute to the various cosmetic deformities associated with the lower eyelid and midface, including underlying bony and ligamentous structure, descent of the midfacial soft tissues, and skin changes due to sun damage and aging [1].

2.1 Bone Structure and Ligamentous Framework

The orbital and midfacial bones, with contributions from the facial osseo-cutaneous ligaments, provide the framework for soft tissue support and divide the facial fat compartments. With aging, there is orbital rim recession and malar bone volume loss, which ultimately leads to tethering of the relatively inextensible orbital and midfacial retaining ligaments (orbitomalar ligament, zygomatic cutaneous ligament, and masseteric ligament) [2, 3]. This phenomenon leads to facial hollowing and worsening of shadowing, particularly in the inferomedial orbit, known as the tear trough region [4]. Additionally, if the patient has an anteriorly positioned globe, this loss of infraorbital rim projection may lead to a negative vector configuration, increasing the risk for lower eyelid retraction following blepharoplasty [5]. Indeed, the underlying genetic configuration of maxillary projection has produces a negative or positive vector that has immense strategic implications for lower eyelid rejuvenation, as well as midfacial and lower facial rejuvenation. Specifically, a positive vector (convex maxillary projection/globe relatively recessed configuration) is supportive of enhanced cosmetic outcomes of lower blepharoplasty, midfacial rejuvenation and perioral rejuvenation from facelifting. In contrast, a negative vector (concave maxillary projection/globe relatively prominent configuration) requires more assertive maneuvers during lower blepharoplasty as well as lower facelifting to produce ideal cosmetic outcomes.

The lateral canthal tarsoligamentous band of the lower eyelid, also referred to as the inferior limb/crus of the lateral canthal tendon, with its attachments to the lateral orbital tubercle, is a crucial structure to the support framework of the lower eyelid. With aging, the ligament becomes lax, which can result in lower eyelid ectropion and retraction. Additionally, the lower eyelid blink mechanics, which are vital to replenish the ocular surface tear film, become altered with lower eyelid laxity, and these changes can lead to increased ocular surface exposure. Identification of lower eyelid laxity preoperatively is crucial, so lower eyelid tightening, and support maneuvers can be utilized intraoperatively to prevent unwanted postoperative complications [4].

2.2 Lower Eyelid and Midface Soft Tissue Anatomy

The eyelid skin is the thinnest of the body, and this transparency allows for prominence of the underlying soft tissues, including the orbicularis muscle [6, 7]. Hypertrophy of the pretarsal orbicularis muscle, more commonly identified in the Asian patient population, may result in an elevated appearance to the pretarsal eyelid with an inferior hollowing and a darkened appearance to the overlying skin. Orbicularis muscle plication/resection maneuvers can be utilized during lower blepharoplasty to address these changes.

There exist three clinically apparent fat compartments in the lower eyelid—the medial, central, and lateral fat compartments. The central fat compartment is divided from the medial by the inferior oblique muscle, and divided from the lateral by the lateral arcuate expansion of the inferior oblique muscle (Fig. 1). Midfacial fat is divided into deep and superficial compartments, separated by the facial retaining ligaments. Pseudoherniation of the suboorbicularis oculi fibroadipose tissue, combined with subcutaneous fat atrophy and volume loss as a result of aging, as well as a tight orbital retaining ligament and negative vector configuration may further accentuate periorbital hollows and infraorbital dark circles [1]. The suborbicularis oculi fat, which lies superficial to the deep facial fascia layer, may be lifted during midfacial rejuvenation maneuvers to provide volume support to the lower eyelid/ tear trough junction.

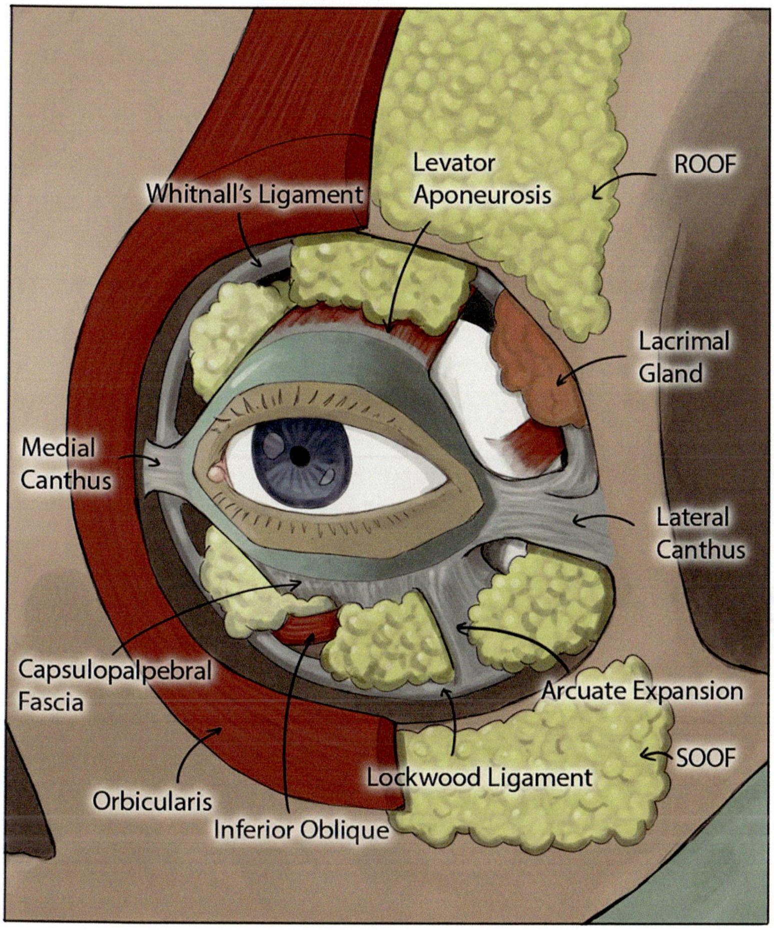

Fig. 1 Inferior orbital fat compartments

The lower eyelid soft tissues have a propensity to retain fluid from both local and systemic processes. Infraorbital eyelid fluid may accumulate as a result of interstitial edema or lead to true festoons. Festoons typically develop in the potential space between the orbitomalar and zygomatic cutaneous ligaments [8]. Festoons are important to recognize preoperatively, as fluid retention may increase following periorbital and midfacial rejuvenation maneuvers. Furthermore, untreated festoons during facial rejuvenation can lead to patient dissatisfaction. Festoon management, an important component of periorbital rejuvenation, can be surgical as well as non-surgical, but is beyond the scope of this chapter [9].

2.3 Facial Nerve Anatomy

The 7th cranial nerve, or the facial nerve, provides innervation to the muscles of facial expression, including the orbicularis oculi. A detailed understanding of its typical anatomic distribution is key during both lower rhytidectomy and midfacial and brow-lifting maneuvers, as damage to the zygomatic and/or temporal branches can lead to impaired blink and subsequent ophthalmic injury. The facial nerve exits the stylomastoid foramen and divides into an upper and lower trunk within the parotid gland, and ultimately into five motor nerve branches: temporal, zygomatic, buccal, marginal mandibular, and cervical branches (Fig. 2). The temporal

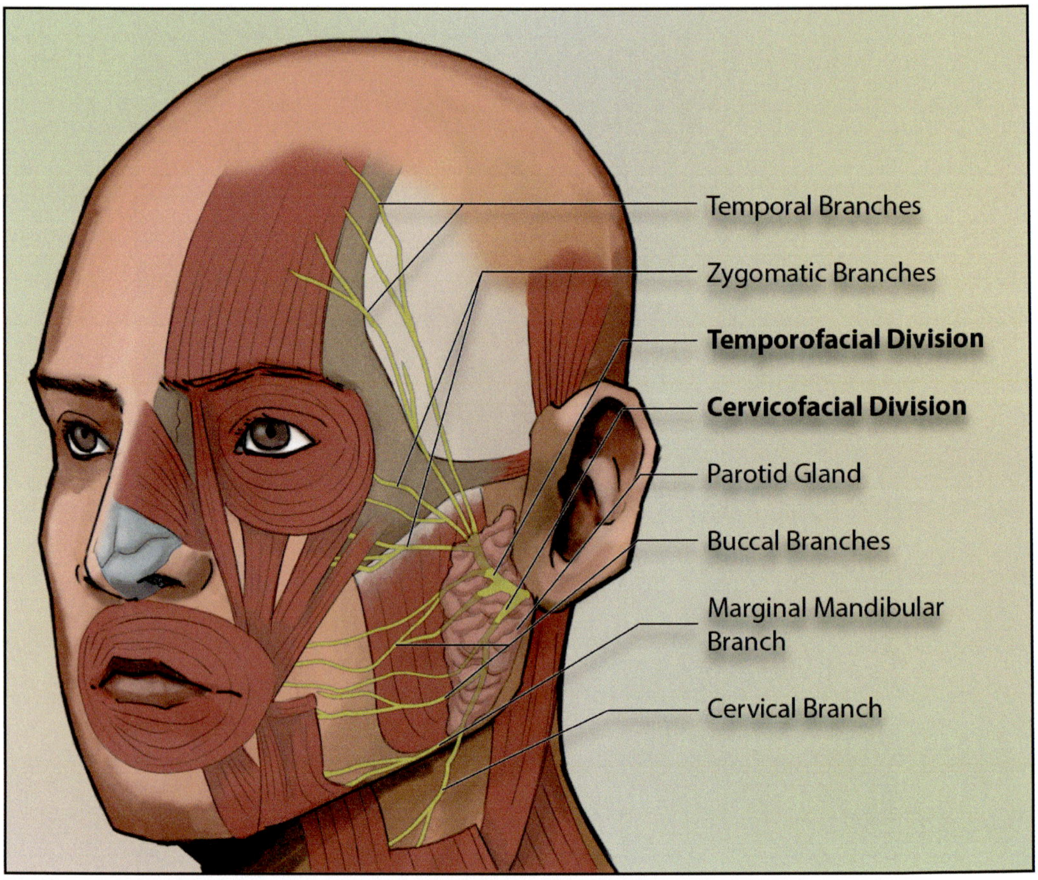

Fig. 2 Facial nerve and its branches

branch of the facial nerve courses over the middle one-third of the zygomatic arch periosteum after exiting the parotid, and then travels within the superficial fascia over the temporal fossa to eventually innervate the frontalis muscle, corrugator supercilii, and superior aspect of the orbicularis oculi muscle. The zygomatic branch exits the parotid gland superolaterally and travels along the zygomaticus muscles inferior border to innervate the inferior orbicularis oculi [10].

2.4 Lower Eyelid and Midface Skin

As the eyelid skin is the thinnest of the body with minimal to no subcutaneous tissue, aging changes are more accentuated in the periorbital region in comparison to the remaining facial skin. Reduced skin elasticity as a result of elastin/collagen loss leads to increased thinning. Thinning of the periorbital skin, in addition to actinic changes secondary to chronic ultraviolet radiation as dictated by underlying genetic alterations, hormonal fluctuations and Fitzpatrick skin type, can lead to visible dyschromia, which are best treated with topical, laser, or chemical therapy as opposed to surgical intervention [11]. Additionally, it is key to differentiate true lower eyelid dermatochalasis versus rhytids. True dermatochalasis can be treated surgically. Dynamic rhytids, distinguished by active orbicularis oculi muscle contraction, are managed better with neurotoxin injection; whereas static rhytids are most addressed with resurfacing or redraping maneuvers [4].

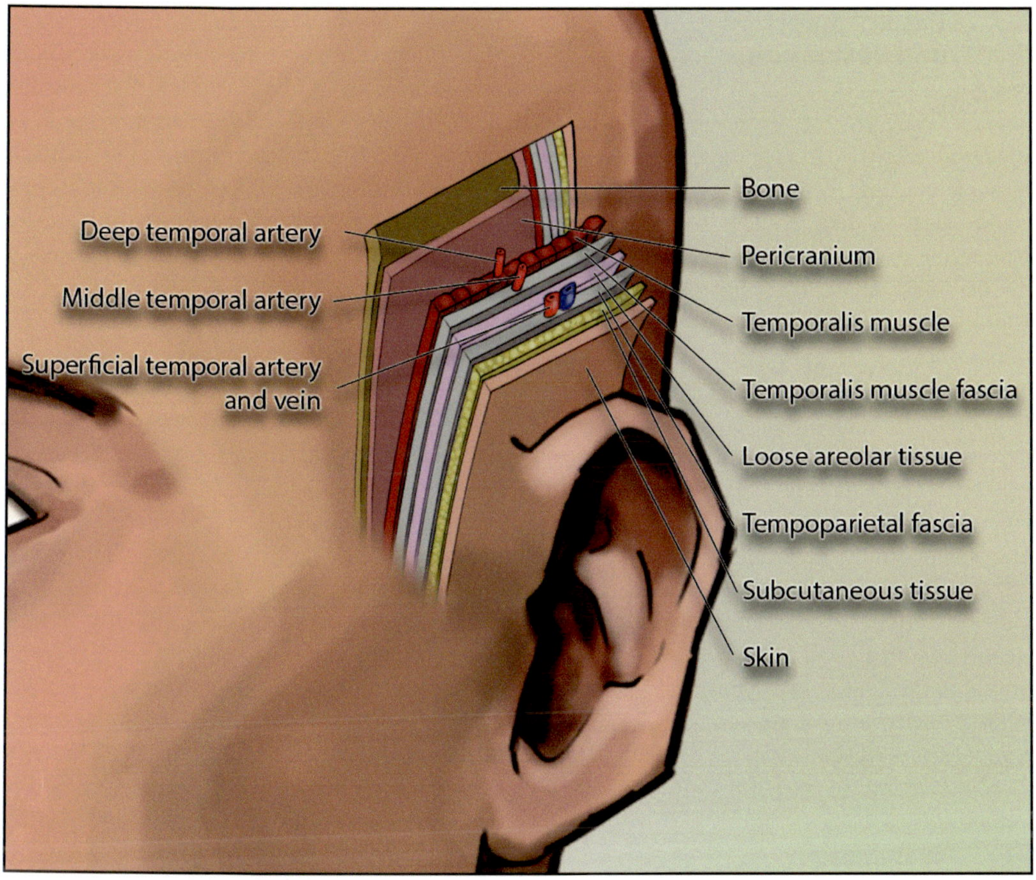

Fig. 3 Layers of the temporalis fossa

2.5 Temporal Fossa Anatomy

As multiple midfacial rejuvenation maneuvers utilize a temporally based approach, an understanding of the anatomy of the temporal fossa is crucial to a successful procedure and the prevention of complications. The temporal fossa is a bony cavitation of the frontal, temporal and zygomatic bones bounded by the superior temporal line, the frontal process of the zygomatic bone anteriorly, housing the temporalis muscle, superficial and deep temporalis fascia, and terminating at the level of the zygomatic arch inferiorly. From superficial to deep, it begins with skin, subcutaneous tissue, the superficial temporoparietal fascia within which lies the superficial temporal artery and temporal branch of CN VII, loose areolar tissue, the deep temporoparietal fascia, the temporalis muscle, and the pericranium [12] Fig. 3. Dissection along the deep temporoparietal fascia is a safe surgical plane, as this will prevent damage to the temporal branch of the facial nerve. The intermediate fat pad (Yasargil fat pad) is a critically important surgical landmark, as staying within or beneath this fat pad will prevent damage to the temporal facial nerve branch during temporal surgical approaches to midface release [13].

3 Patient Selection and Evaluation

Patients often present for cosmetic periorbital rejuvenation at the time of lower facial aging consultation with complaints regarding lower eyelid bags or dark circles. Careful discernment of the underlying etiology is key to selecting the most appropriate treatment approach. Additionally, identification of preoperative conditions such as floppy eyelid syndrome, lower eyelid laxity, and a negative vector eyelid configuration will assist in the prevention of possible complications of lower eyelid retraction and ocular surface exposure [14]. Furthermore, an understanding of the varying anatomic configurations between the periorbital regions of different ethnicities is important. Lastly, screening for body dysmorphic disorder and/or borderline personality disorder is of utmost importance, and referral to the appropriate specialist is necessary in these instances. As always, setting realistic expectations is fundamental.

3.1 Examination

The lower eyelid, midface, and lower face should be carefully assessed and the interplay between the regions appreciated. Lower eyelid orbital fat protrusion and pseudoherniation of each lower eyelid fat pad should be evaluated in primary gaze and in upgaze, in addition to the presence of lower eyelid dermatochalasis, eyelid skin elasticity, evidence of prior surgery, and the presence or absence of festoons or dyschromia. The presence of a tear trough deformity and periorbital hollowing, in addition to the relationship of the inferior orbital rim to the anterior projection of the globe should be noted. In cases of severe negative vectors, realistic expectations must be set, and deeper conversations may be appropriate about the potential benefits of midfacial augmentation with either soft tissue autografting or even alloplastic premaxillary implants. Preoperative eyelid malposition such as retraction, in addition to eyelid laxity assessed with snapback and distraction testing, should be assessed. Midfacial soft tissue volume and descent should be evaluated. A lengthening of the distance of the eyelid margin to the insertion of the orbitomalar ligament is an indicator for midfacial ptosis [4]. An ocular surface and tear film ophthalmic evaluation should be undertaken in the setting of subjective complaints of dry eye disease that may exacerbate during the postoperative healing phase of periorbital rejuvenation with concomitant lower facelifting.

4 Perioperative Considerations

Specific documentation and awareness of any underlying cardiac, pulmonary, hematologic, renal, and autoimmune disease is paramount to safe surgical rejuvenation, especially facelift that is usually performed under general anesthesia and for a longer duration than most isolated eyelid surgeries. Medical testing preoperatively is guided by the patient's age and medical comorbidities, and medical clearance should be obtained if necessary. It is advisable for anticoagulant medications to be held for 7–10 days preoperatively, and smoking cessation is required. Indeed, nicotine urine testing is recommended on the day of surgery for all at-risk rhytidectomy patients. Ocular surface lubrication should be optimized preoperatively. Detailed informed consent including expected outcomes and frank discussion of possible risks, with a discussion of nonsurgical alternatives including observation is mandatory.

In addition to systemic anesthesia, full-strength local anesthetic solution containing epinephrine in the periorbital region with tumescent local anesthetic administration in the temporal and midfacial regions aids in intraoperative hemostasis and visualization. Tranexamic acid (TXA) administered in the local anesthetic or intravenously, has been shown to improve hemostasis and decrease the risk of postoperative hematoma formation during rhytidectomy [15–17]. Corneal protective shields can be utilized intraoperatively for ocular surface protection during surgical periorbital maneuvers, and are required for periorbital laser resurfacing maneuvers. Intraoperative systemic antibiotic and corticosteroid administration is recommended, and deep venous thrombosis prophylaxis is essential. Strict intraoperative blood pressure management and hemostasis, in addition to post-extubation emesis prophylaxis, are key to avoiding hematoma formation. Novel approaches to perioperative pain management can reduce the need for narcotics, and enhance perceived outcomes.

In addition to standard postoperative care associated with lower facelifting, postoperative care with concomitant periorbital rejuvenation is directed at ocular surface protection. Frequent periorbital ice compresses and head elevation decreases postoperative edema, and should be maintained for 48–72 hours postoperatively. Patients should avoid heavy lifting, bending, or exertion for at least the first week postoperatively. Ophthalmic antibiotic ointment with or without corticosteroid, should be administered to the periorbital incision sites for the first week postoperatively. Frequent ocular surface lubrication with tear substitutes and ointments is recommended. Patients should be made aware of the high potential for blurred vision and ocular surface irritation for up to 10 days postoperatively [4].

5 Surgical Techniques

There exist a vast number of described surgical approaches to lower eyelid and midface rejuvenation at the time of lower facelifting (Figs. 4 and 5). Each approach has nuances and specific risks. The timing of particular maneuvers intraoperatively is also as they can affect subsequent maneuvers.

5.1 Lower Blepharoplasty Concomitant with Lower Facelifting

Lower blepharoplasty may be safely performed concurrently with lower facelifting maneuvers. Either transconjunctival and transcutaneous approaches may be utilized as described in other chapters. In general, the authors prefer a transconjunctival approach to manipulating the lower eyelid fat pads with volume preservation via fat redraping versus subtractive fat sculpting maneuvers. Fat remains is an effective maneuver to efface the tear trough deformity, with or without midfacial lifting maneuvers. A skin pinch, chemical peel application, or laser resurfacing may be utilized as an adjunct to address mild lower eyelid skin laxity. Skin and orbicularis muscle redraping via a subciliary incision may be necessary if there is a significant component of lower eyelid dermatochalasis. However, the authors caution the aggressive removal of skin or resurfacing concomitant to lower facelifting, as this can lead to lower eyelid retraction and cicatricial ectropion at a higher rate than staged surgery.

5.2 Lower Blepharoplasty with Midface Lift

Midface release with concurrent elevation of the upper two-thirds of the face including the malar, zygomatic, and orbital regions offer significant benefit to periorbital as well as midface rejuvenation. These procedures are described in other chapters in detail, but in brief, it can release the midfacial ligaments and facilitate more complete mobilization of the lower face during concurrent deep plane rhytidectomy. Subperiosteal release essentially creates a full release of the midfacial ligaments and allows elevation of the midfacial soft tissues en-bloc, providing further volumization of the midface, decreasing the appearance of the tear trough and infraorbital hollow, and potentially decreasing the risk of lower eyelid retraction. The endoscopic forehead and midface lift alone can decrease the vertical height of the lower eyelid while softening infraorbital hollows [18, 19]. When combined with lower blepharoplasty or autologous fat transfer to address the medial tear trough region, this can be an effective adjunctive maneuver to provide complete rejuvenation of the lower eyelid-midface continuum during upper and lower facelifting.

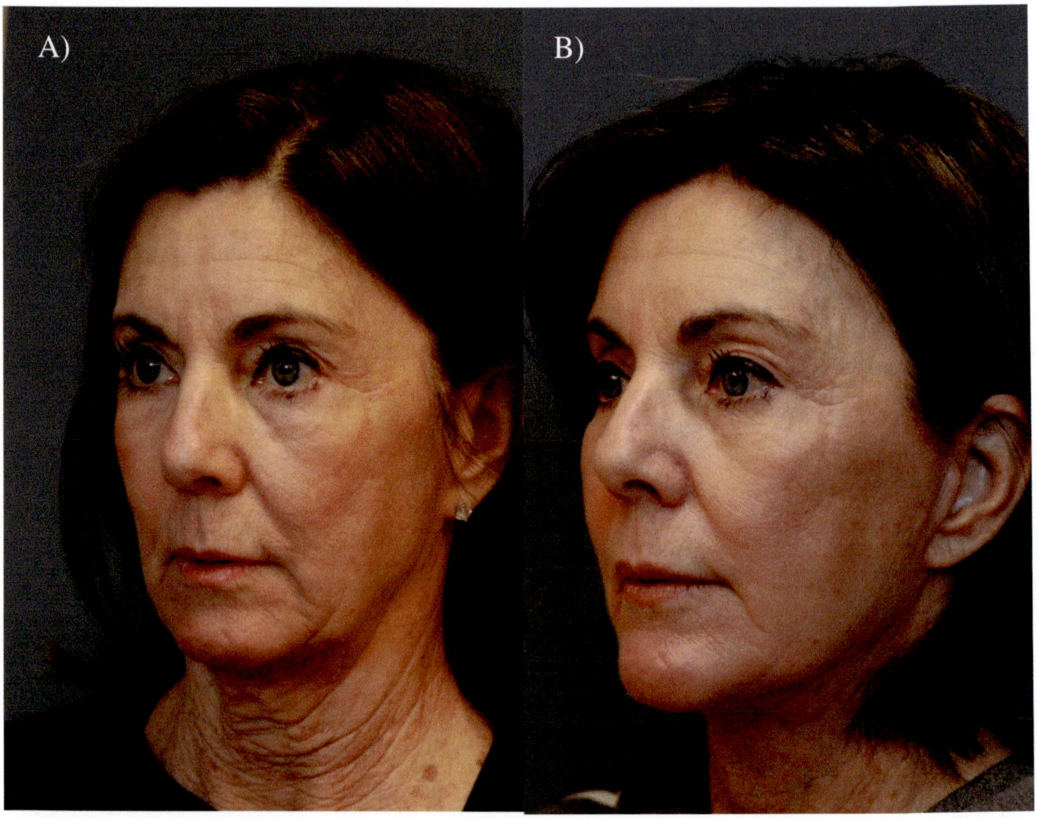

Fig. 4 A) Preoperative photograph demonstrating lower facial descent with jowling and prominent nasolabial fold, in addition to temporal hooding and lower eyelid 'bags' at oblique angle. B) Postoperative 6-month photograph at oblique angle demonstrating satisfactory results with significant improvement in lower facial descent. This patient underwent concomitant endoscopic brow lifting with subperiosteal midfacial release and transconjunctival lower blepharoplasty at the time of lower facelifting

Intraoperatively, the authors recommend performing the subperiosteal midfacial release prior to lower blepharoplasty, as the release of the orbital retaining ligament from the subperiosteal approach makes the subsequent blepharoplasty much easier. Manipulation and/or transposition of the lower fat pads into the midface can be then easily accomplished with complete release of the orbital retaining ligament. Of note, canthoplasty during periorbital periosteal release requires leaving a cuff of periosteum intact or designing fixation of the canthal ligament to the deep temporalis fascia within temporalis fossa or to the upper crus of the lateral canthal ligament.

5.3 Composite Facelift

Though the composite facelift has been described as an approach to provide additional periorbital rejuvenation to the deep plane rhytidectomy, the authors stress that this technique may have greater risks. Touted to provide comprehensive facial rejuvenation, the composite facelift involves a deep plane dissection continued posterior to the orbicularis oculi muscle to provide resuspension of the infraorbital soft tissues. A composite flap with SMAS, orbicularis muscle, and malar fat is then elevated in a superolateral vector to provide rejuvenation [20]. However, inherent to this technique is partial

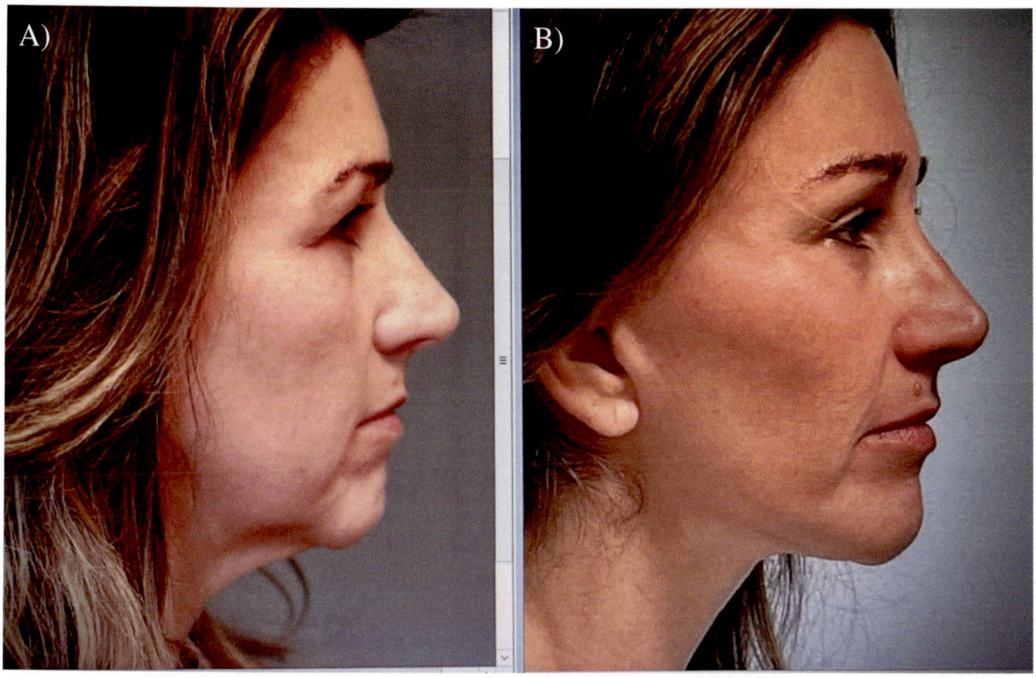

Fig. 5 A) Preoperative photograph demonstrating lower facial descent with jowling and prominent nasolabial fold, in addition to temporal hooding and lower eyelid 'bags'. B) Postoperative 6-month photograph demonstrating satisfactory results with significant improvement in lower facial descent and cervicomental angle. This patient underwent concomitant endoscopic brow lifting with subperiosteal midfacial release and transconjunctival lower blepharoplasty at the time of lower facelifting

orbicularis muscle denervation with dissection to the lateral orbicularis oculi muscle and submalar region (Fig. 6).

5.4 Autologous Fat Transfer

Volume preservation and redistribution is key to cosmetic midfacial augmentation. As described in another chapter, autologous fat transfer is a relatively safe, and effective adjunct to periorbital rejuvenation and it may be performed concomitant to facelift as well [21]. Malar fat atrophy, in addition to midfacial ptosis, progressively lengthens the lower eyelid and leads to the presence of negative vector configuration and increases the risk of lower eyelid retraction during both lower blepharoplasty and lower facelifting maneuvers. With the addition of malar autologous fat grafting to standard blepharoplasty and midfacial lifting techniques, the lower eyelid height can be more effectively shortened, negative vector and eyelid retraction corrected, and the overall rejuvenation of the midfacial and periorbital regions improved. Additionally, facial autologous fat grafting improves tissue quality, including the overlying skin by physical augmentation and the physiologic transplantation of autogenous stem cells [22].

5.5 Skin Resurfacing

Skin textural changes are the final important component to facial aging that may need to be addressed with cosmetic rejuvenation maneuvers. As the periorbital skin is extremely thin, it is particularly susceptible to an aged appearance with chronic ultraviolet damage compounded by collagen, elastin and subcutaneous volume loss. Though historically addressed by excisional

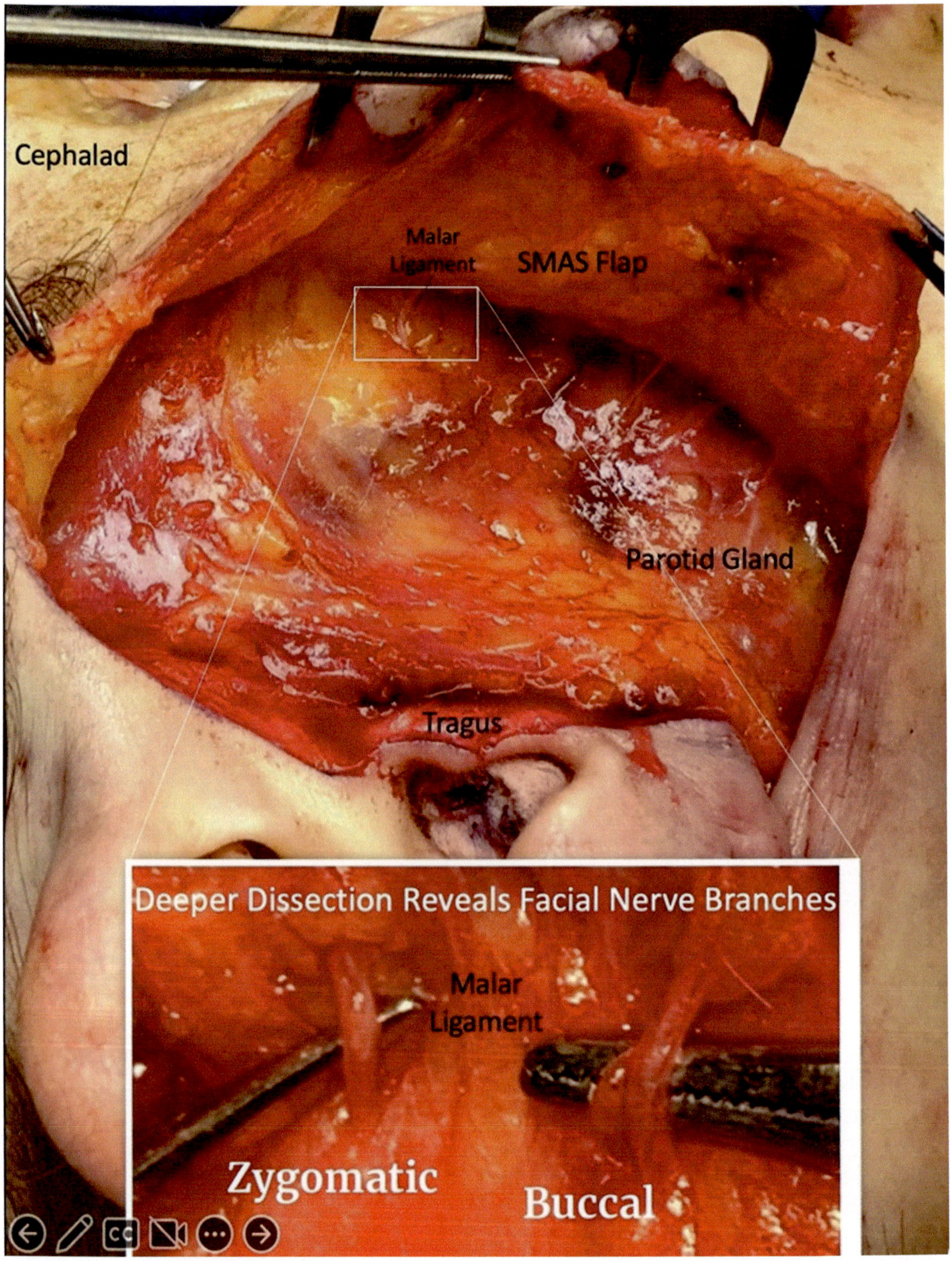

Fig. 6 Intraoperative photo of right side deep-plane facelift dissection with malar ligament visible. Inset demonstrates subsequent intraoperative deeper dissection revealing zygomatic and buccal branches of the facial nerve. Inadvertent injury to a zygomatic branch can result in partial or complete inferior orbicularis oculi paresis and subsequent lower eyelid retraction

maneuvers, lower eyelid skin redundancy presents a unique challenge where aggressive excision can yield lower eyelid malposition and ocular surface compromise. Alternatives to surgical excision include chemical peel application and laser resurfacing. These are described in another chapter, but, in brief adjunctive Er:YAG or CO2 laser resurfacing and chemical peel application have been demonstrated to safely and effectively address lower eyelid skin redundancy and static rhytids without the need for a transcutaneous incisions [23, 24]. Importantly, laser concomitant to lower facelifting definitively increase the risk of postoperative eyelid malposition. As such, less aggressive approaches to treating periorbital skin laxity is recommended during facelifting.

6 Periocular Postoperative Complications

6.1 Vision Loss

Fortunately, vision-threatening complications such as retrobulbar hemorrhage or globe injury are incredibly rare with facelifting and lower blepharoplasty procedures. However, the risk of retrobulbar hemorrhage that leads to orbital compartment syndrome remains present. Intraoperative hemostasis is crucial, as is early recognition and appropriate treatment with drainage to prevent ultimate vision loss. An open globe injury may occur from local anesthetic administration or direct globe injury intraoperatively, and should be managed urgently by an ophthalmic surgeon. Mitigation of the risk of these complications is accomplished by intraoperative ocular shields and/or adhesive ocular barriers (such as Tegaderm, 3M Nexcare, St. Paul, MN) Other adnexal structures at risk of damage include the inferior rectus and inferior oblique muscle, which may be directly damaged or incarcerated during orbital fat pad resection or redraping. Damage to the extraocular muscles can lead to visually debilitating diplopia, and avoidance of inadvertent damage and an intimate knowledge of the anatomy is key to prevention. Local anesthetic myotoxicity can also lead to diplopia in the early postoperative course, and this tends to resolve with observation alone. Patients with diplopia that persists for months postoperatively should be referred to an ophthalmic strabismus specialist [25].

6.2 Dry Eye Syndrome

Lower blepharoplasty at the time of lower facelifting compounds the risk of postoperative ocular surface dryness, as facial nerve stretch injury can temporarily reduce orbicularis oculi muscle function. As such, appropriate patient selection and extensive preoperative counseling is key, in addition to frequent ocular surface lubrication in the early postoperative course. Frequent application of preservative free artificial tear substitutes and ointments are often all that is needed; however, in patients with significantly impaired blink and ocular surface compromise, a temporary suture tarsorrhaphy may be necessary. Additionally, the presence of inflammatory chemosis is significantly greater with the utilization of periorbital rejuvenation maneuvers, particularly lower blepharoplasty, secondary to lymphatic disruption or the presence of lower eyelid retraction postoperatively. Postoperative chemosis typically responds to anti-inflammatory and hypertonic topical medication; however, prolonged conjunctival chemosis may require suture tarsorrhaphy or other surgical interventions [26].

6.3 Lower Eyelid Malposition

Several postoperative changes to eyelid position may occur secondary to periorbital rejuvenation, that are compounded by concomitant lower facelifting, midface lifting, and resurfacing maneuvers. Patients with negative vector morphology or preoperative lower eyelid laxity are at a significantly increased risk of postoperative lower eyelid malposition. Preoperative identification and intraoperative correction of lower eyelid laxity minimizes this risk [14].

Lower eyelid retraction results from middle lamella (orbital septum) shortening from intraoperative septal trauma and postoperative contraction. Patients with negative vector eyelid configuration or preoperative retraction are at a significantly higher risk of developing postoperative eyelid retraction. The authors recommend avoidance of open surgical manipulation of the septum, particularly as volume augmentation maneuvers including autologous fat grafting or subperiosteal lower eyelid fat pad redraping exist to address the tear trough region effectively without the need for orbital septum manipulation. Furthermore, conservative treatment of the orbicularis and skin when blepharoplasty is performed concurrent to rhytidectomy is essential to reduce the risks of retraction. Postoperative lower eyelid retraction management is beyond the scope of this chapter, but generally includes addressing any lower eyelid laxity, release of any contraction, and providing midfacial support with vertical lifting maneuvers and midfacial volume augmentation [27].

Lower eyelid frank ectropion occurs secondary to anterior lamella shortening from aggressive skin removal or resurfacing techniques, as well as orbicularis injury from direct muscle resection or indirect facial nerve branch injury leading to paralytic ectropion. If lower eyelid skin requires excision at the time of lower blepharoplasty and rhytidectomy to adequately address significant skin laxity, the authors recommend lateral canthal support maneuvers with either canthopexy, orbicularis muscle sling construction, or canthoplasty to provide adequate eyelid tightening. Additionally, as aforementioned, any periorbital laser resurfacing should be conservative.

With any transconjunctival incision, cicatricial lower eyelid entropion may result. This typically occurs with poor conjunctival incision technique, either too close to the inferior tarsal border or too deep in the fornix. Excessive cauterization can also injure the conjunctiva/lower eyelid retractors. Clinically significant post-surgical cicatricial entropion is beyond the scope of this chapter, but generally requires posterior lamellar lengthening procedures such as lower eyelid retractor release as well as possible autografting.

Canthal dystopia or rounding may occur secondary to temporal vertical elevation from lower facelifting and temporal midfacial lifting maneuvers if the canthal position is not taken into consideration intraoperatively. Canthoplasty is typically required to reset the canthal position if the patient is bothered by canthal dystopia postoperatively. This may be particularly challenging if any prior eyelid-shortening maneuver has been performed.

7 Conclusion

Lower eyelid and midfacial rejuvenation at the time of lower facelifting can be safe and offer improved cosmesis but requires knowledge regarding the complexities of periorbital anatomy. There exist increased risks for eyelid complications when the lower face is treated concomitantly with the eyelids. With careful planning and sound facelift and blepharoplasty technique iatrogenic complications can be avoided and allow further cosmetic facial enhancements in a single setting.

References

1. Vrcek I, Ozgur O, Nakra T. Infraorbital dark circles: a review of the pathogenesis, evaluation, and treatment. J Cutan Aesthet Surg. 2016;9(2):65–72.
2. Rohrich RJ, Pessa JE. The fat compartments of the face: anatomy and clinical implications for cosmetic surgery. Plast Reconstr Surg. 2007;119:2219–27.
3. Pessa JE, Zadoo VP, Mutimer KL, Haffner C, Yuan C, DeWitt AI, et al. Relative maxillary retrusion as a natural consequence of aging: combining skeletal and soft-tissue changes into an integrated model of midfacial aging. Plast Reconstr Surg. 1998;102:205–12.
4. Nakra T. Biplanar contour-oriented approach to lower eyelid and midface rejuvenation. JAMA Facial Plast Surg. 2015;17:374–81.
5. Serra-Renom JM, Serra-Mestre JM. Periorbital rejuvenation to improve the negative vector with

blepharoplasty and fat grafting in the malar area. Aesthetic Plast Surg. 2009;33(2):163–6.
6. Friedmann DP, Goldman MP. Dark circles: etiology and management options. Clin Plast Surg. 2015;42:33–50.
7. Roh MR, Chung KY. Infraorbital dark circles: definition, causes, and treatment options. Dermatol Surg. 2009;35:1163–71.
8. Goldberg RA, McCann JD, Fiaschetti D, Ben Simon GJ. What causes eyelid bags? Analysis of 114 consecutive patients. Plast Reconstr Surg. 2005;115:1395–402.
9. Chon BH, Hwang CJ, Perry JD. Long-term patient experience with tetracycline injections for festoons. Plast Reconstr Surg. 2020;146(6):737e–43e.
10. Mendelson B, Wong C. Chapter 6.1: Facelift: facial anatomy and aging. Aesthetic surgery of the face. 2012.
11. Gendler EC. Treatment of periorbital hyperpigmentation. Aesthet Surg J. 2005;25:618–24.
12. Demirdover C, Sahin B, Vayvada H, Oztan HY. The versatile use of temporoparietal fascial flap. Int J Med Sci. 2011;8(5):362–8.
13. Goldberg RA. Chapter 5: Mid-face lift. Oculoplastic surgery atlas. 2005. p. 55–62.
14. Hester TR, Douglas T, Szczerba S. Decreasing complications in lower eyelid and midface rejuvenation: the importance of orbital morphology, horizontal lower eyelid laxity, history of previous surgery, and minimizing trauma to the orbital septum: a critical review of 269 consecutive cases. Plast Reconstr Surgery. 2009;123(3):1037–49.
15. Schroeder RJ, Langsdon PR. Effect of local tranexamic acid on hemostasis in rhytidectomy. Facial Plast Surg Aesthet Med. 2020;22(3):195–9.
16. Cohen JC, Glasgold RA, Alloju LM, Glasgold MJ. Effects of intravenous tranexamic acid during rhytidectomy: a randomized, controlled, double-blind piolot study. Aesthet Surg J. 2021;41(2):155–60.
17. Sagiv O, et al. Subcutaneous tranexamic acid in upper eyelid blepharoplasty: a prospective randomized pilot study. Can J Ophthalmol. 2018;53(6):600–4.
18. Marotta JC, Quatela VC. Lower eyelid aesthetics after endoscopic forehead midface-lift. Arch Facial Plast Surg. 2008;10(4):267–72.
19. Ransom ER, Stong BC, Jacono AA. Persistent improvement in lower eyelid-cheek contour after a transtemporal midface lift. Aesthetic Plast Surg. 2012;36(6):1277–82.
20. Hamra ST. Composite rhytidectomy. Plast Reconstr Surg. 1992;90(1):1–13.
21. Serra-Reno JM, Serra-Mestre JM. Periorbital rejuvenation to improve the negative vector with blepharoplasty and fat grafting in the malar area. Ophthalmic Plast Reconstr Surg. 2011;27(6):442–6.
22. Cook T, Nakra T, Shorr N, Douglas RS. Facial recontouring with autogenous fat. Facial Plast Surg. 2004;20(2):145–7.
23. Carter SR, Seiff SR, Choo PH, Vallabhanath P. Lower eyelid CO(2) laser rejuvenation: a randomized prospective clinical study. Ophthalmology. 2001;108(3):437–41.
24. Morgenstern KE, Foster JA. Advances in cosmetic oculoplastic surgery. Curr Opin Ophthalmol. 2002;13(5):324–30.
25. Schwarcz RM, Kotlus B. Complications of lower blepharoplasty and midface lifting. Clin Plast Surg. 2015;42(1):63–71.
26. Prischmann J, Sufyan A, Tin JY, Ruffin C, Perkins SW. Dry eye symptoms and chemosis following blepharoplasty: a 10-year retrospective review of 892 cases in a single-surgeon series. JAMA Facial Plast Surg. 2013;15(1):39–46.
27. Patipa M. The evaluation and management of lower eyelid retraction following cosmetic surgery. Plast Reconstr Surg. 2000;106(2):438–53.

Trans-Eyelid Inferior Orbitotomy

Betina Wächter, Ricardo Mörschbächer and Caroline A. Sue

Abstract

Exposure of the inferior orbit can be achieved through a variety of incisions. These include subciliary, subtarsal, infraorbital or transconjuntival incisions. The ideal approach minimizes the risk for eyelid malposition or conspicuous scars, hence the transconjunctival is generally the preferred. In this chapter, the authors describe transconjunctival and other inferior orbitotomy surgical approaches.

Keywords

Inferior orbitotomy · Orbital floor approach · Orbital surgery · Orbital decompression · Orbital tumor · Transconjunctival approach

Illustrations by Michael Han

Supplementary Information The online version contains supplementary material available at https://doi.org/10.1007/978-3-031-36175-3_30.

B. Wächter (✉) · R. Mörschbächer · C. A. Sue
Santa Casa De Misericordia, Porto Alegre, Brazil
e-mail: betina.w@hotmail.com

1 Introduction

The inferior orbit must be exposed for different surgical treatments including fractures, orbital tumors, and orbital decompression in thyroid eye disease.

The choice of surgical orbital approach is influenced by factors such as tumor location, imaging exam characteristics, previous orbital surgeries and history of orbital trauma. The ideal approach should provide enough exposure and visibility to safely manipulate the orbital structures, with minimal postoperative scar formation and good aesthetic results.

A variety of surgical approaches to the orbital floor and infraorbital rim exist and can be categorized as transcutaneous or transconjunctival. The subciliary, subtarsal, and infraorbital incisions are collectively the transcutaneous approaches to the orbital floor and infraorbital rim. The authors detail the various approaches (Fig. 1).

2 Transcutaneous Incisions

Early descriptions of subciliary incisions to the orbit were in the context of orbital trauma [1]. The incision is placed 1–2 mm inferior to the lower eyelid lash line. The plane of subcutaneous dissection can be superficial to the orbicularis (skin-only flap) or deep to the muscle

J. P. Tao (ed.), *Plastic Surgery of the Lower Eyelids*,
https://doi.org/10.1007/978-3-031-36175-3_30

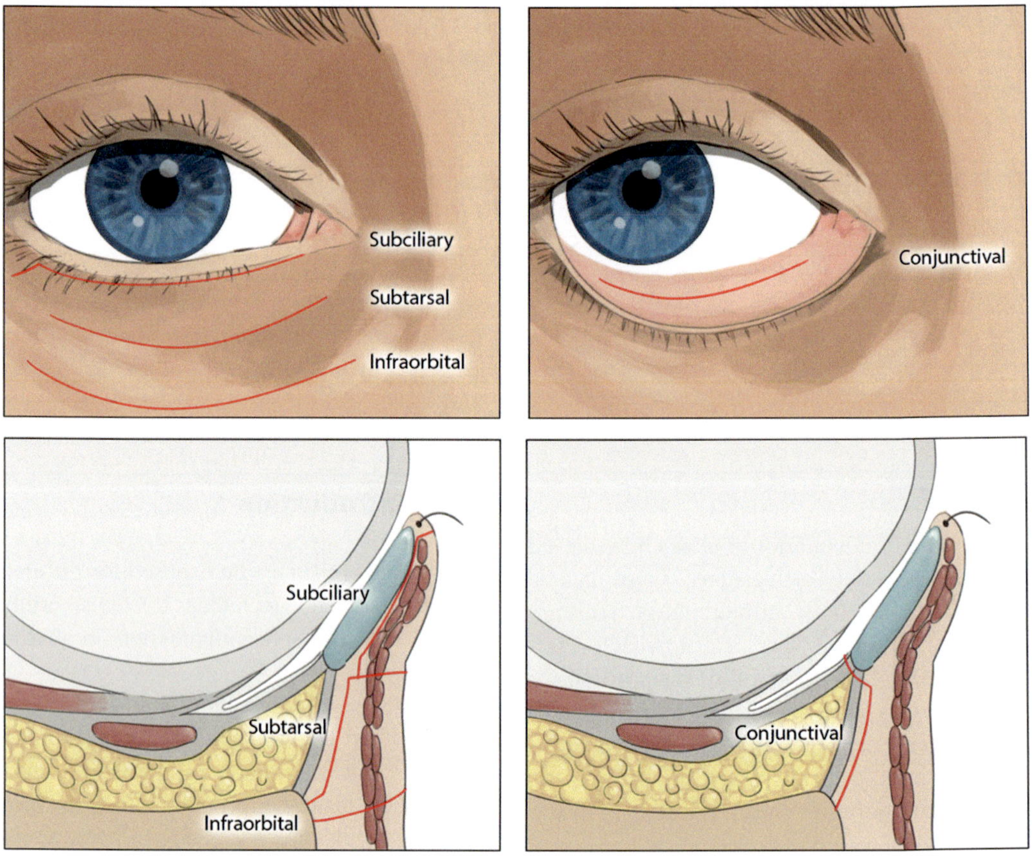

Fig. 1 Various inferior orbitotomy incisions (top) and eyelid dissecion plane (bottom)

(skin-muscle flap). The skin-only technique is associated with risks of necrosis, ecchymosis, and ectropion [2, 3]. Hence the skin-muscle flap approach is preferable. The inital dissection deep to skin is through the orbicularis oculi muscle that may or may not be separated from tarsus.

The dissection then proceeds in the preseptal plane deep to the orbicularis oculi to the level of infraorbital rim. Once the orbital rim is reached, an incision through the periosteum anterior to arcus marginalis is made and subperiosteal dissection exposes the orbital region of interest. The orbital septum is then not disrupted and the anterior orbital fat pads are maintained out of surgical field. There exists some risk of scarring in the plane of the septum that may lead to lower eyelid retraction or ectropion [2, 4–6].

A subtarsal incision or lower eyelid skin incision whereby the incision is placed in the natural fold of the lower lid below the tarsal plate, approximately 5–7 mm below the lower lid margin and above the orbital rim [1]. Following the inicial incision through skin and orbicularis oculi, a preseptal dissection is carried to the level of the orbital rim and the periosteum just below the infraorbital rim is incised to reveal the orbital floor and infraorbital rim. This approach may be more direct than the subcilary approach but is not odeal because the scar is quite visible [7]. Similarly, an infraorbital cutaneous incision at the level of inferior orbital rim leaves a conspicuous scar [3].

3 Transconjunctival Incision

Transconjuntival lower eyelid incision is widely preferred for exposure of the inferior rim, orbital floor. It offers some access to the inferior medial and lateral walls, as well. The benefits are minimal risk of eyelid malposition (with good technique) and no visible scar [8–11]

Transconjunctival surgery can be used to access anterior orbital tumors and fractures, drain inferior orbital abscesses, orbital decompression in thyroid eye disease, aesthetic surgery, congenital malformation and incisional or excisional biopsies [12, 13]. Many posterior orbital tumors can also be reached and excised by this approach.

The transconjunctival approach has been used for lower eyelid blepharoplasty for nearly a century [14]. For a half century, it has been used for facial trauma repair [15, 16]. Today, the transconjunctial inferior orbitotomy is the workhorse for orbital floor fractures as well as orbit floor decompression, among other less common surgeries.

Wider inferior orbital exposure can be achieved with a concomitant lateral canthotomy and inferior cantholysis. Other benefits include more precision in incising only the conjunctiva and lower retractors. The lateral eyelid, when detached can be distracted or swung anteriorly to allow for a lateral to medial incision that preserves the septum and anterior lamella structures. Additionally, resecuring the lateral eyelid to the lateral rim periosteum at the end of the surgery achieves eyelid tightening and stability [17–21]. Compared to a transcutaneous orbitotomy approaches, transconjunctival incisions leave no external scars.

An incision is fashioned at the conjunctiva below the level of the tarsus. A preseptal or postpseptal dissection plane is then followed to the orbital rim. The incision can be placed more inferiorly near the conjunctival fornix but the authors generally favor a position between the fornix and inferior tarsal border. When the incision is too inferior, the bulbar conjunctiva may separate from the underlying sclera, leading to a more tedious closure.

The chief limitations of the transconjunctival orbitotomy, like other anterior orbitotomy approaches is limited access to the orbital apex [20–22]. This procedure is also contraindicated in patients with ocular surface disease, glaucoma, or conjunctival disorders, such as cicatricial pemphigoid [23].

4 Surgical Technique (Video 1)

Usually under general anesthesia, local anesthetic is injected to the lower eyelid. A protective contact lens should be placed with an ophthalmic lubricant for the duration of the procedure. The authors prefer to start with a lateral canthotomy and lower cantholysis [24]. A scalpel is used toc reate a small 1–3 mm horizontal lateral canthal skin incision. A straight scissors completes the canthotomy (Fig. 2). With a toothed forceps, the lateral lower eyelid is distracted anteriorly and inferiorly and the scissors are used to achieve an inferior cantholysis so that the eyelid is free to swing externally and inferiorly (Fig. 3).

A 4-0 silk suture is passed through the gray line of the lower eyelid margin or an eyelid retractor (e.g. skin hook, Desmarres retractor, or Senn retractor) is used to retract the lower eyelid gently and expose the fornix. After the eversion of the eyelid, the transconjunctival incision is performed with scissors between the inferior tarsal border and fornix in the preseptal plane (Fig. 3). The lower eyelid retractors, along with conjunctiva, but no other structures are

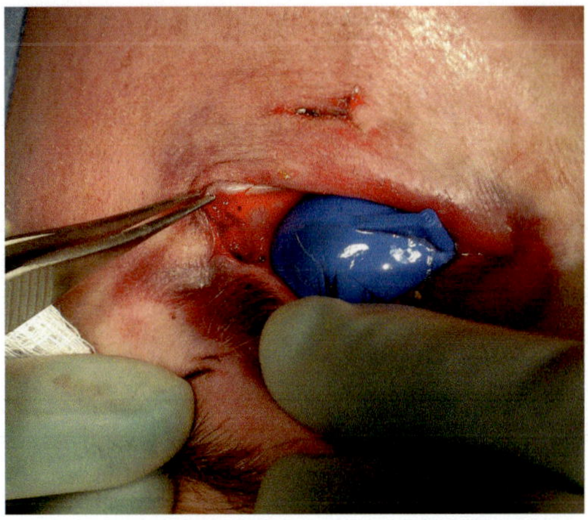

Fig. 2 Lateral canthotomy

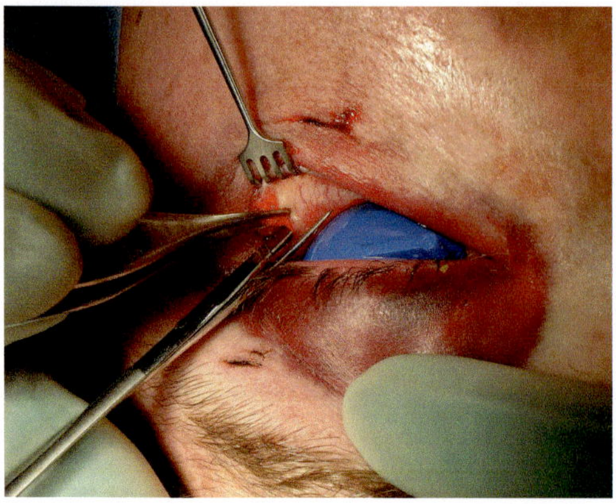

Fig. 3 Inferior cantholyisis and inititiation of conjunctiva/retractor band incision

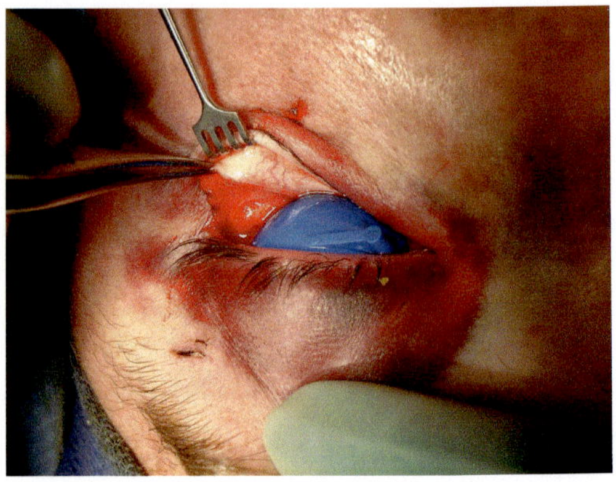

Fig. 5 Eyelid planes evident through conjunctiva/retractor incision (orbital fat posteriorly and orbicularis oculi muscle anteriorly)

incorporated in the scissor incision that proceeds laterally to medial (Fig. 4).

The dissection to the orbital rim can be performed in a preseptal or postseptal plane. The preseptal approach is generally preferred. As such, the rake instruments are repositioned to evert the anterior lamella anteriorly (Fig. 5). The everted eyelid can be draped over the inferor orbital rim. The instruments are further repositioned to ensure orbicularis oculi muscle is anterior. A malleable ribbon retractor is used to move orbital fat and the septum posteriorly (Fig. 6). These maneuvers leave only septum overlying the inferior orbital rim. The septum and periosteum are incised with a scalpel or an elctrosurgical unit. The incision should be external on the maxillary face and not on the crest of the infraorbital rim to improve the access and to avoid inadvetently cutting orbital structures such as the inferior oblique muscle (Fig. 7).

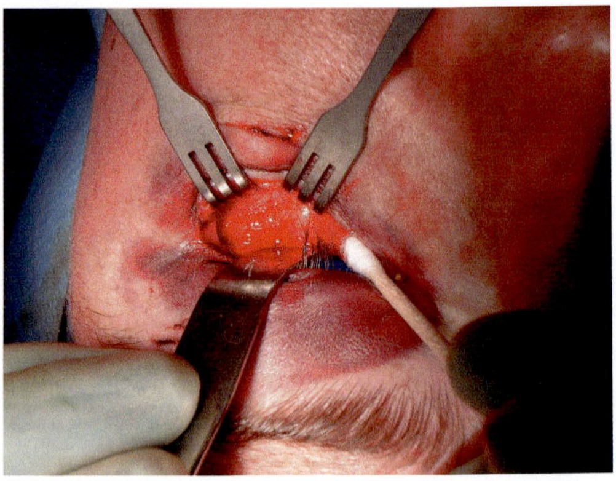

Fig. 6 Anterior lamella tissueds retracted with Senn retractors and orbital fat held within the orbit with a malleable ribbon retractor

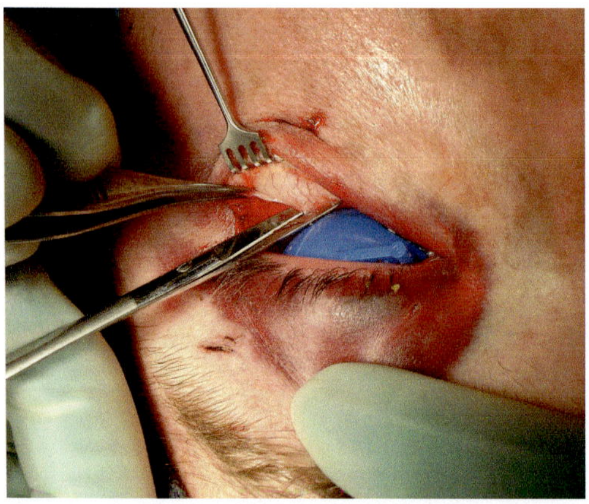

Fig. 4 Conjunctiva and underlying retractor band incised between infratarsal border and fornix

The orbital dissection begins after this lower orbital rim incision. Malleable retractor adjustments are made to hold fat posteriorly with other orbital contentes including the globe. The dissection is then carried out subperiosteally with a Freer or Cottle elevator to expose the orbital floor (Fig. 8).

Hemostasis is achieved with electrocautery. Commonly a large orbit floor perforating artery

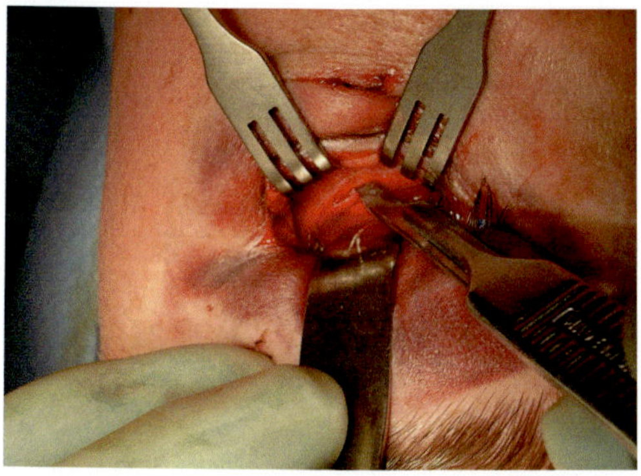

Fig. 7 With only septum folded on the rim, an incision is made down to the orbital rim boné (through epstum and periosteum)

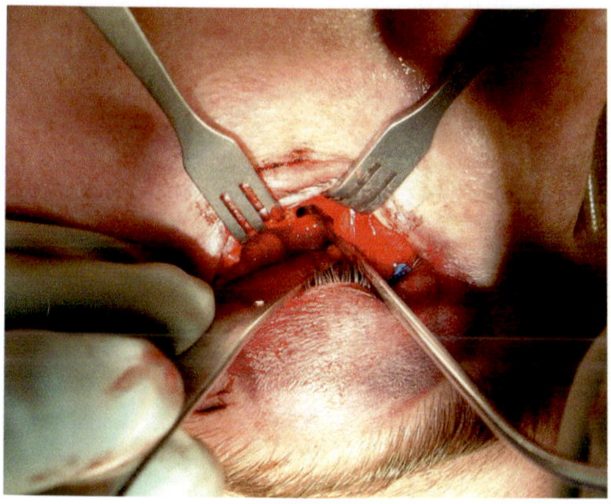

Fig. 8 Exposure of inferior orbit (for orbital fracture repair in this case)

on the mid floor, 1–2 cm posterior to the rim requires cautery. Orbit surgery can then commence (Fig. 9).

Once the orbit surgery (e.g. fracture repair or decompression) is completed and hemostasis is verified, the wounds are closed. Some surgeons close periosteum but the authors believe this step is uneccessary. The conjunctival and retractor band incision is closed with absorbable 6-0 sutures. The sutures are placed with special attention to not incorporate the orbital septum.

Next, the lateral canthotomy and lower cantholysis are repaired [3]. Specifically, the free lateral tarsus is anchored to the lateral rim periosteum using a 4-0 or 5-0 polyglactin or braided

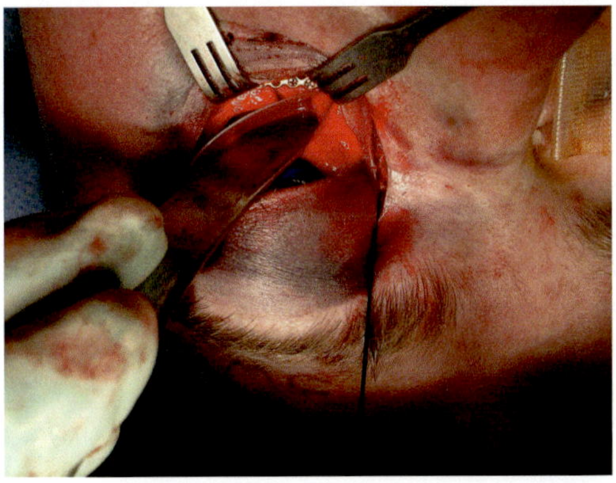

Fig. 9 Inferior orbitotomy nylon implant fracture repair in this case. Note that extraorbital rim fractures were also approached and plated through this approach

polyester suture (Fig. 10). The skin is sutured with 6-0 plain suture.

When medial or inferomedial orbit access is required, a concomitant transcutaneous or transcaruncular incision can be created [25]. In the transcutaneous approach, an incision can be fashioned just anterior to the medial canthal tendon. In the transcaruncle approach, a retrocaruncular incision is created with scissors. In either approach, dissection proceeds towards the posterior lacrimal crest. Stevens scissors are used to

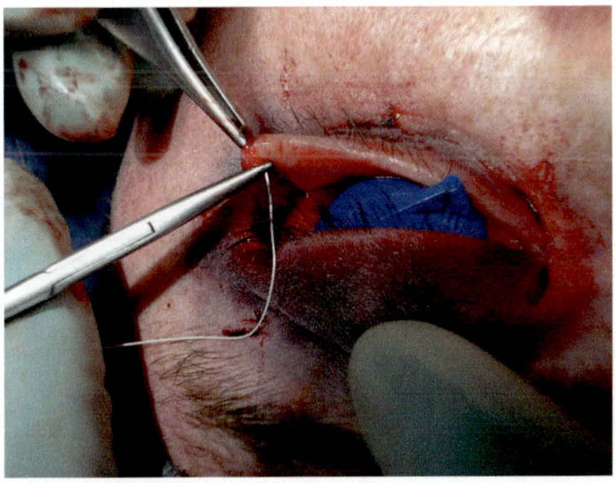

Fig. 10 Closure of transconjunctival inferior orbitotomy. Interrupted 6-0 chromic sutures to close the conjunctiva/retractor incision. The free lateral tarsos is secured to the lateral inner rim periosteum with 4-0 polyglactin sutures

dissect a plane to the medial orbital wall immediately posterior to the posterior lacrimal crest with care to not damage the lacrimal drainage system. After the periosteum at the medial wall is identified, it is opened and elevated to widely expose the medial orbital wall with help of malleable retractors and a periosteal elevator. Suture to the periostium is not necessary and conjunctival incision can be closed with 6-0 sutures, but sutures are generally not necessary (Figs. 11, 12, 13 and 14).

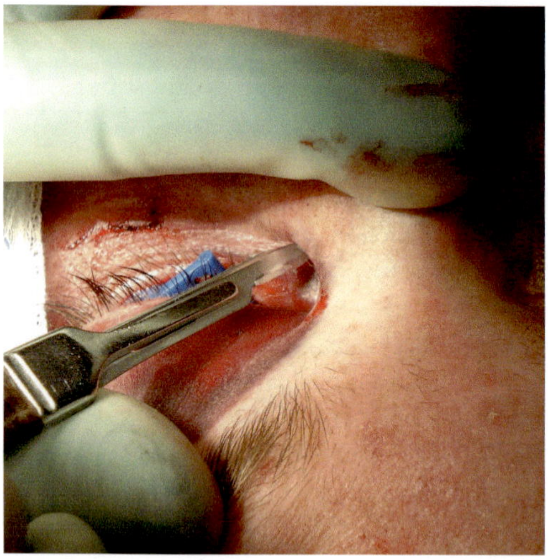

Fig. 11 Medial orbitotomy through a transcutaneois incision fashioned just anterior to the medial canthal tendon

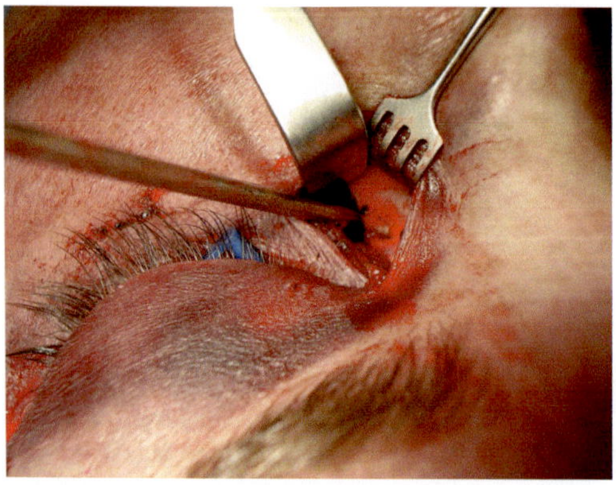

Fig. 12 Anterior orbital rim exposed through medial orbitotomy

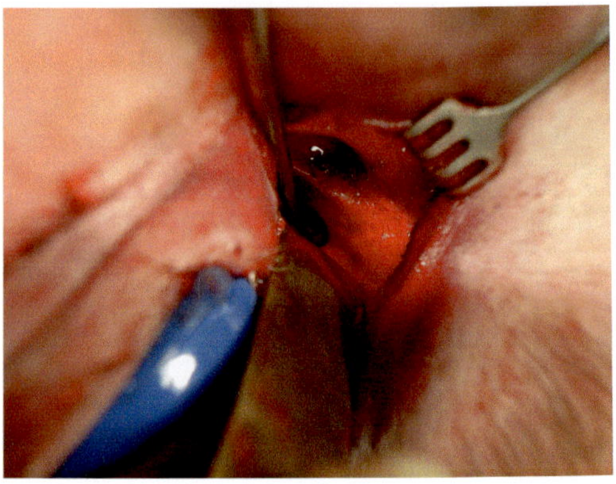

Fig. 13 Lacrimal fossa and anterior medial orbit exposed

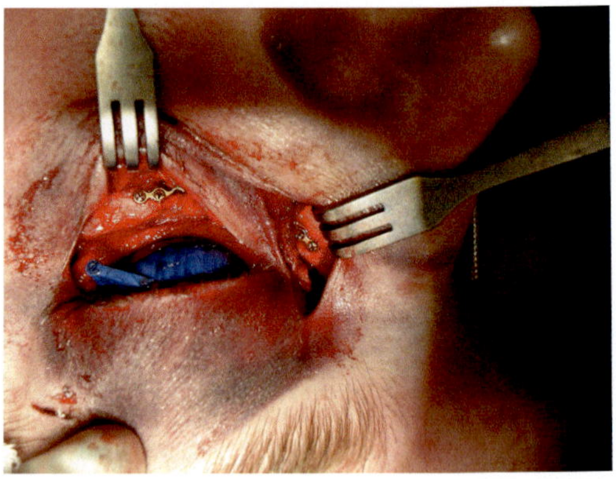

Fig. 14 Medial orbitotomy wound used to aid in inferomedial rim exposure for facial fracture repair in this case

5 Discussion

The transconjunctival inferior orbitotomy is an ideal approach to the inferior orbit.

A combined canthotomy and cantholysis increases orbitotomy exposure and may allow for better preservation of eyelid during the approach [2, 5, 28, 29].

The transconjunctival technique, when performed correctly, minimizes the risk of eyelid malpositon [9, 12, 23, 30–32]. Compared to other incisions, the transconjunctival approach has lower overall complications rates [2, 4, 23, 30]. This approach may be combined with medial orbitotomy to further access the inferomedial orbit.

There exist some postoperative transient complications, such as chemosis, lid swelling, tearing and diplopia, all resolved without treatment [4, 10, 33]. Conjunctival granuloma may be the most common complication of the transconjunctival technique. These may be treated with topical corticosteroids or excision [33, 34]. Entropion is a rare complication due toscarring of the posterior lamella and conjunctival shortening trichiasis [32, 36].

6 Conclusion

The transconjunctival inferior orbitotomy is an excellent choice for inferior orbit exposure [22]. Inferior orbitotomy may be combined with other approaches, such as medial orbitotomy, if necessary. Transcutaneous options to the inferior orbit are available, but generally less desirable, but can be safe and effective with good technique. Subtarsal and infrorbital cutaneous incisions are generally not preferred owing to the conspicuous resultant scar. Evaluation for risk factors for eyelid retraction and malposition, including horizontal laxity or cicatrix, is important when performing inferior orbitotomy [5, 8].

References

1. Converse JM. Severe trauma and extensive comminuted fracture. Arch Ophthalmol. 1944;31(4):323–5.
2. Wray RC, Holtmann B, Ribaudo JM, Keiter J, Weeks PM. A comparison of conjunctival and subciliary incisions for orbital fractures. Br J Plast Surg. 1977;30(2):142–5.
3. Bähr W, Bagambisa FrB, Stom D, Schlegel G, Schilli W. Comparison of transcutaneous incisions used for exposure of the infraorbital rim and orbital floor: a retrospective study. Plast Reconstr Surg. 1992;90:585–91.
4. Ridgway EB, Chen C, Colakoglu S, Gautam S, Lee BT. The incidence of lower eyelid malposition after facial fracture repair: a retrospective study and meta-analysis comparing subtarsal, subciliary, and transconjunctival incisions. Plast Reconstr Surg. 2009;124(5):1578–86.
5. Appling DW, Patrinely JR, Salzer TA. Transconjunctival approach vs subciliary skin-muscle flap approach for orbital racture repair. Arch Otolaryngol Head Neck Surg. 1993;119:1000–7
6. Holtmann B, Wray RC, Little AG. A randomized comparison of four incisions for orbital fractures. In: *Plastic and reconstructive surgery*, vol. 67. 1981. p. 731–35.
7. Feldman EM, Bruner TW, Sharabi SE, Koshy JC, Hollier Jr LH. The subtarsal incision: where should it be placed? J Oral Maxillofac Surg. 2011;69:2419–423. https://doi.org/10.1016/j.joms.2011.02.008
8. Ho VH, Rowland JP, Linder JS, Fleming JC. Sutureless transconjunctival repair of orbital blowout fractures. Ophthal Plast Reconstr Surg. 2004;20(6):458–60.
9. Goldberg RA, Lessner AM, Shorr N, Baylis HI. The transconjunctival approach to the orbital floor and orbital fat. Ophthal Plast Reconstr Surg. 1990;6(4):241–6.
10. Kim DW, Choi SR, Park SH, Koo SH. Versatile use of extended transconjunctival approach for orbital reconstruction. Ann Plast Surg. 2009;62(4):374–80.
11. Santosh BS, Giraddi G. Transconjunctival preseptal approach for orbital floor and infraorbital rim fracture. J Maxillofac Oral Surg. 2011;10(4):301–5.
12. Kushner GM. Surgical approaches to the infraorbital rim and orbital floor: the case for the transconjunctival approach. J Cranio-Maxillofacial Surg. 2006;64(1):108–10.
13. Westfall CT, Col L, Mc U, Shore JW. Operative complications of the transconjunctival inferior. Ophthalmology. 1991;98:1525–528. https://doi.org/10.1016/S0161-6420(91)32094-3
14. Bourguet J. Les hernies graisseuses de l'orbite: notre traitement chirurgical. Bull Acad Nat Med. 1924;92:1270–2.
15. Converse JM, Firmin F, Wood-Smith D, Friedland JA. The conjunctival approach in orbital fractures. Plast Reconstr Surg. 1973;52(6):656–7.
16. Tessier P. The conjunctival approach to the orbital floor and maxilla in congenital malformation and trauma. J Max-Fac Surg. 1973;1:8–12.
17. Kiratli H, Bulur B, Bilgiç S. Transconjunctival approach for retrobulbar intraconal orbital cavernous hemangiomas. Orbital surgeon's perspective. Surg Neurol. 2005;64(1):71–4.
18. Barkhuysen R, Nielsen CCM, Klevering BJ, Van Damme PA. The transconjunctival approach with lateral canthal extension for three-wall orbital decompression in thyroid orbitopathy. J Cranio-Maxillofacial Surg. 2009;37(3):127–31. https://doi.org/10.1016/j.jcms.2008.10.010
19. Bernardini FP, Nerad J, Fay A, Zambelli A, Cruz AA V, Paulo S. The revised direct transconjunctival approach to the orbital floor. Ophthal Plast Reconstr Surg. 2016;XX(Xx):1–8.
20. Cheng JW, Wei RL, Cai JP, Li Y. Transconjunctival orbitotomy for orbital cavernous hemangiomas. Can J Ophthalmol. 2008;43(2):234–38. https://doi.org/10.3129/i08-005
21. Cho KJ, Paik JS, Yang SW. Surgical outcomes of transconjunctival anterior orbitotomy for

intraconal orbital cavernous hemangioma. Korean J Ophthalmol. 2010;24(5):274–8.
22. Park SJ, Yang JW. The transconjunctival approach a minimally invasive approach to various kinds of retrobulbar tumors. J Craniofac Surg. 2013;24(6):1991–5.
23. Novelli G, Ferrari L, Sozzi D, Mazzoleni F, Bozzetti A. Transconjunctival approach in orbital traumatology: a review of 56 cases. J Cranio-Maxillofacial Surg. 2011;39(4):266–70. https://doi.org/10.1016/j.jcms.2010.06.003
24. Bronstein JA, Bruce WJ, Bakhos F, Ishaq D, Joyce CJ, Cimino V. Surgical approach to orbital floor fractures: comparing complication rates between subciliary and subconjunctival approaches. Craniomaxillofac Trauma Reconstr. 2020;13(1):45–8.
25. Lee CS, Jin SY, Sang YL. Combined transconjunctival and transcaruncular approach for repair of large medial orbital wall fractures. Arch Ophthalmol. 2009;127(3):291–6.
26. Ishida K. Evolution of the surgical approach to the orbitozygomatic fracture: from a subciliary to a transconjunctival and to a novel extended transconjunctival approach without skin incisions*. J Plast Reconstr Aesthetic Surg. 2016;69(4):497–505. https://doi.org/10.1016/j.bjps.2015.11.016
27. Hadeed H, Ziccardi VB, Sotereanos GC, Patterson GT. Latheral canthotomy transcojunctival approach to the orbit. Oral Surg Oral Med Oral Pathol. 1992;73:526–30.
28. Ilankovan V. Transconjunctival approach to the infraorbita: l a cadaveric and clinical study. Br J Oral Maxillofac Surg. 1991;29:169–73.
29. Waite PD, Carr DD. The transconjunctival approach for treating orbital trauma. J Oral Maxillofac Surg. 1991;49:499–503.
30. Bonawitz S, Crawley W, Shores JT, Manson PN. Modified transconjunctival approach to the lower eyelid: technical details for predictable results. Craniomaxillofac Trauma Reconstr. 2016;9(1):29–34.
31. Jacono AA, Moskowitz B. Transconjunctival versus transcutaneous approach in upper and lower blepharoplasty. Facial Plast Surg. 2001;17(1):21–7.
32. Yoon SH, Lee JH. The reliability of the transconjunctival approach for orbital exposure: measurement of positional changes in the lower eyelid. Arch Craniofacial Surg. 2017;18(4):249–54.
33. Mullins JB, Holds JB, Braham GH, Thomas JR. Complications of transconjunctival approach. a review of 400 cases. Arch Otoryngol Head Neck Surg. 1997;123:385–88.
34. Schmäl F, Basel T, Grenzebach UH, Thiede O, Stoll W. Preseptal transconjunctival approach for orbital floor fracture repair: ophthalmologic results in 209 patients. Acta Otolaryngol. 2006;126(4):381–9.
35. Al-Moraissi EA, Thaller SR, Ellis E. Subciliary vs. transconjunctival approach for the management of orbital floor and periorbital fractures: a systematic review and meta-analysis. J Cranio-Maxillofacial Surg. 2017;45(10):1647–654. https://doi.org/10.1016/j.jcms.2017.07.004
36. Kesselring AG, Promes DDSP, Strabbing DDSEM, Wal KGH Van Der Koudstaal MJ. Lower eyelid malposition following orbital fracture surgery : A retrospective analysis based on 198 surgeries. Craniomxillofac Trauma Reconstr. 2016;9:109–112.

Light and Thermal Devices for Lower Eyelid and Facial Rejuvenation

Melanie Ho Erb

Abstract

There exist many energy-based technologies for facial rejuvenation. These include lasers as well as light and thermal devices. This chapter will describe intense pulsed light, radiofrequency micro needling, radiofrequency, and ultrasound. Indications, contraindications, expected outcomes and complications of these technologies are discussed.

Keywords

Laser · Rejuvenation · Intense pulsed light · Radiofrequency microneedling · Broadband light · Cryotherapy · Nonsurgical blepharoplasty

Energy-Based devices for facial rejuvenation Table 1.

M. H. Erb (✉)
Private Practice, Irvine, CA, USA
e-mail: MelanieHoErb@gmail.com

1 Light Treatments

1.1 Intense Pulsed Light (IPL) Also Called Broadband Light (BBL)

Intense pulsed light (IPL), also known as broadband light (BBL) emits a strong pulse of light in the visible spectrum and a filter is placed to restrict the other wavelengths and allow just one wavelength to go through. This one wavelength that goes through mimics a laser wavelength of the non-ablative laser. The IPL device has many filters available which gives IPL the flexibility to treat a wide range of conditions.

IPL/BBL has minimal downtime, but the results are modest, and usually require multiple treatments and re-treatments. IPL reduces brown pigment, reduces red pigment, and reduces hair follicles which reduces unwanted hair growth. (Fig. 1) Browns caused by sun damage will go away but will always come back with time, thus necessitating periodic retreatments. IPL works best on Fitzpatrick skin types I, II, III while Fitzpatrick IV, V, VI risk getting hyperpigmentation which may be worse than the original lesion. Patient must be asked if they have recently tanned (or gone on vacation) because tanned skin risks hypopigmentation from IPL if the increase in skin melanin gets targeted.

J. P. Tao (ed.), *Plastic Surgery of the Lower Eyelids*,
https://doi.org/10.1007/978-3-031-36175-3_31

Table 1 Light and thermal devices for facial rejuvenation

Light Treatments	
Intense pulsed light (IPL) or broadband light (BBL)	Emits a strong flash of light in the visible spectrum and a filter is placed to restrict the other wavelengths and allow one wavelength to go through which mimics a laser wavelength of the non-ablative laser. The IPL device has many different filters available which gives IPL the flexibility to treat a wide range of conditions. Improve, reduce browns, reduce reds, reduce unwanted hair growth. Mild to moderate results with no downtime
Thermal treatments to tighten dermis	
Radiofrequency (RF) and/or Ultrasound	Uses energy to bulk heat up the dermis and the collagen, while leaving the epidermis cooler. Shrinks and contracts the collagen which improves texture and tone. Might induce neo-collagenesis. Usually safe for all Fitzpatrick skin types. Scant results with no downtime
Radiofrequency (RF) microneedling	Uses microneedles to drive through the epidermis and the dermis and then delivers radiofrequency to the needle tips to heat up the dermis. This tightens the collagen by both mechanical injury and heat. Increases collagen, improves texture and tone, improves acne scars, improves fine wrinkles. Mild to moderate results with very short downtime. (There also exist small, AC or DC, handheld microneedling devices without the addition of radiofrequency energy.)
Thermal reduction of fat	
Freezing/cryolipolysis, laser diode 1060, radiofrequency ultrasound	Uses cold or laser or radiofrequency or ultrasound to injure/kill fat which leads to fat reduction below the chin or on the body. Mild results with very short downtime
Thermal breakdown of fat with internal probe which assists with liposuction	
Laser assisted liposuction, ultrasound assisted liposuction	Uses a probe placed in the subcutaneous fat which delivers energy in the form of laser or ultrasound which helps melt the fat for ease of removal with liposuction
RF assisted lipolysis	Uses one internal electrode probe placed in the subcutaneous fat and one external electrode probe placed atop the skin. The RF stimulates the collagen in the skin between the probes for slight tightening and melts the fat near the internal probe which helps with fat removal during liposuction

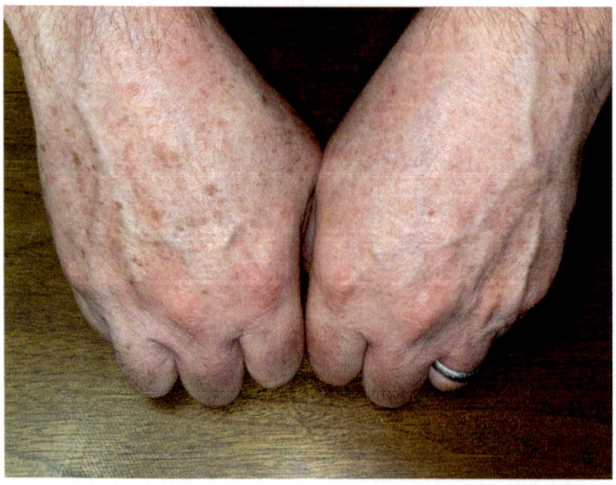

Fig. 1 Intense pulsed light results. Left hand had three treatments with IPL for for brown spots. Right hand was untreated

IPL/BBL is first used to correct dyschromia with higher power based on patient's concerns. After the skin color is more uniform, then maintenance treatment can be with lower power and multiple filters, every few months to maintain the skin's more uniform color and texture. Facial IPL treatment has been referred to as a "photofacial."

IPL/BBL: Procedure in Detail

The face is cleaned. Topical anesthetic cream may or may not be applied then removed. The patient's eyes are protected with metal goggles that sit atop the eyelids, or disposable foam and metal stickers that sit atop the eyelids, or with metal ocular shields that sit atop the globe. Eye protection is critical because the pigment in the iris can react with the IPL light causing iris atrophy and deformation. Ultrasound/IPL gel is thinly applied as a coupling agent. The pulsed light is transmitted through a continuously cooled applicator which helps with pain control.

The appropriate wavelength filter and IPL energy are selected. The applicator is lightly placed on the skin. Too much force can drive the red blood cells out of the vascular lesions thus making the target less visible to the IPL. The provider and others in the room wear appropriate protective eyewear from the intense light.

The light administration feels like a rubber band snap. The firing creates a super bright light that is seen by the patient despite complete eye protection. The treatment settings are titrated so that the skin turns just a faint pink. After treatment, the face will be slightly pink. The browns will later look like coffee grounds and then fall off. The reds will reduce and then come back and need retreatments in 2 steps forward and 1 step back effect. The results are noted so that adjustments can be made to the settings for the subsequent treatment.

IPL for Meibomian Gland Disease (MGD) and Dry Eye Disease (DED): Procedure in Detail

Although this chapter is focused on energy-based devices for facial rejuvenation, the author will briefly describe IPL for MGD and DED. As with all IPL, Fitzpatrick I, II, III are best candidates. IPL may be applied to the eyelids and periocular region in the following method [1–7].

Proparacaine drops, lubricant drops, then laser grade metal ocular shields are placed on the eyes. A thin amount of IPL/ultrasound coupling gel is placed on the face. The coupling gel is carefully placed on the eyelids to prevent the gel from getting onto the ocular shields and eyes which can cause significant irritation.

First the whole face is treated using a larger standard handpiece. A few test shots to the face are applied and the area is assessed for settings that achieve faint pinkness. Once the settings are satisfactory, the whole face is treated in standard fashion, 10% overlap, single pulse, single pass. A second pass is then made from tragus to tragus along V2 with the same settings with handpiece oriented vertically (superior/inferior).

The IPL settings are lowered and a pass is made from tragus to tragus along V2 vertically orienting handpiece (superior/inferior) covering the cheeks and lower eyelids. Settings are 590 nm filter, 5–6 ms pulse 50 ms rest, triple pulse, energy can range from 10 to 14 mJ, overlap by 10%, and do double pass (2 passes).

The handpiece is changed to the small light guide. With the same settings: 590 nm filter, 5–6 ms pulse 50 ms rest, triple pulse, energy can range from 10 to 14 mJ, the upper eyelids are treated with care to avoid lashes and brow by 2 mm. Typically 3–4 pulses are made and a double pass is administered. The patient should be asked to look down while raising the eyebrows to increase access the upper eyelid skin.

Next, the lower eyelids are treated, again avoiding lashes by 2 mm. 3 pulses and a double pass are performed with the patient looking up while opening the mouth to increase access the lower eyelid skin.

Upon completion of the therapy, the gel is cleaned, with care to not get the gel onto the ocular shield or eye. The ocular shields are removed. An optional drop of Lumify may be placed onto the eyes.

2 Thermal Tightening of Dermis

Radiofrequency (RF)
Ultrasound
Radiofrequency (Rf) Microneedling

2.1 Radiofrequency

Radiofrequency uses energy to bulk heat the dermis while leaving the epidermis cooler. It attempts to get the dermis to a temperature between 50 and 75 °C whereby collagen will denature and then contract and shrink. This improves texture and tone. Then the processes lead to tissue repair response, dermal remodeling, and presumed neocollagenesis. Zelickson demonstrated, through abdominal skin biopsies, there is an induction of new collagen synthesis at 8 weeks [8].

The RF device heats the dermis while cooling the epidermis. When applying RF, the epidermis is warmed to 40–46 °C. The deeper dermis is presumed to be heated to approximately 65 °C, a temperature that should denature the collagen. Once the temperature of the epidermis is 40–46 °C, this temperature must be maintained for over 3 min. The RF handpiece is moved across the skin at a fast enough rate so it does not become unbearably hot for the patient, however, if moved too fast then the temperature at the epidermis drops.

Trying to get the dermis to a consistent heated temperature based on the temperature at the epidermis is challenging. Differences in skin thickness, hydration and the composition of collagen and fat can lead to placement of the energy at unknown or variable depths. If the energy is placed too deep, then fat necrosis and fat loss may occur. If the energy is placed too superficial, then skin burns, and hyperpigmentation may occur. Also, if the critical temperatures are not reached and are not maintained for the prescribed length of time, then collagen may not denature, contract, and shrink and neocollagenesis may not be initiated. All cutaneous RF devices have the problem with unpredictable heating of the dermis and therefore unpredictable results.

Radiofrequency Handheld Bulk Heating: Procedure in Detail

RF makes the tissue feel very warm, which can range in the level of pain depending on patient sensitivity and pain tolerance. No anesthesia is used. During the treatment, the skin can look pink with warmth, but this resolves after stopping the treatment. Ice and cold should NOT be used to cool down the skin because the heat should stay captured within the dermis for as long as possible. After the skin cools down naturally and without ice, the skin looks normal. RF has no downtime. RF does result in a small amount of immediate plumping of the skin, which lasts a variable amount of time. Neocollagenesis is slight. Thus, RF can be used just prior to social events if some slight fullness is desired with no downtime.

2.2 Ultrasound

Ultrasound works in a similar manner as radiofrequency but using ultrasound energy instead of radiofrequency energy. And like RF, cutaneous ultrasound devices may unpredictably heat the dermis and have unpredictable results.

2.3 Radiofrequency (RF) Microneedling (MN)

Radiofrequency (RF) microneedling (MN) uses microneedles to drive through the epidermis and into the dermis and then delivers RF energy to the needle tips to heat up the dermis. This tightens the collagen and skin by both mechanical injury and thermal injury (Figs. 2 and 3). The needles can be coated or uncoated and vary in length/depth. With coated needles, the base of the needle is coated, which protects the epidermis from the RF energy, which is then delivered only to the needle tips at the prescribed depth. This epidermis protection allows treatment to Fitzpatrick I, II, III, IV, V. The needles provide good treatment to deep acne scars. If the base of the needle is uncoated, then the epidermis also receives the RF energy with improves skin tightening. RFMN increases collagen, improves texture and tone, improves acne scars, and slightly tightens skin. Downtime is usually 2 days. Risks

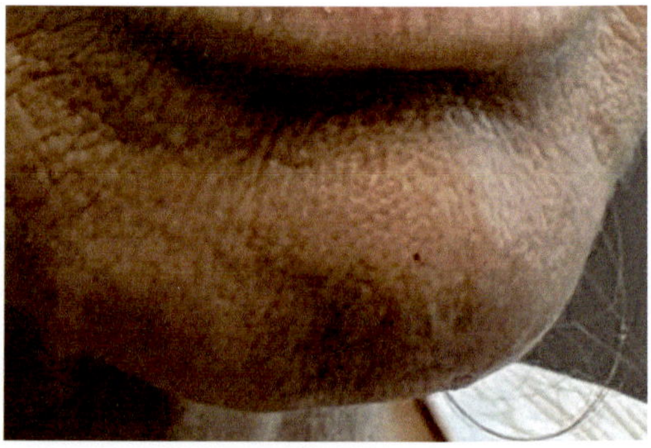

Fig. 2 Chin before radiofrequency microneedling

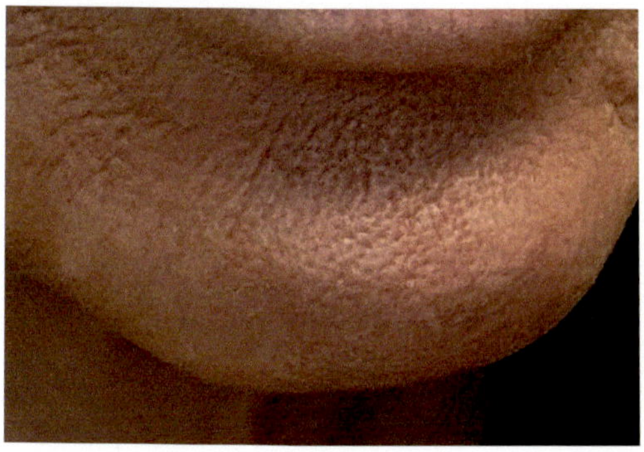

Fig. 3 Chin of patient in Fig. 2 after one treatment of radiofrequency microneedling with improved texture and tone

include scars, irregular skin texture with little holes, subcutaneous fat loss, or burns.

Separate from RF microneedling, there are also small, handheld microneedling devices that deliver microneedling alone without the addition of radiofrequency energy. These microneedling devices range from rollers to manual stampers to electric pens that rapidly and continuously insert and remove the microneedles.

Radiofrequency Microneedling: Procedure in Detail

Patient selection:
Fitzpatrick skin types I, II, III, IV, V

Pre-procedure: Consider prophylaxis with oral valacyclovir 500 mg po BID starting 1 day before laser and continue until 5 days after. Oral acetominophen for pain and oral benzodiazepines for sedation may be necessary.

Procedure:

Makeup is removed and the face is washed. Topical compounded anesthetic cream is applied and once the face is anesthetized, the cream is removed and the skin is cleaned with alcohol. Local anesthetic nerve blocks are administered around supraorbital, supratrochlear, infraorbital, paranasal, and mental nerves. Local anesthetic infiltration or tumescent is administered around the lateral periphery of the face.

Deliver 2 pulses of energy (double stack) with 30% overlap and double pass (2 passes).

The patient's facial muscles occasionally may contract upon delivery of RF.

Patient may develop pinpoint bleeding from a few of the microneedles.

Post procedure: Triple antibiotic ointment is applied. Later, the patient applies triple antibiotic ointment 4 times per day for 3 days or until the microneedle holes are no longer visible. The patient is usually red for 1 day and the skin may show microneedle holes for a few days.

3 Thermal Reduction of Fat

Freezing cryolipolysis
Laser Diode 1060 nm
Radiofrequency
Ultrasound

There are many devices which are applied externally to the skin to reduce unwanted fat. These devices use either cold or laser or radiofrequency or ultrasound to injure the fat cells which leads to fat cell apoptosis which leads to fat reduction. These devices are often used on submental fat or on unwanted fat on the body such as the abdomen, thighs, flanks, back, and elsewhere.

4 Thermal Breakdown of Fat with Internal Probe Which Assists with Liposuction

4.1 Internal Probe to Breakdown Fat

Laser Assisted liposuction
Ultrasound assisted liposuction

These devices employ a probe that is placed internally though a skin incision. The probe is placed directly into the unwanted fat. The device delivers energy in the form of laser or ultrasound which helps melt the fat which allows for ease of fat removal with liposuction.

4.2 Internal Probe Breakdown Fat and External Probe to Tighten Skin

RF assisted lipolysis

This device uses two electrode probes. One internal electrode probe is placed internally though a skin incision and into the unwanted fat. Once external electrode probe is placed atop the skin. The RF passes through the skin from one electrode to the other electrode which stimulates collagen production in the skin between the probes for slight skin tightening. The internal probe also melts the fat which allows for ease of fat removal with liposuction.

5 Conclusions

Intense pulsed light, radiofrequency micro needling, radiofrequency, and ultrasound offer nonsurgical facial rejuvenation. These energy-based devices add to lasers (described in the next chapter) and the overall armamentarium of aesthetic treatments for the eyelids and midface region. Understanding their scope and context with surgical alternatives is important.

References

1. Toyos R, Toyos M, Willcox J, Mulliniks H, Hoover J. Evaluation of the safety and efficacy of intense pulsed light treatment with meibomian gland expression of the upper eyelids for dry eye disease. Photobiomodul Photomed Laser Surg. 2019;37(9):527–31.
2. DryEyeMaster. Periman IPL Protocol – Video 1 of 6. In: YouTube. 2018. https://www.youtube.com/watch?v=oCCDVgFB3Lg. Accessed 7 July 2022.
3. DryEyeMaster. Periman IPL Protocol: Pearls and Preparation - Video 2 of 6 In: YouTube. 2018. https://www.youtube.com/watch?v=2fVl22vTfsA. Accessed 7 July 2022.
4. DryEyeMaster. Periman IPL Protocol: Rosacea Treatment - Video 3 of 6 In: YouTube. 2018. https://www.youtube.com/watch?v=nBqq0xNMt6Q. Accessed 7 July 2022.
5. DryEyeMaster. Periman IPL Protocol: The Toyos Settings - Video 4 of 6 In: YouTube. 2018. https://www.youtube.com/watch?v=e2w0ENfXBoQ. Accessed 7 July 2022.
6. DryEyeMaster. Periman IPL Protocol: How to Treat the Eyelids - Video 5 of 6 In: YouTube. 2018. https://www.youtube.com/watch?v=6Yvq3QzQr0w. Accessed 7 July 2022
7. DryEyeMaster. Periman IPL Protocol: The Aesthetic Clean Up - Video 6 of 6 In: YouTube. 2018. https://www.youtube.com/watch?v=JVcB-xwPcvQ. Accessed 7 July 2022.
8. Zelickson BD, Kist D, Bernstein E, Brown DB, Ksenzenko S, Burns J, Kilmer S, Mehregan D, Pope K. Histological and ultrastructural evaluation of the effects of a radiofrequency-based nonablative dermal remodeling device: a pilot study. Arch Dermatol. 2004;140(2):204–9.

Periocular Rejuvenation with Lasers and Other Energy-Based Devices

S. Tammy Hsu, Gabriel Scott, Melanie Ho Erb and Julie Woodward

Abstract

Lasers offer an effective tool in periocular rejuvenation. Different lasers achieve different purposes, such as performing the incisions for a blepharoplasty, tightening periocular skin by selectively vaporizing tissue. This chapter will describe different laser and other energy-based options for periocular skin rejuvenation.

Keywords

Laser resurfacing · CO_2 laser · Er;YAG laser · Radiofrequency · Micro needling · Laser blepharoplasty

1 Introduction

Lasers and energy-based devices useful tools in the surgeon's armamentarium to rejuvenate the periocular area. LASER is an acronym for Light Amplification by Stimulated Emission of Radiation. Because lasers emit coherent light at a single wavelength, their effects can be focused to that specific wavelength that will be absorbed by specific tissue.

The theory of selective photothermolysis is key in understanding laser-tissue interaction [1, 2]. Human tissue contains light-absorbing substances called chromophores. The main chromophores in tissue are hemoglobin, melanin, and water, each of which has a different absorption curve: visible light around 300–600 nm is best absorbed by hemoglobin and melanin, whereas near and far infrared is best absorbed by water. For example, the CO_2 laser emits a 10,600 nm wavelength best absorbed by water. When the laser energy is specifically absorbed by the water, less of the laser energy is absorbed by the adjacent proteins and fat. This aspect of laser-tissue interaction is important in choice of laser for procedures: because the CO_2 laser is not as specific for water as the Er: YAG laser, more of its laser energy is absorbed by the surrounding proteins and fat, increasing heat, leading to more coagulation and less bleeding. When the exposure time of the laser to the tissue is less than the time it takes for the heat to diffuse to surrounding tissues (thermal diffusivity), the target area is selectively vaporized without damage to the surrounding tissues. Thus, different lasers can be used for many different purposes, such as performing the incisions for a blepharoplasty,

Illustrations by Michael Han

S. Tammy Hsu · G. Scott · J. Woodward (✉)
Duke University, Durham, USA
e-mail: juliewoodward1@mac.com

M. Ho Erb
Irvine, CA, USA

J. P. Tao (ed.), *Plastic Surgery of the Lower Eyelids*,
https://doi.org/10.1007/978-3-031-36175-3_32

tightening periocular skin by selectively vaporizing tissue.

This chapter will focus on different options for periocular skin rejuvenation via absorption of laser energy by water rather than vascular lasers that are preferentially absorbed by hemoglobin and hair removal lasers that are preferentially absorbed by melanin.

2 Anatomy of the Periocular Skin

Familiarity with the anatomical features of the lower eyelids, particular of the periocular skin, is also important for understanding the options, indications, contraindications, and potential complications for periocular rejuvenation with lasers and other energy-based devices. These anatomical differences and the imminent presence of the eyeball require that the lower eyelids be treated differently from the rest of the face to optimize surgical outcomes and avoid damage to the eye.

The lower eyelids have 4 major layers in the superior 5 mm: skin, orbicularis oculi muscle, tarsal plate, and palpebral conjunctiva. The inferior 5 mm of the lower eyelid has 7 major layers: skin, orbicularis oculi muscle, orbital septum, orbital fat, inferior sympathetic muscle, capsulopalpebral fascia, and palpebral conjunctiva [3, 4]

Eyelid skin is the thinnest skin of the human body. The periocular skin can be divided into 2 main layers: the epidermis and dermis (Table 1, Fig. 1). These layers contain important pilosebaceous appendages that serve a reservoir of new epithelial cells for re-epithelization and healing. These layers sit above the subcutaneous connective tissue layer also known as the hypodermis. A unique aspect of the eyelid is that it does not contain any subcutaneous fat in comparison to the remainder of the face that has distinct subcutaneous fat pads.

The epidermis consists of layers of keratinocytes, melanocytes, Langerhan cells, and Merkel cells. The dermis consists of collagen and includes important appendages, including eyelashes, blood vessels, nerves, and glands.

Table 1 Layers of the periocular skin

Layers	Sub-layers	Thickness (mm)* [5]
Epidermis	Stratum corneum	0.02
	Living epidermis	0.07
Dermis	Papillary dermis	0.15
	Reticular dermis	1.55

*Average thicknesses based on a 55-year-old

3 Laser Skin Resurfacing and Energy Based Devices

Laser skin resurfacing is an important option to discuss with patients considering rejuvenation of their lower eyelids. Many different types of lasers and energy-based devices are available. This chapter will focus mostly on the ablative lasers as they are often preferred for periocular rejuvenation. The ablative lasers are available as carbon dioxide (CO_2) 10,600 nm and Erbium YAG 2940 nm. Both types have peaks for water absorption. The Er: Yag is nearly 20 times more specific for water than the CO_2. This allows the Er: Yag to vaporize tissue very precisely with minimal heat dissipation, hence less coagulation and potentially more bleeding. CO_2 is less specific for water so more heat is created when surrounding proteins absorb more laser energy, thus there is more heat and so more coagulation and less bleeding. There is potentially more skin contraction at the price of possibly prolonged post-operative erythema. The increased coagulation with the CO_2 beam makes laser incisional surgery possible with the CO_2 beam, but not an Er: Yag beam.

3.1 Ablative Laser Skin Resurfacing

Ablative laser skin resurfacing is a useful adjunct for lower eyelid blepharoplasty. It can be used to treat photodamaged skin with rhytids in a uniform manner and contract festoons. It can also be used to tighten upper eyelid skin in patients with mild dermatochalasis. Fractional lasers can even release contracted scars such as from acne or burns to improve ectropion.

The pre-operative evaluation for ablative laser skin resurfacing should include assessment of Fitzpatrick skin pigmentation scale 1–6, and Glogau photodamage/wrinkle scale 1–4. Higher Fitzpatrick skin types may be more prone to pigmentary disturbances. A thorough medical history should be taken. Retinoids may be used up until the day of the procedure but should be stopped for 3–4 weeks afterwards. Topical antioxidants may be used up to the day of the procedure and continued daily throughout the immediate post-operative healing. Patients with a history of keloids should know that keloid formation are extremely rare on the face, but an infection or severe allergic reaction to the topical emollients used after laser could cause scarring. Patients with severe itching with wool sweaters could have allergy to lanolin that is included in some emollients. Previous aggressive chemical peels such as phenol could result in loss of appendages and hence delayed healing after laser.

Making sure that the patient understands and can tolerate the expected post-operative healing process is paramount, as even a light fractional treatment can require a week to re-epithelialize and is followed by weeks of redness. Typically, patients are told not to wear makeup for 10 days and to expect mild erythema for 4–6 months. Patients should understand that erythema is expected.

Patients should be counseled that festoons are often reduced but may not eliminated with lasers and energy-based devices. Additional passes of laser may be necessary and prolonged erythema, hypopigmentation, and scarring are risks with more aggressive laser. They may be best treated by more than one session of laser spaced apart by 6 or more months.

Relative contraindications to ablative laser skin resurfacing include collagen vascular disease (scleroderma, systemic lupus erythematosus) and recent use of oral tretinoin, and some darker Fitzpatrick type skin types.

In cases of patients with uncorrected lower eyelid laxity or prior lower eyelid transcutaneous blepharoplasty, care must be taken to avoid lower eyelid ectropion. In patients with prior treatments that may damage dermal appendages, such as isotretinoin use or history of deep dermal peels, proceed with caution as they can have delayed healing and increased risk of scarring.

Absolute contraindications include active infections, herpes lesions, and unrealistic expectations. Active herpes simplex is an absolute contraindication. All full-face laser patients should be treated with oral valacyclovir 1000 mg/day until post-operative day 10. The dose should be doubled or tripled if the patient breaks through with an infection.

Dysplastic nevi or other lesions that could have malignant potential should be recognized and biopsied prior to laser. Lasers are also contraindicated in melasma.

Ablative laser types can be divided into the traditional and fractional types. The traditional ablative laser removes 100% of the epithelium but vaporizes only 50–75 microns of tissue in depth as it provides heat and coagulation to another 250 microns deep. Fractional ablative lasers vaporize micro-ablative columns (MACs) up to 700–1000 microns in depth into the tissue while leaving non-lasered tissue between the MACs. This undisturbed tissue allows for faster healing with less post-operative erythema than traditional ablative lasers. Depending on the device, the columns are usually 120–300 microns in diameter. The 120-micron lasers can penetrate deeper because they concentrate more energy into a smaller spot. Most lasers allow the computer pattern generators to be set to vary the density of spots per cm^2. Additional passes can be placed to increase the density. For patients with diffuse superficial pigment such as lentigos, the traditional ablative laser is preferred to strip off the pigment in the epithelium. Both the traditional and fractional ablative lasers are available in CO_2 and Er: YAG. The chromophore for both is water. The CO_2 laser induces less bleeding because it is absorbed by proteins and fat, increasing heat and thus coagulation. The Er: YAG laser is more specific for water, and thus less is absorbed by the adjacent proteins.

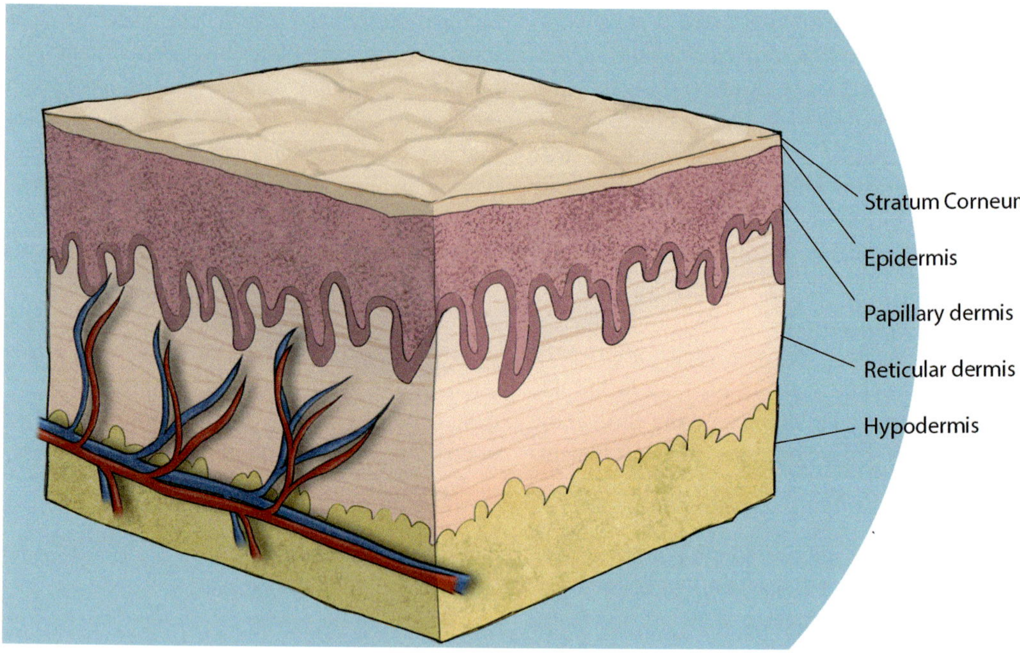

Fig. 1 Layers of the skin

Anesthetic options include topical, regional nerve blocks, or general anesthesia. Topical anesthesia with lidocaine cream can be applied to the surgical areas and then removed prior to the procedure. Subcutaneous infiltration with local anesthetic is usually sufficient for periocular resurfacing, but the introduction of water with this injection may require higher settings with the laser because the hydrated tissue will absorb more laser energy. Alternatively, treatments done just with topical anesthetic may utilize lower laser energy settings. Regional nerve blocks can be applied to the supraorbital, supratrochlear, infraorbital, nasal, zygomaticotemporal, zygomaticofacial, and mental nerves. Local infiltration from the modiolus to the jawline may be necessary. For patients with low pain thresholds for full-face treatments with ablative CO_2 laser, intravenous sedation or general anesthesia can be helpful.

Prior to starting the laser treatment, a couple precautionary steps should be followed. OSHA rules require laser safe drapes and a warning laser sign on the door of the laser room. Eye protection for the patient and staff is also required. Eye protection for the patient can consist of a stainless-steel David-Baker eyelid clamp/retractor, a Jagger plate, or laser-protective contact lens. Supplemental oxygen should be turned off. The laser should be tested on a wet tongue depressor to ensure coaxial beam and correct settings. The patient's skin should be prepared in a sterile manner.

The laser settings depend on the brand of laser used so detailed settings are beyond the scope of this chapter. Shallow rhytids usually require only a single pass, whereas moderate to deep rhytids may require double or even triple passes. Festoons and the perioral area can usually be resurfaced with 2–4 passes. Only one pass should be applied on the inferior tarsal plate to avoid ectropion. After each pass, exfoliation is performed for the traditional laser resurfacing prior to the next pass. To avoid demarcation lines, deliver the laser in a feathered fashion meaning subsequent passes are placed within the borders of previous passes. At the end of the procedure, a bland emollient ointment is applied to the treated areas. Figure 2 shows an example of a patient before and after

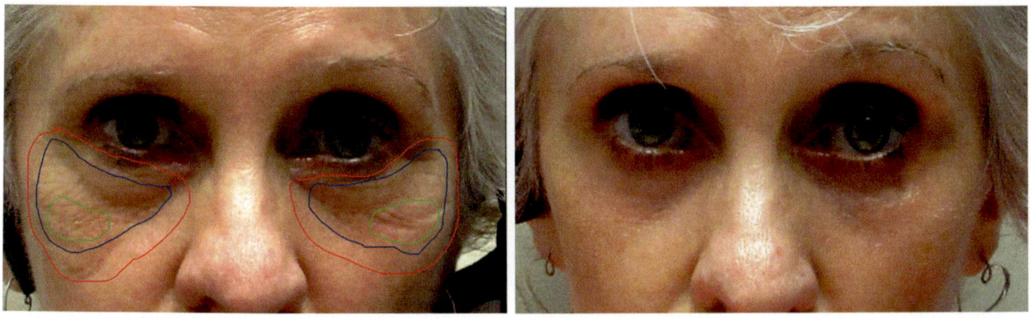

Fig. 2 The pre-operative (left) and post-operative (right) photo of a patient before and after a lower eyelid blepharoplasty with laser skin resurfacing. The markings in the pre-operative photo show the areas to deliver the first (red), second (blue), and third (green) passes of laser in a feathered fashion

a lower eyelid blepharoplasty with laser skin resurfacing; the markings in the pre-operative photo show the areas to deliver the first, second, and third passes of laser in a feathered fashion.

Post-operative care for ablative laser treatment includes using vinegar soaks (1 teaspoon distilled white vinegar to 1 cup distilled water) with reapplication of topical Aquaphor every 2 hours to help prevent infection for the first week. The vinegar water mixture provides weak acetic acid that is anti-bacterial. It is used on a gauze to gently wipe off the old ointment so fresh ointment can then be applied every 2–3 hours while the patient is awake. It is decreased to 4 times per day at the 7-day mark and mineral sunblock is applied instead of the emollient. Makeup can be applied starting 10 days post-operatively when soaks are stopped.

3.2 Non-ablative Skin Resurfacing

Non-ablative can be divided into fractional and non-fractional types. The fractional lasers use thousands of microthermal zones to create columns of coagulated tissue, rather than ablated tissue. Compared to ablative lasers, the healing is faster because the zones of unheated tissue start the repair rapidly. However, less effect is noted, and multiple treatments are often required. The indications and contraindications are like those for ablative laser.

3.3 Energy-Based Devices

The goal of energy-based devices is to tighten tissue by stimulating new collagen and elastin through the creation of a sub-epidermal wound. The advantages of energy-based devices include the ability to use with any Fitzpatrick skin type because the low risk of post-inflammatory hyperpigmentation. The results are subtle, and thus not meant as a replacement for those who need surgery.

The energy-based devices are mainly categorized into radiofrequency, microfocused ultrasound, plasma resurfacing and most recently, micro-coring technologies. Safety-wise, currently no eye shields exist that can protect the eyes from ultrasound energy, so it is not recommended for use on the eyelids. The FDA approvals are to lift rather than to resurface. Radiofrequency can be monopolar without needles but with a grounding device applied, or bipolar with microneedling where the positive and negative poles are introduced at preset depths into the skin before their energy is applied to create heat.

Plasma pens create a series of individually applied 1 mm spots of electrostatic energy through a probe where oxygen and nitrogen gases are combined to create an arc of plasma which heats the skin without direct contact. It is technically FDA approved for cutting tissue, but for not for skin rejuvenation, so its use is considered off-label.

Micro-coring is now a treatment with no heating that removes tiny columns of tissue with hollow needles that are too small to leave scars. Reviews of this novel treatment in the periocular area are still pending.

Broad Band Light (BBL) and Intense Pulsed Light (IPL) are also commonly used as part of plastic surgery of the lower eyelids. These are described in chapter "Light and Thermal Devices for Lower Eyelid and Facial Rejuvenation".

4 Combination Devices

Some machines combine non-ablative 1470 nm lasers with broad band light delivered simultaneously for optimal results. Also, 1927 nm lasers are combined with the 1550 nm laser emitted simultaneously for more dramatic results than either laser alone.

5 Potential Complications of Lower Eyelid Laser Skin Resurfacing

Complications that can occur with laser skin resurfacing performed as part of lower eyelid surgery include the following: scar, infection, ectropion, ocular injury, pigmentary changes, contact dermatitis, acne, milia, and more [6, 7].

Scarring or infection can occur due to an overly aggressive and deep laser treatment, or due to infection or severe contact dermatitis during the time that the skin is re-epithelizing which can take about 7–10 days for a fully ablative laser treatment. The epithelium is replenished from the hair follicles and pores, and thus, the areas of the face with fewer of these appendages, such as the angle of the jaw and neck, are more prone to scarring. In a study by Kim et al., 0.9% of patients had a small scar that resolved after local steroid injections. When scarring causes severe contraction of the anterior and middle lamella of the eyelid, ectropion can occur. Kim et al. revealed no cases of ectropion out of 424 cases. Severe ectropion may require surgery such as a full thickness skin graft with a tarsal strip to correct. Infections such as atypical mycobacterium and fungus can be difficult and may require prolonged treatment.

The proximity of the eyeball to the treatment area puts ocular injury high on the list of potential side effects. CO_2 and Erbium lasers can penetrate the cornea and create a hole in the eye. Thus, steel eye shields should be used for eye protection.

Hyper- and hypopigmentation can occur with any laser or energy-based device. Hyperpigmentation is common, whereas hypopigmentation is uncommon and usually due to fibrosis. Patients with Fitzpatrick skin type 3 or darker are at increased risk for post-inflammatory hyperpigmentation (PIH), which can start around 3–4 weeks after treatment. Kim et al. reported that PIH occurred in 9.4% of patients of whom 89.9% were Fitzpatrick skin types 2–3 [6].

Treatment of hyperpigmentation can involve topical and oral agents. Topical agents such as hydroquinone 2–8%, tranexamic acid, antioxidants, kojic acid, and others can be introduced at 3–4 weeks after laser treatment. Oral tranexamic acid 325 mg daily or twice a day can also be used, although patients should be screened for increased risk of clotting prior to starting treatment.

6 Conclusions

Overall, periocular laser and energy-based device treatments add to the therapeutic armamentarium of the aesthetic eyelid and facial surgeon. These devices produce results that are associated with high patient satisfaction with low complication rates when performed properly.

References

1. "Laser-tissue interaction: Interaction of the laser beam with living tissue." Laser Safety Training Program for Health Professionals. Leonardo da Vinci programme. URL: http://www3.univ-lille2.fr/safelase/english.html Last accessed: 30 Jul 2022.
2. Zahra A, Alhabee M. Laser dental treatment techniques. Oral Cancer. IntechOpen; 2019;2–16. https://www.intechopen.com/chapters/64030
3. Korn BS, et al. Chapter 9: facial and eyelid anatomy. Oculofacial Plastic and Orbital Surgery. Basic and Clinical Science Course, 2020–2021 ed. American Academy of Ophthalmology; 2020;151–171.
4. Goodman, RL. Orbit, eyelids, and ocular adnexa. Ophtho Notes. Thieme 2003:38–9.
5. Campbell CL, et al. 3D Monte Carlo radiation transfer modelling of photodynamic therapy. *Biophotonics South America*, vol. 9531. SPIE, 2015.
6. Kim JS, et al. Patient satisfaction and management of postoperative complications following ablative carbon dioxide laser resurfacing of the lower eyelids. Ophthalmic Plast Reconstr Surg. 2021;37(5):450–6.
7. Metelitsa AI, Alster TS. Fractionated laser skin resurfacing treatment complications: a review. Dermatol Surg. 2010;36(3):299–306. https://doi.org/10.1111/j.1524-4725.2009.01434.x. Epub 2010 Jan 19 PMID: 20100273.

Neurotoxins to the Lower Eyelids

Zahra A. Markatia, Shanlee M. Stevens, Christopher R. Dermarkarian, Steve Yoelin and Wendy W. Lee

Abstract

Repeated contraction of periorbital muscles over time can contribute to aging via the formation of hyperkinetic facial lines better known as wrinkles. Superficial injection of neurotoxin such as botulinum toxin A (BTX-A) into the lower eyelid transiently corrects these hyperkinetic facial lines or a mounded, redundant pretarsal orbicularis oculi muscle. Lower eyelid injections can also be used to widen the palpebral fissure. Caution must be taken with the administration techniques of these injections to prevent potential adverse complications from treatment. This chapter describes neurotoxin use in the lower eyelids.

Supplementary Information The online version contains supplementary material available at https://doi.org/10.1007/978-3-031-36175-3_33.

Z. A. Markatia · S. M. Stevens · W. W. Lee (✉)
Bascom Palmer Eye Institute, Miami, FL, USA
e-mail: wlee@med.miami.edu

Z. A. Markatia
e-mail: zahra.markatia@med.miami.edu

S. M. Stevens
e-mail: sms415@miami.edu

C. R. Dermarkarian · S. Yoelin
University of California Irvine, Irvine, CA, USA
e-mail: cdermark@hs.uci.edu

Keywords

Neurotoxin · Botulinum · Hyperkinetic lines · Wrinkles · Injectable · Lower eyelid · Aging

1 Introduction and Clinical Evaluation

Visible signs of aging such as the gradual appearance of hyperkinetic facial lines, better known as wrinkles, under the eyes arise mainly from repeated contraction of facial muscles over time. Specifically, the action that contributes most to under-eye wrinkles is contraction of the orbicularis oculi muscle. Simple movements including smiling, talking, and even laughing can cause these changes. Hyperkinetic lines, in comparison to younger skin, represent changes in the elastic properties of the dermis layer of the skin, in which ultraviolet B radiation can cause deterioration of intermediate fibers [1, 2]. A thickened pretarsal orbicularis oculi muscle can appear as a raised fold, also described as a jelly roll, (Video 1) These infraorbital wrinkles and folds for may be targeted with injection of neurotoxin both to to smoothen existing lines and prevent the formation of additional fine lines.

Botulinum toxin A (BTX-A) injection is a type of neurotoxin treatment that treats

J. P. Tao (ed.), *Plastic Surgery of the Lower Eyelids*,
https://doi.org/10.1007/978-3-031-36175-3_33

under-eye wrinkles by targeting the orbicularis oculi muscle. BTX-A acts on the muscle by temporarily inducing paralysis by blocking acetylcholine release from cholinergic nerve endings, relaxing the surrounding skin and widening the eye. In addition to its cosmetic use, BTX-A can also be used to treat conditions such as blepharospasm, cervical dystonia, and strabismus. These injections, although effective, are not permanent, as the impact on skin only lasts between four and six months [3].

While BTX-A is commonly implemented for peri- and supraorbital skin changes such as crow's feet, forehead lines, and frown lines between the eyebrows, it is less commonly used to treat infraorbital wrinkles. This is mainly because the muscle movement under the eye is often less significant than the forehead. As well, weakening this muscle puts patients at risk for dry eyes and tear pump function abnormalities.

Higher doses of neurotoxin injections can cause a variety of side effects, ranging from ptosis or fat bulges near the injection site to more serious side effects such as shortness of breath, facial asymmetry, and/or blurry vision [4]. For this reason, the choice of dose, dilution, and placement is critical for each individual toxin. Studies show that conservatively dosed lower-eyelid BTX-A injections have proven to be the most safe and effective overall [5] Pilot studies have also indicated that only patients with brisk lower-lid snap test results serve as strong candidates for infraorbital botulinum toxin injections, as the rest are more likely to face unwanted outcomes due to increased eyelid laxity. On the other hand, patients with a history of lower eyelid puffiness can present with worsened symptoms after neurotoxin treatment and are therefore contraindicated to infraorbital injections. A history of lower eyelid blepharoplasty may be contraindication as well. Patients with dry eye are advised to avoid BTX-A injections because dry eye syndrome is a potential complication of this treatment [6]. Lastly, younger patients tend to demonstrate better responses to BTX-A injections than older patients [7].

2 Technique/Procedure Steps

To mitigate discomfort with needle injections, an ice pack and/or the delivery of topical anesthesia prior to injection can be helpful. Caution must be taken in the infraorbital region to avoid contact with the eye because these creams can be toxic to or irritate the ocular surface.

The snap test should be performed to measure muscle tone by pulling the lower eyelid inferiorly while the patient looks straight ahead and releasing it to observe the recoil [6]. After confirming a brisk response, the surface of the skin should be cleaned with rubbing alcohol or hypochlorous acid. The patients should be seated comfortably with good head support, laying at a degree that allows the provider proper visualization of and access to the skin of the lower eyelid. The patient can be asked to close his or her eyes tightly to help visualize the muscle fibers of the orbicularis oculi and the associated hyperkinetic facial lines. The patient is then asked to look up to expose the lower eyelid and put the skin on stretch.

The non-injecting hand should then gently tighten the surrounding skin so that vessels below the skins surface can be visualized and the needle can penetrate the skin without tension. A ½ inch 30-gauge needle (some practitioners use a ½ inch, 31-guage, 32-guage or 33-gauge needle) is inserted in the subdermal plane parallel to the eyelid margin at the mid-pupillary line. Either 1 central injection or 2 paramedian injections can be given. (Video 2) To avoid risk of bruising or injury, insert the needle from the side rather than directly at the lower eyelid [6] (Fig. 1). Superficial injection of two to six units of botulinum toxin in the infraorbital rhytids is recommended to soften hyperkinetic facial lines as well as reduce bruising. After the injection is complete, the needle can be withdrawn, creating expected, raised wheels just under the skin [8] (Fig. 2).

Minimal compression can then be exerted with a cotton swab, with a particular avoidance of rubbing or pushing the areas of swelling to

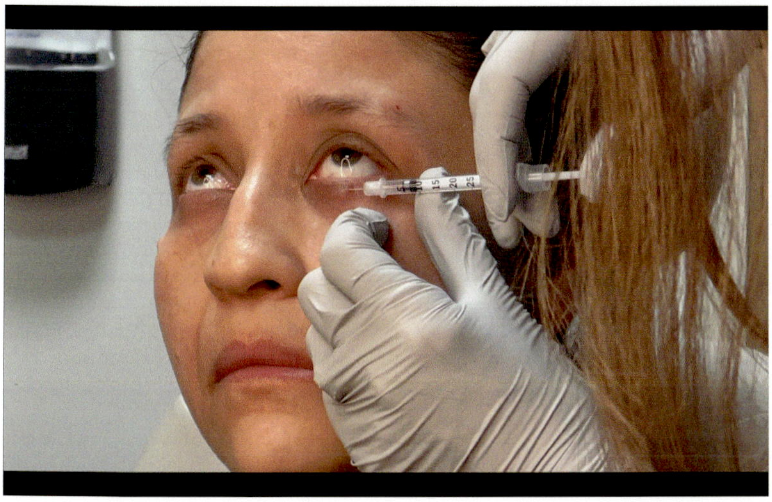

Fig. 1 Neurotoxin injection to the pretarsal orbicularis oculi muscle to reduce a pretarsal jelly roll. Note needle axis away from the globe

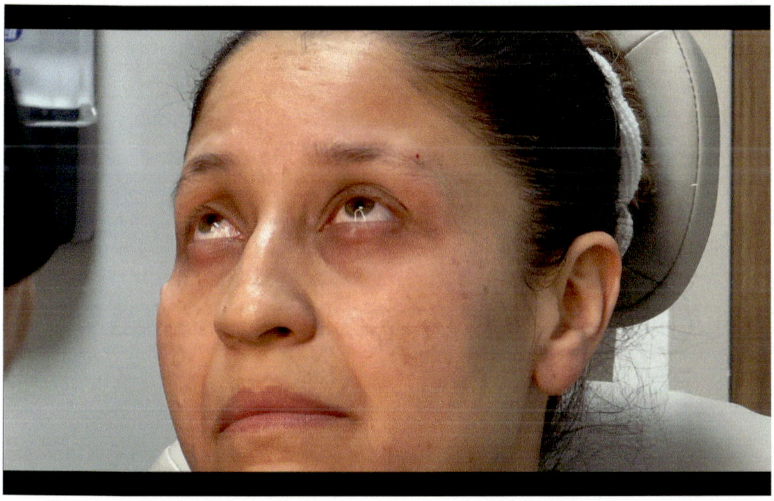

Fig. 2 Immediately post neurotoxin injection with small wheal at injection site

avoid a stronger diffusion of the neurotoxin. Ice packs may be applied over the next twenty-four hours to reduce swelling, so long as the patient is advised not to apply pressure to the injection points and increase the spread. A follow-up appointment can be made in two weeks to allow for the provider to assess the patient's response to treatment and provide additional touch-ups, if necessary.

It is important to avoid injecting too laterally and too deeply along the cheek because this can cause a smile deformity due to zygomaticus major paralysis. A consequence of injecting too large of a dose or promoting spread of the toxin could be a lack of synchrony between the movement of the periorbital skin and the raising of the cheek, creating a shelf look. It's important to note, therefore, that administration of BTX-A along with other neuromuscular agents such as curare may increase the magnitude of the toxin's effect from the start. Dry eye is another common complication of BTX-A injections, led to by the lower eyelid falling away from the eye resulting in reduced eyelid closure. To avoid this, the snap test should be used to assess the elasticity of the skin under the eye before performing injections [8]. Adequate research on the effect of botulinum toxin on pregnant mothers has not been performed, for which reason it is contraindicated in this population [3]. In all patients, extreme side effects including muscle weakness, vision problems, or dizziness after injection warrant emergent referral to an ophthalmologist for further treatment.

3 Conclusion

Neorotoxins offer a non-surgical rejuvenation to the lower eyelids. Its effects for transient improvement of lateral crow's feet are well known. Neurotoxin given conservatively and carefully to the lower eyelid may soften fine lines, reduce a prominent pretarsal orbicularis mound, or subtly widen the palpebral aperture effectively in select patients with good eyelid tone and no dry eye.

References

1. Kim EJ, Reeck JB, Maas CS. A validated rating scale for hyperkinetic facial lines. Arch Facial Plast Surg. 2004;6(4):253–6. https://doi.org/10.1001/archfaci.6.4.253.
2. Sano T, Kume T, Fujimura T, et al. The formation of wrinkles caused by transition of keratin intermediate filaments after repetitive UVB exposure. Arch Dermatol Res. 2005;296(8):359–65. https://doi.org/10.1007/s00403-004-0533-9.
3. Flynn TC, Carruthers JA, Carruthers JA, et al. Botulinum A toxin (Botox) in the lower eyelid: dose-finding study. Dermatol Surg. 2003;29(9): 943–50; discussion 950–1. https://doi.org/10.1046/j.1524-4725.2003.29257.x.
4. Jia Z, Lu H, Yang X, et al. Adverse events of botulinum toxin type a in facial rejuvenation: a systematic review and meta-analysis. Aesthetic Plast Surg. 2016;40(5):769–77. https://doi.org/10.1007/s00266-016-0682-1.
5. Lowe NJ, Shah A, Lowe PL, et al. Dosing, efficacy and safety plus the use of computerized photography for botulinum toxins type A for upper facial lines. J Cosmet Laser Ther. 2010;12(2):106–11. https://doi.org/10.3109/14764170903480013.
6. Ozgur O, Murariu D, Parsa AA, et al. Dry eye syndrome due to botulinum toxin type-a injection: guideline for prevention. Hawaii J Med Public Health. 2012;71(5):120–3 PMID: 22737648.
7. Flynn TC, Carruthers JA, Carruthers JA. Botulinum-A toxin treatment of the lower eyelid improves infraorbital rhytides and widens the eye. Dermatol Surg. 2001;27(8):703–8. https://doi.org/10.1046/j.1524-4725.2001.01038.x.
8. Kaplan JB. Consideration of muscle depth for botulinum toxin injections: a three-dimensional approach. Plast Surg Nurs. 2017;37(1):32–8. https://doi.org/10.1097/PSN.0000000000000178.

Injectable Fillers for Lower Eyelid Rejuvenation

Shanlee M. Stevens, Zahra A. Markatia, Christopher R. Dermarkarian, Steven G. Yoelin and Wendy W. Lee

Abstract

Correction of the lower eyelid hollows is one of the most common cosmetic patient requests. Over time, volume loss, tissue descent and bony resorption in this area can cause a prominent tear trough deformity and a discrepancy between the eyelid and cheek, either from a sunken and excavated appearance of the lower eyelid. Orbital fat prolapse can accentuate the transition between these two areas. This chapter describes non-surgical rejuvenation of the lower eyelids with dermal fillers.

Illustrations by Michael Han

Supplementary Information The online version contains supplementary material available at https://doi.org/10.1007/978-3-031-36175-3_34.

S. M. Stevens · Z. A. Markatia · C. R. Dermarkarian · S. G. Yoelin (✉)
Private Practice, Newport Beach, CA, USA
e-mail: syoelinmd@gmail.com

Z. A. Markatia
University of Miami, School of Medicine, Miami, FL, USA

C. R. Dermarkarian
Gavin Herbert Eye Institute, University of California, Irvine, Irvine, CA, USA

S. M. Stevens · W. W. Lee
Bascom Palmer Eye Institute, University of Miami, Miami, FL, USA

Keywords

Rejuvenation · Filler · Injectable · Tear trough · Lower eyelid · Hyaluronic acid

1 Introduction and Clinical Evaluation

The youthful eye has a short, full lower eyelid with a smooth transition to the cheek. With age, volume loss in the periorbital tissues and lengthening of the lower eyelid can creates a tired and hollowed appearance. Descent of the cheek and thinning of the skin can also contribute to an aged look. The goal with dermal filler is to restore youthful volume and contour.

Careful evaluation of the lower eyelid will help determine if a patient is a good candidate for lower eyelid filler. The first aspect to evaluate is skin quality. Thick, smooth skin will have a better result than thin, wrinkled, or inelastic skin [1]. Significant rhytidosis can accentuate the depth of the trough and marked laxity may lead to excess product use. Skin pigmentation should also be considered as hyperpigmentation can create an illusion of trough depth. The lower eyelid has a rich vascular plexus and may be a site of venous pooling. Filler can improve shadowing from venous blood but will not improve eyelid skin hyperpigmentation [1, 2].

J. P. Tao (ed.), *Plastic Surgery of the Lower Eyelids*,
https://doi.org/10.1007/978-3-031-36175-3_34

Other factors to consider are lower eyelid edema and fat prolapse. Certain materials such as some hyaluronic acids are hydrophilic and can cause fluid accumulation and retention. Filler may also compress lymphatic structures, worsening lower eyelid edema [2]. The orbital fat pads are difficult to correct non-surgically, and injection can exacerbate puffiness. The higher degree of fat pad prolapse decreases the likelihood of achieving a good result with filler [2] Lastly, some patients complain of a jelly roll or prominent orbicularis oculi that may be amenable to neurotoxin but not filler [3].

Hyaluronic acid (HA) fillers are the mainstay of treatment for the infraorbital hollows, as they have proven to be safe, effective, produce high patient satisfaction, and are easily reversible [4, 5]. An important property to consider is the G′ (G prime) of the product, which defines the stiffness of the gel. A product with higher G′ is more resistant to deformation and, if over-injected, may cause lumpiness or blue discoloration under the thin skin of the tear trough [6]. For this reason, products such as Juvederm® (Abbvie, North Chicago, IL, USA), Volbella® (Abbvie, North Chicago, IL, USA), or Belotero® (Merz, Raleigh, NC, USA) have been used. Their lower G′ allows easier spread and molding. The varying particle size of Belotero® may decrease the chances of Tyndall effect, a light bluish gray discoloration of the skin. Some injectors prefer a high G′ product such as Restylane L because of its ability to stay where it is put.

Contraindications to lower eyelid filler include unrealistic patient expectations, known allergy to the material, active dermatologic conditions, infections at or near the injection site, and pregnancy or lactation. It is important to obtain any history of prior permanent fillers such as silicone or acrylic polymers as these can alter the anatomy. If able, patients should hold non-steroidal anti-inflammatory drugs, aspirin, vitamin E, gingko biloba for five days prior to injection to prevent excessive bleeding and bruising [2].

2 Technique/Procedure Steps

An ice pack may be applied to the lower eyelid and cheek a few minutes prior to injection, as well as a topical anesthetic cream for 15 min. Rarely is an injected anesthetic necessary. Care should be taken not to alter the tear trough hollow with such injections. The skin should be appropriately cleansed with a sterilizing solution that is non-toxic to the cornea, such as hypochlorous acid, isopropyl alcohol or povidone iodine. Chlorhexidine should be avoided or used very cautiously near the eyes as it can cause keratopathy. The patient should be positioned sitting up so that the area is subject to full gravitational forces, and the lighting is sufficient to identify anatomic landmarks.

The non-injecting hand can be used to support and balance the syringe, without creating tension on the area and obliterating the contour deformities. Injections can be done with a cannula or with a needle. Some products are packaged with a 30- or 32-gauge needle, which is appropriate for this area. Some injectors prefer to backload the product into an insulin syringe as well. The advantage of using a needle in this area is it provides better precision but tends to lead to more bruising. Aspirating prior to injection will help confirm the needle is not in a blood vessel, although vascular compromise in the region is rare. Whether using a needle or cannula, the product is injected into the pre-periosteal plane. Deeper injection is important to reduce visibility of product and Tyndall effect which can cause bluish discoloration [2]. Injection is continued in a linear fashion while withdrawing the needle, careful not to inject too superficially. It is important to inject cautiously when around the infraorbital foramen to avoid injury to the neovascular bundle [2]. Utilizing low volumes per injection can forestall irregularities or inadvertent vascular occlusion.

Alternatively, the needle can be inserted at the mid-pupillary line about 1.5 cm below the orbital rim (Fig. 2A, B). Inserting below the

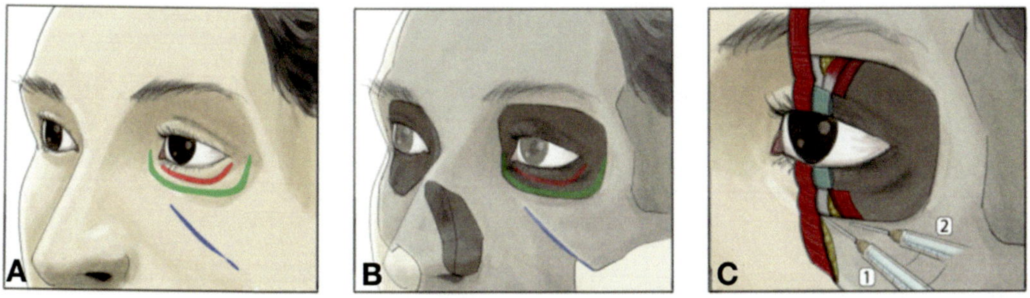

Fig. 1 A and B. The three periorbital hollows include the septal confluence (red), the orbital rim (green), and the zygomatic (blue). C. Dissected tissue layers of the face showing needle entry into the (1) preperiosteal and (2) subperiosteal planes

tear trough reduces risk of bruising by avoiding the rich vascular plexus of the lower eyelid. The needle is directed diagonally toward the medial canthus and inserted fully into the preperiosteal (Fig. 1C) plane. It is important to protect the globe by palpating the inferior orbital rim with the non-injecting hand. A depot of filler is deposited until the deformity is corrected or even slightly under-corrected. Additional depots can be injected by directing the needle towards the pupil and lateral canthus as needed. It is better to err on the side of under-correction than over-correction.

Tear trough deformities can also be corrected with a 25- or 27-gauge cannula, which may have less risk of neurovascular injury and bruising. However, it may be more difficult to stay in the supraperiosteal plane with a cannula compared to a needle. The entry point is determined by the intersection of two imaginary lines: one from the lateral canthus downward and one directed inferolateral along the nasojugal fold, although the port location depends on the location of the area to be filled (Fig. 2C). The skin is pierced at a 90-degree angle with a needle that is 1 or 2 gauges larger than the cannula. The cannula is inserted until it reaches the periosteum. The cannula is rotated until it is directed towards the medial canthus, and filler is deposited in a retrograde manner until the depression is corrected. Additional lines are added moving laterally in a fan-shape until the cannula is directed vertically, in-line with the mid-pupillary line. If the injector also wishes to access the eyelid/cheek transition, an entry point in the upper malar tissue below the orbital rim in line with the center point of the upper eyelid could also be considered [7].

A combined needle and cannula approach may be used to tailor the amount of product used and individualize the technique. Jaishree Sharad described injecting with a needle using a vertical subperiosteal depot technique at the mid-pupillary line and lateral tear trough. This reduces the hollow and stretches the skin over the medial tear trough, which helps to deposit less product in this less-forgiving area. A 23-gauge needle is then inserted 2 cm below the orbital rim in line with the lateral canthus, and a blunt-tipped cannula can be inserted and advanced towards the medial canthus (Fig. 2D). Filler is injected in a retrograde fashion in this area until the defect is corrected [8].

Volume injected per eyelid can range from 0.1 to 0.5 mL, but most patients need 0.2–03 mL [2]. The product is then gently massaged either with fingertips or a cotton-tipped applicator to contour the gel and disperse irregularities. Ice packs may be used for the next 24 h. A follow-up appointment should be made 2 weeks post-injection to determine the need for a touch up.

One advantage of HA fillers is their ease of reversibility with hyaluronidase. Hyaluronidase is an enzyme that breaks down hyaluronic acid and may be used to dissolve HA in the setting of lumps, asymmetries, overcorrection, migrated filler, or adverse events [6, 8] There are two commercially available hyaluronidases, Hylenex (Halozyme, San Diego, CA, USA) and Vitrase

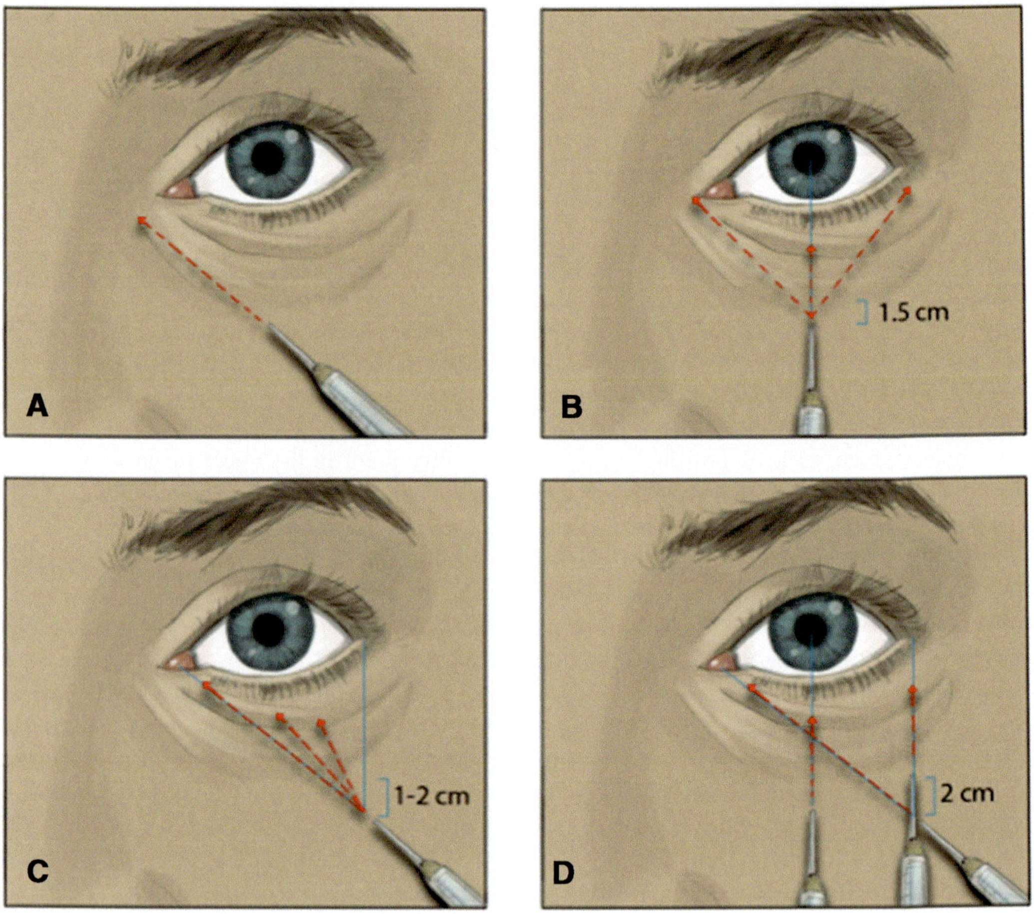

Fig. 2 A. The insertion point for lower eyelid filler with needle technique is found 1.5 mm below the orbital rim at the mid pupillary line. B. The needle can be directed upwards towards the pupil and lateral towards the lateral canthus as needed to correct the deformity. C. The entry point for the cannula technique is found at the intersection of a line running inferiorly from the lateral canthus and a line running along the nasojugal fold. Filler is then deposited in a fan technique. D. Entry points for the combined needle and cannula technique are shown here

(Bausch & Lomb, Bridgewater, NJ, USA) [1]. Hyaluronidase may be reconstituted with saline or water with a range in volume between 1 and 10 mL depending on the amount of product and surface area requiring treatment [9]. A consensus opinion in the literature has recommended five units of hyaluronidase to break down 0.1 mL of 20 mg/mL HA [10] however other studies have shown a wide range of required amount and dose–response depending on the specific product [11]. The amount of hyaluronidase may be varied to dissolve some or all of the filler [1].

Filler injection is a relatively safe procedure with a low complication rate. However, it is important to be aware of potential complications. Adverse events of soft tissue fillers can be divided into early and late categories.

Bruising is one of the most common immediate/early-onset complications and is more commonly seen after fanning and threading techniques. The risk of bruising can be reduced by injecting slowly and compressing the area if bruising appears. Patients should discontinue anticoagulants 7–10 days prior to injection if able. After the procedure, bruising may be treated with cold compresses, or vitamin K cream. Swelling, another common early complication, may also be treated with cold compresses. Moderate swelling may benefit from NSAIDs or streptokinase/streptodornase (10,000/2500 U: 2 pills every 8 h for 3–6 days), and severe swelling can be treated with prednisone 1 mg/kg/day for 3 days. Some patients may develop a hypersensitivity reaction to the material resulting in angioedema within hours of and up to months after an injection. This should be treated with oral steroids and antihistamines [12]. It is also important to dissolve any inciting material.

Injection-site infections, although rare, are a risk with any procedure that breaks the skin surface. Common pathogens include normal skin flora such as *Staphylococcus aureus* and *Streptococcus pyogenes*. Mild infections can be treated with a two-week course of oral antibiotics, while more severe infections may require hospital admission for intravenous antibiotics. Injection of dermal filler may also lead to reactivation of herpes virus infections. Patients with a history of 3 + episodes of cold sores may be prescribed anti-herpetic medication as prophylaxis, and injection should be delayed in patients with active herpetic lesions [12].

Dysesthesias and paresthesia can be the result of direct trauma or injection to a nerve or from nerve compression by the product. The most common site of injury is the infraorbital nerve during periorbital injection. It is essential to have a knowledge of facial anatomy to avoid these complications.

Lumps and bumps can also be avoided with good technique to avoid overfill, superficial placement, and incorrect product for the indication. Lumps occurring in the early post-treatment period may be amenable to massage, however they may also require dissolution with hyaluronidase [12].

The most severe immediate complication is vascular compromise due to inadvertent intravascular injection [12] Arterial occlusion may present with immediate, disproportional pain and blanching of the skin. Venous occlusion presents with less severe, dull, or delayed pain. If vascular occlusion is suspected, the injection should be stopped immediately. An injection of high-dose hyaluronidase (200–300U) should be repeated hourly until resolution. Other vasodilators can be considered, such as nitroglycerin paste and hot packs. If the patient reports sudden, painless vision loss, therapeutic measures to treat a central retinal artery occlusion should be implemented immediately, as occlusion for more than 60–90 min can cause permanent blindness. Medical treatment is unproven, but some advise administration of topical timolol 0.5% and/or 500 mg acetazolamide to lower the intraocular pressure. 325 mg sublingual aspirin or 0.6 mg nitroglycerin can also be considered. Digital ocular massage with repeated firm pressure for 5–15 s and quick release for five minutes aims to release any embolic obstruction. If there is no visual recovery within 20 min, anterior chamber paracentesis or a retrobulbar injection of hyaluronidase can be considered [12]. Importantly, the evidence for the efficacy of these interventions is very limited and outcomes of treatments for filler induced ocular ischemia are poor. Avoidance is key. Importantly, anterior chamber paracentesis or retrobulbar injection introduces risk for iatrogenic eye injury.

Edema may also be seen as a late/delayed-onset complication. This is typically non-antibody-mediated and doesn't respond to antihistamines. The best approach is to remove or dissolve the product. Late-onset infections may also be seen causing erythema and edema, possibly due to atypical organisms such as *Mycobacteria*. If infection is suspected, a culture should be obtained to determine antibiotic coverage, and steroids should be avoided until infection is ruled out [12].

Skin discoloration weeks to months after dermal filler is another late-onset complication. Neovascularization causing reddish discoloration may result from tissue trauma and expansion and is usually amenable to laser. The Tyndall effect is a form of bluish discoloration seen when product is implanted into the superficial dermis. This can be avoided with good technique and treated by dissolving the filler with hyaluronidase. Hyperpigmentation, more

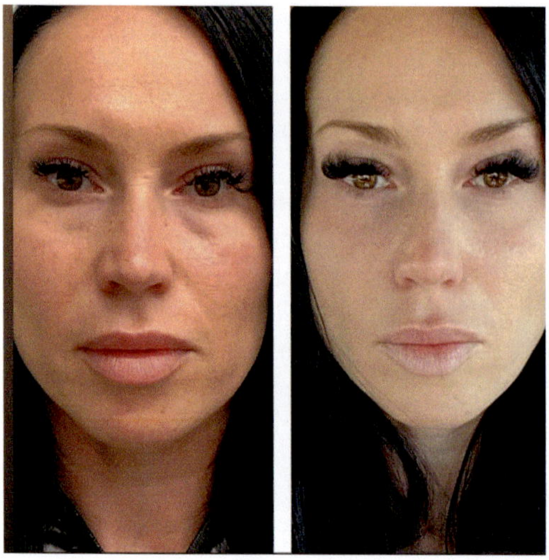

Fig. 3 Before (left) and after hyaluronic acid filler to the tear trough (photo courtesy of Maria Belen Camacho)

commonly occurring in patients with Fitzpatrick skin types IV–VI may be treated with bleaching agents such as hydroquinone or tretinoin. If resistant, chemical peels, intense pulsed light, or fractional laser may be used [12].

3 Conclusion

Injection of dermal filler is a quick, non-surgical procedure used to correct hollowing of the lower eyelid, with a goal to replace volume loss and restore a youthful contour (Fig. 3). Hyaluronic acid is preferred in the periocular region because it has been shown to be safe, result in high patient satisfaction, and is easily reversible. Knowledge of lower eyelid anatomy is important prior to injecting this region to achieve a good cosmetic result and avoid complications.

References

1. Hwang CJ, Golan S, Goldberg R. Chapter 9 - Nonsurgical brow and eyelid rejuvenation. In: Master techniques in facial rejuvenation, 2nd ed. Elsevier Inc; 2018. p. 101–6.e1. https://doi.org/10.1016/B978-0-323-35876-7.00009-1.
2. Sharad J. Dermal fillers for the treatment of tear trough deformity: A review of anatomy, treatment techniques, and their outcomes. J Cutan Aesthet Surg. 2012;5(4):229–38. https://doi.org/10.4103/0974-2077.104910.
3. Naik MN. Hills and valleys: understanding the under-eye. J Cutan Aesthet Surg. 2016;9(2):61–4. https://doi.org/10.4103/0974-2077.184048.
4. Morley AMS, Malhotra R. Use of hyaluronic acid filler for tear-trough rejuvenation as an alternative to lower eyelid surgery. Ophthalmic Plast Reconstr Surg. 2011;27(2):69–73. https://doi.org/10.1097/IOP.0b013e3181b80f93.
5. Lambros VS. Hyaluronic acid injections for correction of the tear trough deformity. Plastic and Reconstructive Surgery (1963). 2007;120(6 Suppl):74S-80S. https://doi.org/10.1097/01.prs.0000248858.26595.46.
6. Rohrich RJ, Bartlett ELm Dayan E. Practical approach and safety of hyaluronic acid fillers, plastic and reconstructive surgery. Global Open 2019;7(6):e2172. https://doi.org/10.1097/GOX.0000000000002172.
7. Anido J, Fernández JM, Genol I, Ribé N, Pérez SG. Recommendations for the treatment of tear trough deformity with cross-linked hyaluronic acid filler. J Cosmet Dermatol. 2021;20(1):6–17. https://doi.org/10.1111/jocd.13475.
8. Sharad J. Treatment of the tear trough and infraorbital hollow with hyaluronic acid fillers using both needle and cannula. Dermatologic Therapy. 2020;34(3):e13453-n/a. https://doi.org/10.1111/dth.13453.
9. Rzany B, Becker-Wegerich P, Bachmann F, Erdmann R, Wollina U. Hyaluronidase in the correction of hyaluronic acid-based fillers: a review and a recommendation for use. J Cosmet Dermatol. 2009;8(4):317–23. https://doi.org/10.1111/j.1473-2165.2009.00462.x.
10. King M, Convery C, Davies E. This month's guideline: The use of hyaluronidase in aesthetic practice (v2.4). J Clin Aesthet Dermatol. 2018;11(6):E61–8.
11. Quezada-Gaón N, Wortsman X. Ultrasound-guided hyaluronidase injection in cosmetic complications. J Eur Acad Dermatol Venereol. 2016;30(10):e39–40.
12. Urdiales-Gálvez F, Delgado NE, Figueiredo V, et al. Treatment of soft tissue filler complications: expert consensus recommendations. Aesthetic Plast Surg. 2018;42(2):498–510. https://doi.org/10.1007/s00266-017-1063-0.

Platelet Rich Plasma to the Lower Eyelids

Dan Georgescu

Abstract

Platelet Rich Plasma (PRP) injections are an emerging nonsurgical modality in facial rejuvenation. They are purported to modulate wound healing through the release of growth factors. They may be used as a standalone procedure to improve skin rhytids and color or they may improve the results of other procedures, such as micro needling or fat grafting. This chapter describes PRP for lower eyelid and facial rejuvenation.

Keywords

Platelet rich plasma · PRP

Platelet Rich Plasma (PRP) is a minimally invasive procedure that has been described for lower eyelid rejuvenation. It has been described as a stand-alone treatment or, as an adjuvant procedure to other eyelid rejuvenation treatments [1, 2].

As the name implies, platelet rich plasma is a volume of plasma that has a high concentration of platelet cells, typically above 1,000,000 per microliter. Normal blood concentration of platelets is between 150,000 and 350,000. Recent studies have shown that, although a platelet concentration of at least 1,000,000 is necessary to achieve any clinically meaningful result, higher concentrations of platelets do not correlate with improved wound healing [3].

Because PRP is derived from autologous blood, it is free of transmissible diseases and is relatively safe, although allergic reaction has been reported [4]. PRP handling can risk transmittable diseases, such as HIV and Hepatitis, if using faulty PRP devices, or those that are not FDA approved.

There are dozens of commercially available, FDA-approved devices that can produce pyrogen-free and sterile PRP of more than 1,000,000 platelets/microliter. Most but not all use the double centrifugation technique, which is considered crucial for obtaining the high platelet concentration. This involves a first (hard) spin that separates the red blood cells from the plasma, which contains the platelets, the white blood cells, and the clotting factors, and a second (soft) spin that separates the platelets and white blood cells together with a few red blood cells from the plasma.

Due to the high number of platelets in PRP, a higher concentration of growth factors is theoretically released into the surrounding tissues. There are seven known growth factors present in PRP: platelet-derived growth factor aa, bb

D. Georgescu (✉)
Uptown Clinique, Fort Lauderdale, FL, USA
e-mail: dan.oculoplastics@gmail.com

J. P. Tao (ed.), *Plastic Surgery of the Lower Eyelids*,
https://doi.org/10.1007/978-3-031-36175-3_35

and ab (PDGFaa, PDGFbb, PDGFab), epithelial growth factor (EGF), vascular endothelial growth factor (VEGF), transforming growth factor beta one (TGF-b1) and transforming growth factor beta two (TGF-b2). These growth factors are found in the PRP clot in the same native blood proportions and are surrounded by various cell adhesion molecules such as fibrin, fibronectin, and vitronectin. The blood used to produce PRP is anticoagulated immediately after harvesting (required for PRP processing) and hence the highly concentrated platelets are not activated. Clotting is required for platelet activation which happens immediately after the PRP is injected into the tissue and lasts for up to 8 days, when the platelets are depleted and disintegrated. Activated platelets release 70% of their stored growth factors in the first 10 min and 100% in the first hour. After that, the activated platelets continue to synthesize and release growth factors that stimulate cellular growth and angiogenesis.

There is a paucity of controlled studies of PRP treatment in the periocular area. Intradermal PRP application for periocular hyperpigmentation has been shown to improve infraorbital color homogeneity although it did not significantly change the melanin content, stratum corneum hydration, wrinkle volume, and visibility index [4, 5]. In addition, there seems to be a positive effect of PRP treatment on lower eyelid wrinkles, skin tone and actinic keratosis [6]. PRP purportedly hastens recovery after lower blepharoplasty by promoting wound healing although no statistically significant difference in the overall result was found in one study [7].

PRP may have optimal utility for lower eyelid rejuvenation in two settings. The first and most common use of PRP is in conjunction with micro-needling for skin rejuvenation. The

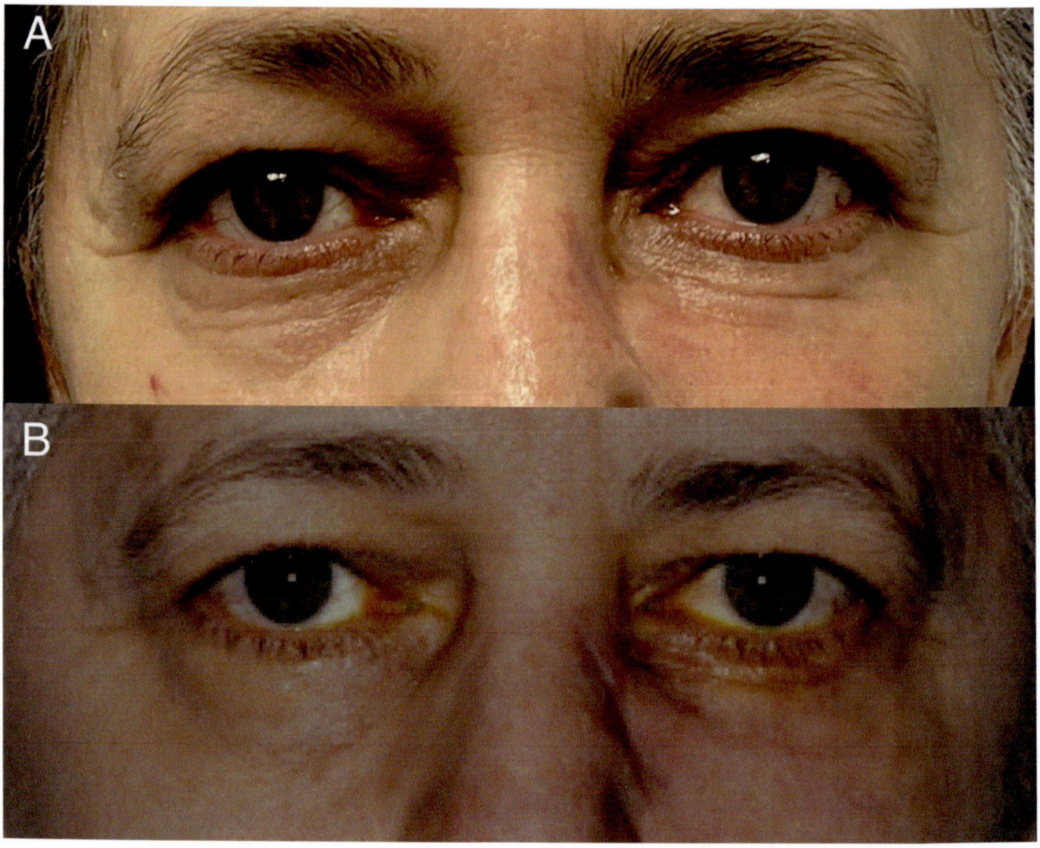

Fig. 1 A patient before (A) and after (B) several sessions of PRP injections to the lower eyelids

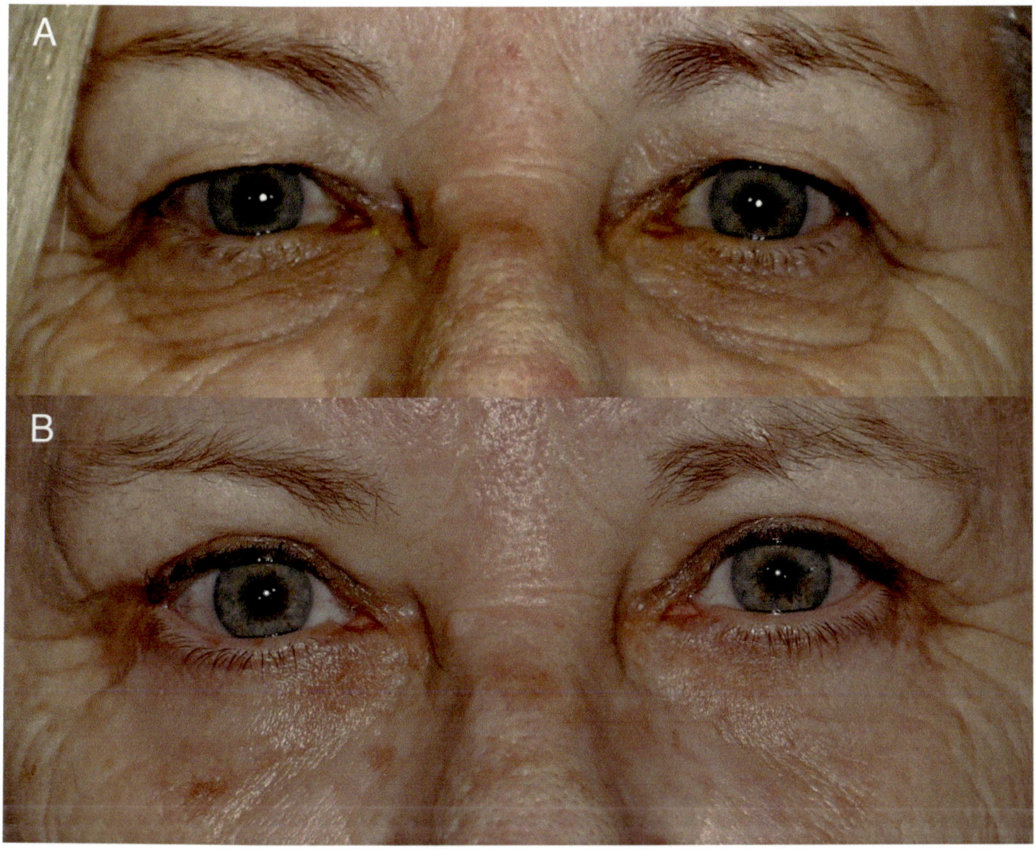

Fig. 2 A patient before (A) and after (B) fat transfer to the lower eyelid-cheek junction combines with PRP injectionsto this zone

advantage of using micro-needling for PRP skin application is the uniformity of treatment (500 micron to 1 mm deep) and patient comfort.

Five monthly sessions are typically used although, in selected cases, the monthly treatments can be extended beyond the fifth session if continued benefits are observed (Fig. 1). A synergistic effect of PRP with micro-needling as opposed to each treatment used alone has been reported [8]. The five monthly sessions may be repeated every year and a half, although some patients do return earlier. The second use of PRP is in conjunction with autologous fat transfer (AFT) to the lower eyelid-cheek junction. Multiple studies have shown the benefit of mixing the PRP with the microfat in order to increase fat uptake [9]. A ratio of PRP to microfat of 1:10 is typically used. Fat retention may be improved with adjuvant PRP (Fig. 2).

In conclusion, although the evidence surrounding its efficacy is limited, platelet-rich-plasma injection is a minimally invasive procedure that may introduce or elaborate growth factors that might enhance lower eyelid rejuvenation. Like other non-invasive approaches, PRP effects may be subtle and it may be an adjuvant to other interventions, such as fat grafting or micro needling. Further research and experience will elucidate PRP's optimal role.

References

1. Vick VL, Holds JB, Hartstein ME, Rich RM, Davidson BR. Use of autologous platelet concentrate in blepharoplasty surgery. Ophthalmic Plast Reconstr Surg. 2006;22(2):102–4.
2. Leo MS, Kumar AS, Kirit R, Konathan R, Sivamani RK. Systematic review of the use of platelet-rich

plasma in aesthetic dermatology Leo. J Cosmet Dermatol. 2015;14:315–23.
3. Robert E. Platelet-Rich Plasma (PRP): What is PRP and what is not PRP? Marx. DDS. Implant Dent 2001;10:225–8.
4. Latalski M, Walczyk A, Fatyga M, Rutz E, Szponder T, Bielecki T, Danielewicz A. Allergic reaction to platelet-rich plasma (PRP): Case report. Medicine (Baltimore). 2019;98(10):e14702.
5. Mehryan, P., Zartab, H., Rajabi, A., Pazhoohi, N., Firooz, A. Assessment of efficacy of platelet-rich plasma (PRP) on infraorbital dark circles and crow's feet wrinkles. J Cosmet Dermatol. 2014;13(1):72–8.
6. Michelle L, Pouldar Foulad D, Ekelem C, Saedi N, Mesinkovska NA. Treatments of Periorbital Hyperpigmentation: A Systematic Review. Dermatol Surg. 2021 Jan 1;47(1):70–74.
7. Aust M, Pototschnig H, Jamchi S, Busch KH. Platelet-rich plasma for skin rejuvenation and treatment of actinic elastosis in the lower eyelid area. Cureus. 2018;10(7):e2999.
8. Kang BK, Shin MK, Lee JH, Kim NI. Effects of platelet-rich plasma on wrinkles and skin tone in Asian lower eyelid skin: preliminary results from a prospective, randomised, split-face trial. Eur J Dermatol. 2014;24(1):100–1.
9. Parra F, Morales-Rome DE, Campos-Rodríguez R, Cruz-Hernández TR, Drago-Serrano ME. Effect of platelet-rich plasma on patients after blepharoplasty surgery. Orbit. 2018;37(2):81–6.

Management of Festoons

Roberto Murillo Limongi, Marisa Novaes de Figueiredo Rassi and Carlos Gustavo Romeiro Santiago Cavalcante

Abstract

Festoons represent a combination of fluid collection and soft tissue laxity in the superolateral cheek region. Festoons contribute to an unsatisfactory appearance for which many patients seek correction. This chapter details surgical and non-surgical treatment options for festoons.

Keywords

Festoons · Malar mounds · Malar edema · Midface Rhytids · Under eye bags

1 Introduction

Festoons represent a combination of fluid collection and soft tissue laxity in the superolateral cheek region [1, 2]. Many patients seek treatment because festoons contribute to an unsatisfactory facial appearance. Concomitant dermatochalasis and other facial aging processes such as malar edema, and malar mounds may be seen together with festoons [3, 4]. It is useful to consider three entities within the spectrum of festoons, as proposed by Kpodzo et al.: (1) malar edema, (2) malar mounds, and (3) festoons (Fig. 1) [4].

Malar edema is fluid that collects over the malar eminence, below the level of the infraorbital rim. It often varies in coloration, and it may be more noticeable in the morning time or after a salty meal. It can be caused by systemic diseases, allergies, postsurgical procedures, or periorbital cosmetic injections. On digital palpation, it appears as pitting edema [4].

Malar mounds are chronic swelling of soft tissues over the malar eminence located between the infraorbital rim and the cheek (mid-cheek). The transition between malar edema and malar mound can be subtle; the characteristic factor of this condition is the permanent presence of redundant tissue [4].

True festoons are laxity of the skin and redundancy of the orbicularis muscle, which appears with a hanging aspect between the medial and lateral corners, below the infraorbital rim, and may also contain edema and herniation of adjacent fatty tissue. The term festoon originates from the Italian festive adornments that were posted on walls in the seventeenth century [4].

Recognition of these midface alterations and differentiation within their clinical spectrum is important in proper management. In this chapter, the classification, anatomy, and

Illustrations by Michael Han

R. M. Limongi (✉) · M. N. de Figueiredo Rassi · C. G. R. S. Cavalcante
Division of Oculoplastic Surgery, Department of Ophthalmology, Federal University of Goiás, Goiás, Brazil
e-mail: rmurillousp@hotmail.com

J. P. Tao (ed.), *Plastic Surgery of the Lower Eyelids*,
https://doi.org/10.1007/978-3-031-36175-3_36

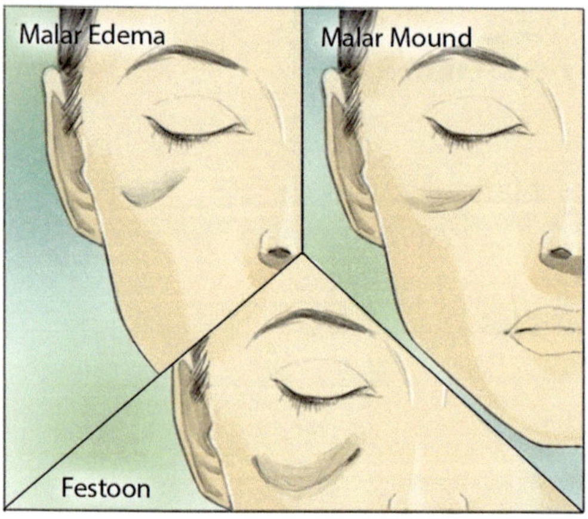

Fig. 1 Classification of festoons: malar edema, malar mound, and true festoon

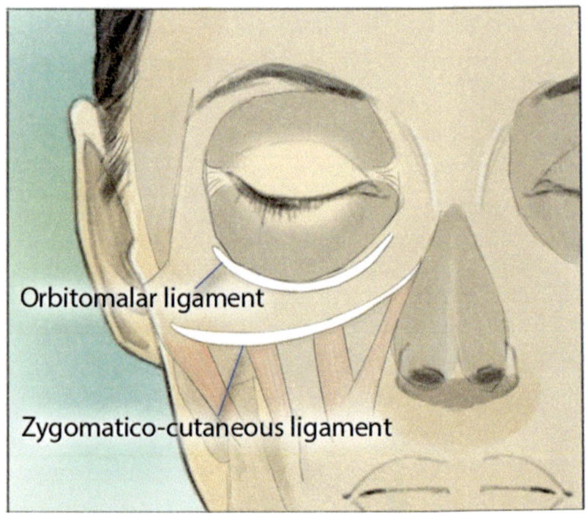

Fig. 2 Orbitocutaneous ligaments of the prezygomatic space

pathophysiology of these alterations are described, as well as surgical and nonsurgical treatments.

2 Anatomy

Anatomy is essential to understand festoons. The prezygomatic space or festoon space is marked superiorly and inferiorly at the palpebromalar junction and the middle third, respectively. The superior rim is marked by the orbitomalar ligament (OML), and the inferior rim by the zygomatic cutaneous ligament (LZC) (Fig. 2). Malar bags/festoons are consistently found approximately 2.5–3 cm below the lateral canthus [2].

3 Pathophysiology

Alterations secondary to age, degenerative factors, imbalance of the local lymphatic system, and the action of gravity, culminate in the weakening of the orbicularis muscle and stretching of the dermis, giving rise to festoons. Anatomical studies on cadavers point to OML elongation and palpebromalar junction drooping as the

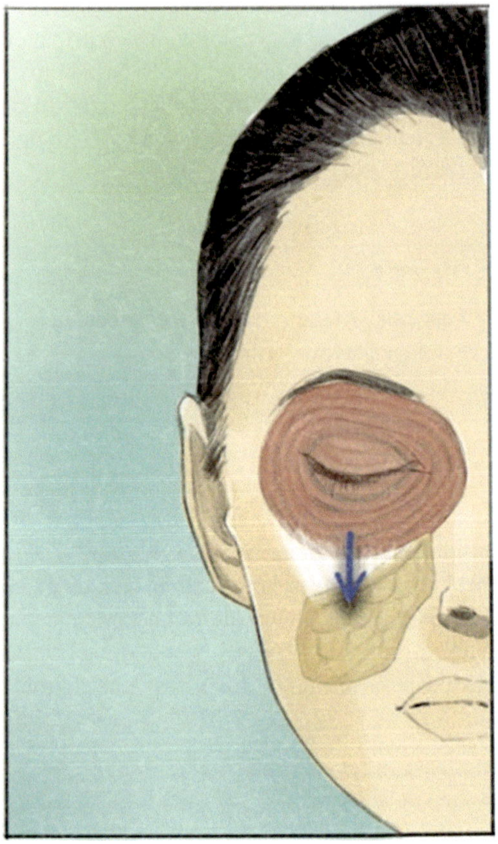

Fig. 3 Elongation of the LOM and palpebromalar junction drooping

basis for the aging process and emergence of malar edema, malar bags, and festoons (Fig. 3). However, the presence of these alterations in younger patients is consistent with the theory that chronic malar edema, occurring on more resistant lower structures, such as the impermeable malar septum, can cause malar mounds, with chronic distension and consequent attenuation of the orbicularis musculature and skin, resulting in festoons [5, 6]. The appearance of transient festoons in a patient after periocular botulinum toxin application reinforces this theory.

Festoons may act like a sponge. Patients with malar edema tend to be predisposed to prolonged postoperative swelling, suggesting a lymphatic origin for festoons.

4 Clinical Evaluation

Malar mounds appear as excess tissue in the prezygomatic space, forming a triangle below the infraorbital rim, with a medial apex. Unlike eyelid bags, they do not undergo major changes when looking up/down.

Several clinical, local, and systemic conditions may trigger periorbital edema. Allergy, rosacea, thyroid eye disease, liver disease, heart diseases, renal disease, and lymphoma are examples. In addition, periorbital edema may be iatrogenic from prior injection of fillers. The inflammatory condition most associated with festoons is ocular rosacea. Ocular rosacea is a chronic inflammation of the periocular skin, associated with erythematous and thickened skin with telangiectasias, papules and pustules [7, 8].

4.1 Squinch Test

The patient is asked to frown, bringing the eyebrows close together, in order to potentiate the action of the orbicularis muscle, allowing the surgeon to assess the muscular contribution to a festoon. If there is orbicularis laxity, an improvement in the appearance of the festoon will occur during this facial expression. The behavior of the fat during the kinetic evaluation (obliteration or just positional variation) will also guide whether or not to excise fat during a surgical procedure.

4.2 Pinch Test

The patient is asked to perform facial movements while the surgeon pinches different regions of the festoon, in order to allow the assessment of tissue resistance and estimate the composition of the mound (skin, muscle, skin-muscle and/or fat) and consequently propose the best treatment technique.

5 Clinical Treatment

The management of festoons spans medical and surgical interventions. The following details some of these approaches.

5.1 Intralesional Tetracycline or Doxycycline Injection

Intralesional applications of tetracycline or doxycycline have been shown to be improve malar mounds. The mechanism of action is a sclerosing action, not antibiotic effects. These medications may stimulate local fibroblast proliferation. It has also been shown to inhibit the matrix metalloproteinases of various cellular tissues to promote collagen and fibrin deposition [9, 10].

Injections of 0.2–1 ml of 2% tetracycline are performed between the subcutaneous and suborbicularis planes, to act on the subcutaneous and suborbicularis fat/edema, in addition to stimulating fibrosis between the orbicularis and deep fascia. Maximal effect is expected around 3 months, after which repeat injections can be considered if required (Fig. 4).

Perry et al. described 11 patients undergoing injection of up to 0.75 ml per side of 2% tetracycline. Before and after injection photos were randomized and then graded on a scale from

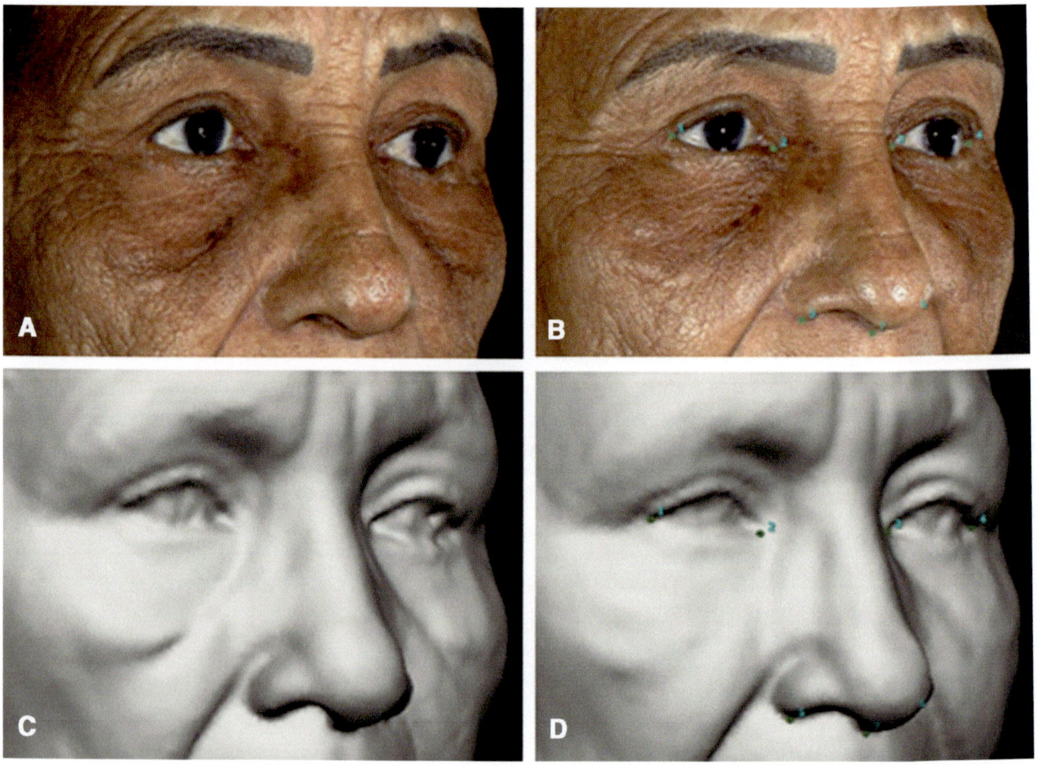

Fig. 4 Female patient with right malar mound side reduced by 0.5 ml on the right side and 0.4 ml on the left side after tetracycline injection. Pre-procedure 3D image (top left); post-procedure 3D image (top right); pre-procedure non-textured image (bottom left); post-procedure non-textured image (bottom right)

0 (no festoons) to 4 (severe festoons) by 4 different oculoplastic observers [9]. The results showed that the mean score dropped from 2.1 to 1.2 and no significant side effects were reported with the injection.

Godfrey et al. reviewed the results of 10 mg/dl doxycycline injections of 15 patients using photographic records before and after application. Patients were graded by two examining physicians who graded them from 0 (no festoon) to 3 (large festoon) [10]. The results showed an average grade reduction from 2.5 to 0.9 with an average of 0.72 ml of injected volume per side and there were no severe side effects.

Initial evidence suggests that doxycycline, in addition to having a greater sclerosing action, promotes less discomfort than tetracycline in the first hours after application. Both drugs have been associated with favorable results in the treatment of festoons in small series, but controlled studies with a greater number of cases are necessary. Pain and discomfort remain chief limitations.

5.2 Fillers

In cases with mild/moderate edema or when there is mild midface and lower eyelid ptosis component, viscous fillers such as calcium hydroxyapatite or hyaluronic acid can be injected deeply to create a posterior support belt, with a lifting effect of the ptotic malar structures. Thinner hyaluronic acid fillers can be used around small swellings and mounds to create a camouflage effect. Such application requires care, as prominent edemas/mounds may not be camouflaged by the filler or, even, worsened (especially in patients with lymphatic involvement and fillers with greater water affinity, which will culminate in an increase in edema) [11, 12].

6 Surgical Treatments

A wide variety of surgical procedures exist for festoons. These include direct excision, extended blepharoplasty and midface lifting. Each is described hereafter.

6.1 Direct Excision

Direct excision is an option in select patients. The benefits of this approach is definitive and direct removal of festoons or malar bags. The amount of skin excised is limited since it may cause eyelid malposition. Elderly patients with extensive skin-redundancy associated with festoons may be the best candidates [13]. However, direct excision should be avoided in those with extensive orbicularis hypertrophy/attenuation or ptotic midface.

Several steps should be taken to optimize the scar's appearance. First, the incision should remain within the thin eyelid skin, avoiding thicker skin over the malar region and follow the relaxed skin tension lines. Second, the edges should be meticulously reapproximated. Finally, patients tendency to pigment or form hypertrophic scars should be excluded.

The procedure can be performed under local anesthesia with or without sedation. Using a skin-pinch technique with the patient in an upward gaze, the greatest amount of skin is drawn-up for excision while ensuring the absence of traction on the lower-lid margin. Subcutaneous undermining is then performed to further allow closure without lower eyelid tension. Skin and subcutaneous tissue are typically excised, but if there is hypertrophic subcutaneous fat or SOOF, it could be removed directly or after delicately spreading apart the orbicularis fibers, respectably. Presumably, if there is attenuated orbicularis, excision, until a thin layer of muscle is left to protect the facial nerve, followed by muscle-plication could improve results; however, with more extensive excisions, postoperative scarring may be more evident. Of note, an eyelid-anchoring procedure should be considered in all patients prior to excision, especially in those with preoperative eyelid laxity signs or symptoms such as foreign body sensation. As this technique does not significantly address orbicularis attenuation and midface ptosis, concomitant orbicularis suspension should be considered [14].

In two studies including over 60 patients, there was no ectropion and minimal to no visible scarring noted. However, proper patient selection and good technique are keys. Scar revision may be necessary. Direct excision is overall not an ideal procedures.

6.2 Midface-Lift

Direct vertical elevation and midface soft tissue fixation provides arguably the most complete and natural correction of infraorbital and eyelid aging. A superolateral muscle-ligament flap sutured directly to the lateral periosteum of the orbital rim and temporalis muscle fascia may be achieve optimal lift [15, 16]. However, suture fixation of SOOF or other fibrofatty tissues to the inferior orbital rim (periosteum or drill holes) or the temporal fascia are alternatives [17]. These concepts are consistent with many well-established lower face and forehead rejuvenation techniques, which also rely on the release of the osteocutaneous ligaments to allow the mobilization and repositioning of loose tissues such as orbicularis and SMAS, both involved in the etiopathogenesis of festoons.

Traditional midface lifts often include subciliary incisions, wide dissection planes, canthotomies, and canthal re-anchoring [18]. The authors have described a minimal incision technique for releasing the orbitomalar ligament and directly suturing a SMAS/orbicularis flap to the periosteum of the lateral orbital rim (Figs. 5, 6, 7, and 8) [19]. (see also chapter "Midface Lift").

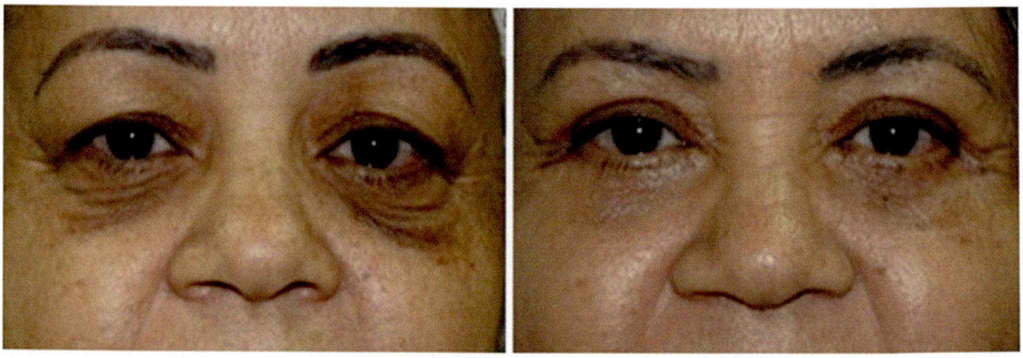

Fig. 5 Preoperative image of a 52 years-old female patient before (left) and after a midface-lift (right) with improvement in malar mounds and dermatochalasis

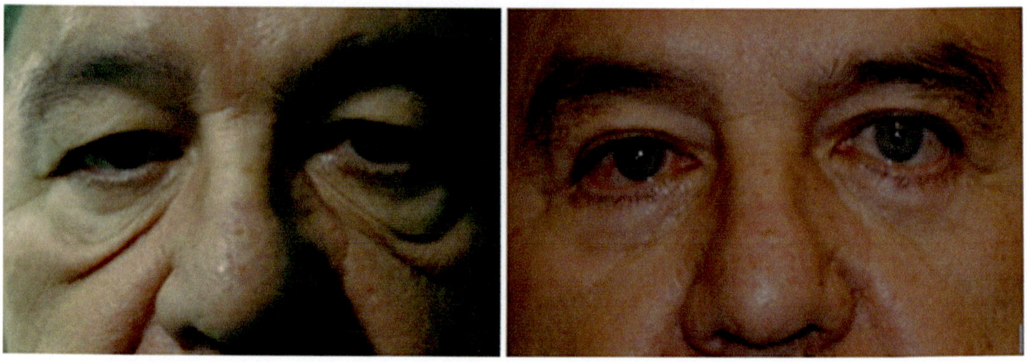

Fig. 6 Preoperative image of a 56 years-old male patient before (left) and after an external midface-lift (right). He has excellent improvement in festoons but had mild lower eyelid retraction that was medically managed with eye lubricating drops

6.3 Subcutaneous Microsuction

Excess subcutaneous fat can be aspirated through a small-caliber liposuction cannula (2.3 mm) until the fold disappears and the fat cannot be palpated. Then, a compressive dressing is applied to promote the adhesion of excess skin. It can be associated with the removal of excess skin and lateral suspension of the orbicularis. This technique is restricted to cases with discreet excess skin, with limited effect on festoons [20, 21].

7 Conclusion

Festoons are a frequent aesthetic complaint. They are a challenge to treat but options include both medical and surgical interventions. Injections of tetracycline and doxycycline are non-surgical options. These are limited in efficacy and are associated with pain. Surgical treatment includes direct excision (rarely) or more ideally midface lifting. Importantly, even with more invasive approaches, recurrence of festoons occurs in a high percentage of patients.

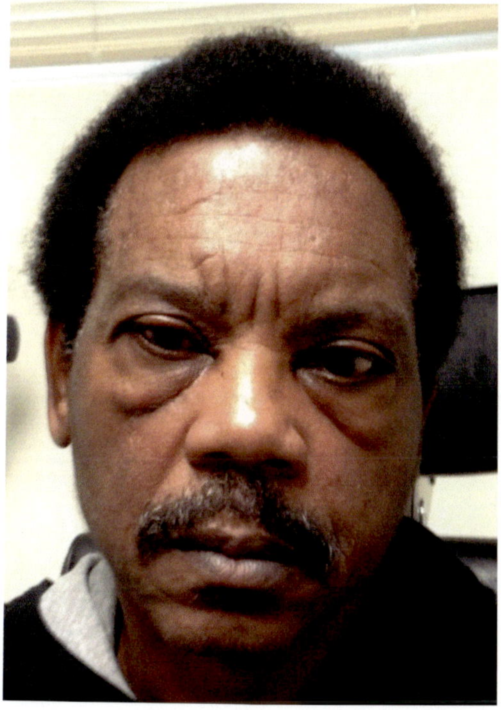

Fig. 7 Preoperative appearance of a patient with malar mounds festoons and right canthal dystopia (after prior orbit decompression for thyroid eye disease)

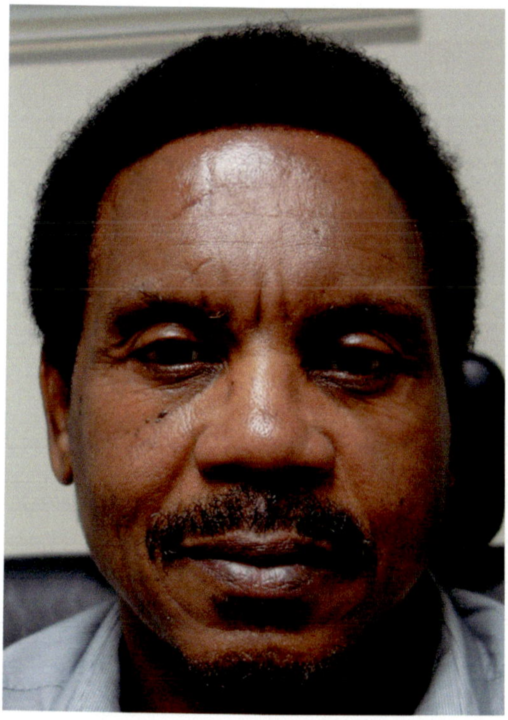

Fig. 8 Patient in Fig. 7 after external midface lift with excellent reduction of malar mounds and festoons.

References

1. Furnas DW. Festoons of orbicularis muscle as a cause of baggy eyelids. Plast Reconstr Surg. 1978;61(4):540–6.
2. Alghoul M, Codner MA. Retaining ligaments of the face: review of anatomy and clinical applications. Aesthet Surg J. 2013;33(6):769–82.
3. Akaishi P, Limongi, RM, Pereira F, Pieroni A. Blefaroplastia. 1. ed. Goiânia: Conexão Propaganda e Editora, 2019. v. 1. 108p. 1° Manual de Condutas Blefaroplastia.
4. Kpodzo DS, Nahai F, McCord CD. Malar mounds and festoons: Review of current management. Aesthet Surg J. 2014;34(2):235–48.
5. Goldberg RA, McCann JD, Fiaschetti D, Ben Simon GJ. What causes eyelid bags? Analysis of 114 consecutive patients. Plast Reconstr Surg. 2005;115(5):1395–1402; discussion 1403–1394.
6. Lam Kar Wai P, Md. The troublesome triad: festoons, malar mounds, and palpebral bags. J Cosmet Med. 2017;1(1):1–7.
7. Scheiner AJ BS, Massry GG. Laser management of festoons. In: Masters Techniques in Blepharoplasty and Periorbital Rejuventation. New York: Springer; 2011, p. 211–21.
8. Roberts TL 3rd. Laser blepharoplasty and laser resurfacing of the periorbital area. Clin Plast Surg. 1998;25(1):95–108.
9. Perry JD, Mehta VJ, Costin BR. Intralesional tetracycline injection for treatment of lower eyelid festoons: a preliminary report. Ophthalmic Plast Reconstr Surg. 2015;31(1):50–2.
10. Godfrey KJ, Kally P, Dunbar KE, Campbell AA, Callahan AB, Lo C, Freund R, Lisman RD. Doxycycline injection for sclerotherapy of lower eyelid festoons and malar edema: Preliminary results. Ophthalmic Plast Reconstr Surg. 2019;35(5):474–477. https://doi.org/10.1097/IOP.0000000000001332. PMID: 30882591.
11. Endara M, Oh C, Davison SP, Baker SB. The management of festoons. Clin Plast Surg. 2015; 42(1):87–94.
12. Jeon H, Geronemus RG. Successful noninvasive treatment of festoons. Plast Reconstr Surg. 2018;141(6):977e–8e.
13. Newberry CI, Mccrary H, Thomas JR, Cerrati EW. Updated management of malar edema, mounds, and festoons: a systematic review. Aesthet Surg J. 2020;40(3):246–58. https://doi.org/10.1093/asj/sjz137.
14. Einan-Lifshitz A, Hartstein ME. Treatment of festoons by direct excision. Orbit. 2012;31(5):303–6.
15. Adamson PA, Tropper GJ, McGraw BL. Extended blepharoplasty. *Arch Otolaryngol Head Neck Surg.* 1991;117(6):606–609; discussion 610.
16. Little JW, Hartstein ME. Simplified muscle-suspension lower blepharoplasty by orbicularis hitch. Aesthet Surg J. 2016;36(6):641–7.
17. Krakauer M, Aakalu VK, Putterman AM. Treatment of malar festoon using modified subperiosteal midface lift. Ophthalmic Plast Reconstr Surg.

2012;28(6):459–62. https://doi.org/10.1097/IOP.0b013e3182696902. PMID: 23138206.
18. Limongi, Roberto Murillo; Tao, Jeremiah, Feijó, Eduardo Damous; Lift terço médio da face, *Estética periocular.* 2018; 96–100.
19. Tao JP, Limongi RM. Short-incision midface-lift in lower blepharoplasty. JAMA Facial Plast Surg. 2016;18(4):313–4. https://doi.org/10.1001/jamafacial.2016.0148. PMID: 27077484.
20. Rosenberg GJ. Correction of saddlebag deformity of the lower eyelids by superficial suction lipectomy. Plast Reconstr Surg. 1995;96(5):1061–5.
21. Liapakis IE, Paschalis EI. Liposuction and suspension of the orbicularis oculi for the correction of persistent malar bags: description of technique and report of a case. Aesthetic Plast Surg. 2012;36(3):546–9.

GPSR Compliance

The European Union's (EU) General Product Safety Regulation (GPSR) is a set of rules that requires consumer products to be safe and our obligations to ensure this.

If you have any concerns about our products, you can contact us on ProductSafety@springernature.com

In case Publisher is established outside the EU, the EU authorized representative is:

Springer Nature Customer Service Center GmbH
Europaplatz 3
69115 Heidelberg, Germany

Batch number: 10383170

Printed by Printforce, the Netherlands